Saida Apsalyamova
Saida Maikoparova
Bella Hashir

# Aspects of medico-environmental technologies of carbon neutrality

Saida Apsalyamova
Saida Maikoparova
Bella Hashir

# Aspects of medico-environmental technologies of carbon neutrality

## Screening of healthy lifestyles using natural resources

ScienciaScripts

Cover image: www.ingimage.com

This book is a translation from the original published under ISBN 978-620-7-64088-1.

Publisher:
Sciencia Scripts
is a trademark of
Dodo Books Indian Ocean Ltd. and OmniScriptum S.R.L publishing group

120 High Road, East Finchley, London, N2 9ED, United Kingdom
Str. Armeneasca 28/1, office 1, Chisinau MD-2012, Republic of Moldova, Europe
Managing Directors: Ieva Konstantinova, Victoria Ursu
info@omniscriptum.com

Printed at: see last page
**ISBN: 978-620-8-59068-0**

## Contents

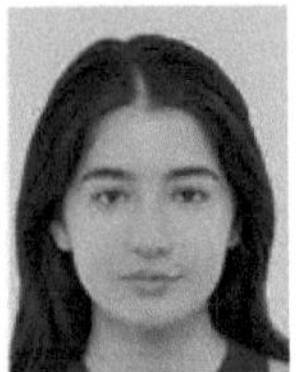

Khashir Esma Aslanovna, Lomonosov Moscow State University

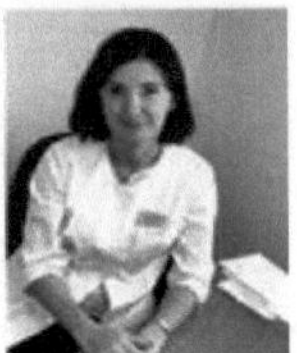

Apsalyamova Saida Olegovna, Candidate of Medical Sciences, KubGMU

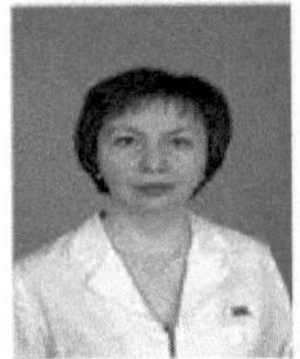

Saida Chelechbievna Maikoparova, Candidate of Medical Sciences, "Forest Institute"

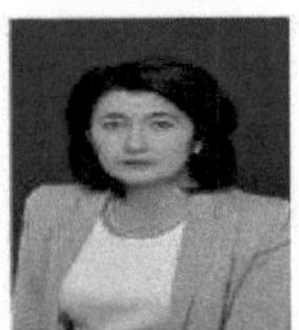

Bella Olegovna Khashir, Professor, Doctor of Economics, KubGTU

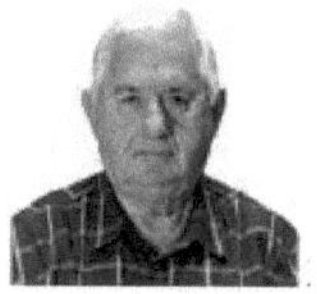

Huazh Olege Zachirievich, Prof. Dr. Sci, "Institute of Forestry"

The research is aimed at the formation of technologies of healthy lifestyle of the population, taking into account social methods of epidemiological analysis in medical and ecological research of the system "human health - habitat", based on the totality of theoretical, methodological, methodological and practical aspects of the development of the concept of sustainable management of the organisation of systems of medical and ecological services of effective environmental management.

The results of the study are that the methodological tools, techniques and methods of accounting for the volume of medical, environmental, their social assessment and performance indicators provide an opportunity for the formation of sustainable management of innovation systems of the cluster, investment programmes of the sphere of medical ecology, social and preventive services provided, create a basis for state regulation of entrepreneurship in the field of effective environmental management

## Introduction

International calls for the creation of urban green spaces, including the planting of urban trees and forests on the assumption that by 2050 more than two-thirds of humanity will live in cities, which already account for about 75 per cent of global CO2 emissions. As a consequence, cities are at the forefront of the fight against climate change. Sustainable urban forestry is a nature-based, integrated and cost-effective solution that promotes greener, healthier and more resilient cities.

Trees and forests in urban and peri-urban areas provide important benefits for health and well-being and are vital for sustainable development, climate change adaptation and mitigation, biodiversity and disaster risk reduction. This contributes not only to sustainable development at the local level, but also to the achievement of national goals and most of the United Nations Sustainable Development Goals (SDGs). The importance of urban green spaces is specifically recognised in the SDGs. Target 11.7 of Goal 11 is to ensure universal access to safe, accessible and inclusive green spaces and public spaces, especially for women and children, older people and people with disabilities. However, significant efforts are needed to achieve this goal, as only approximately 47% of the world's population currently lives within walking distance of public open spaces. The Urban Agenda also highlights the many benefits of "safe, inclusive, accessible, sustainable and quality public spaces for social interaction and inclusion, the promotion of human health and well-being, economic exchange, and cultural expression and dialogue among a wide diversity of people and cultures".

Urban ecosystems are also a priority area, with recent attention being paid to preventing, halting and reversing ecosystem degradation worldwide, which in turn can help end poverty, combat climate change and prevent mass extinctions. The UN Forum on Forests lists forests and trees in urban contexts as thematic priorities under its Global Objective 2 on forests to increase the benefits of forests. In addition, numerous UN organisations and platforms have over time increased their focus on urban forests and green spaces.

An example is the publication by the World Health Organization (WHO) Regional Office for Europe of the publication Urban Green Spaces: A Quick Guide to Action. The Food and Agriculture Organization of the United Nations (FAO) issued 5

"Guidelines for Urban and Peri-urban Forestry". In addition, the Geneva Ministerial Statement on Sustainable Housing and Urban Development, adopted by the Heads of Delegation of the Member States of the United Nations Economic Commission for Europe (UNECE), calls for the promotion of green, compact and resilient cities and emphasises the importance of green infrastructure The importance of inclusive access is highlighted in the UN Geneva Charter on Sustainable Housing, which calls for "universal access to safe, inclusive and accessible housing".

The European Union (EU) Biodiversity Strategy 2030 aims to improve the planning, management and conservation of urban green spaces. The EU Forestry Strategy 2030 envisages expanding forest areas and planting an additional 3 billion trees by 2030, with urban forestry as a priority area. Urban green spaces are also an integral element of Europe's ambitious climate and carbon neutrality targets, which are the focus of the European Green Deal and initiatives such as the European Covenant of Mayors. National Governments have also become more active in incorporating urban trees into their policies and programmes, emphasizing the role of trees and other vegetation in mitigating the effects of extreme heat events. As part of a broader approach to finding nature-based solutions to climate change, for example, the Government of Canada has committed to planting an additional 2 billion trees over the next 10 years, with cities as priority planting areas. In the United Kingdom, endeavours such as the Tree Planting Strategy for England also demonstrate a national focus on urban trees and urban green spaces. Central Asian countries have launched reforestation campaigns to halt land degradation and combat natural disasters, including on the outskirts of cities. However, urban forests and green spaces are often the responsibility of city authorities.

Urban authorities also typically have an integrated mandate across a range of sectors and, in parts of other sectors, are direct beneficiaries of many of the multiple benefits that urban forests and green spaces provide. Creating urban forests and green spaces for all citizens can therefore be an investment in a key public service that delivers these multiple benefits across sectors and facilitates the fulfilment of the multiple responsibilities of urban authorities through a single service delivery mechanism. Recovery from the COVID-19 pandemic on a 'better-than-it-was' basis provides an opportunity to develop and strengthen sustainable urban and peri-urban forestry (SFU). This opportunity was recognised in the Geneva Declaration of Mayors, in which mayors of cities in the UNECE region committed to make cities greener, more equitable, resilient and inclusive, to promote urban biodiversity and to take ambitious action on climate change. The implementation of this declaration represents an important opportunity, but given the challenges cities face, they need more support from other levels of government and other partners in order to fully utilise the potential of UGPLH.

Review of the regular environmental assessment, the environmental assessment framework provides an overview of the regular environmental assessment, as well as a mandate for an information study on national reporting and progress on the SEIS, and a review of environmental policy.

The following subregions are mentioned throughout the assessment, where possible and relevant:

a) European Union of 27 member states;

b) Western Europe - Israel, Iceland, Liechtenstein, Norway, UK and Switzerland;

c) Central Asia - Kazakhstan, Kyrgyzstan, Tajikistan, Turkmenistan and Uzbekistan;

d) Eastern Europe - Armenia, Azerbaijan, Belarus, Georgia, Moldova, Russia,

Ukraine;

e) South-Eastern Europe - Albania, Bosnia and Herzegovina, Macedonia, Montenegro, Serbia and Turkey.

The WHO Health Economic Assessment Tool (HEAT) for Walking and Cycling is designed to allow users without expertise in impact assessment to conduct an economic evaluation of the health impacts of walking or cycling.

HEAT estimates the cost of reduced mortality resulting from a certain amount of walking or cycling, Answering the following question:

If X person walks or *cycles* regularly*, what is the* health impact of premature mortality and its economic significance, while alongside the health benefits of physical activity, HEAT also allows the effects of mortality from exposure to polluted air and road traffic accidents while walking or cycling to be taken into account.

HEAT can further assess the impact on carbon emissions of switching from motorised modes of transport to walking or cycling.

The tool is based on the best available evidence and transparent assumptions. It can be used by a wide range of professionals at both national and local levels. These include primarily Transport Planners, Traffic Engineers and special interest groups working on transport, walking, cycling or the environment.

HEAT can be used for a variety of assessments, e.g.:

- An estimate of current (or past) levels of cycling or walking, for example, showing what cycling or walking is worth in one's city or country.
- Evaluating changes over time, e.g. comparing "before and after" situations, or "scenario A (with measures taken) and scenario B" (without measures taken).
- The evaluation of new or existing projects, including benefit-cost calculations.

HEAT can be used as a stand-alone or to contribute to more comprehensive economic evaluation, or prospective health impact assessments

See examples of results you can work with our local data or script http://www.euro.who.int/HEAT

CHAPTER 1

## 1 Sustainable urban and peri-urban forestry based on natural principles integrated and inclusive solution for the benefit of nature-based integrated and inclusive solution for green restoration and sustainable, healthy and resilient "green regeneration and sustainable, healthy and resilient cities

Addressing urban development through urban and peri-urban forestry at:

A. What is urban and peri-urban forestry urban and peri-urban forestry is one of the many urban green space concepts and approaches that have received increased attention in recent years. It differs from other urban green space concepts in that forests and trees occupy a key place in it. Urban and peri-urban forestry can be a nature-based solution and is integrative, i.e. linking the components of urban and peri-urban green formations and tree-dominated areas into a coherent whole. It is also closely related to the green infrastructure planning approach, which reflects the need to take into account the entire network of green and blue spaces (such as lakes, rivers and wetlands) in a city or metropolis. This requires shifting attention from individual zones to the entire network. This is because a properly connected, well-functioning network of green and blue areas can provide many ecosystem services. Urban areas function as ecosystems, or rather socio-ecological systems, and through the presence of trees and other vegetation they can become more resilient to the effects of climate change and include not only forest ecosystems and woodlands, but also the whole complex of trees and associated vegetation, including street trees, urban parks, cemeteries, trees in private gardens and other urban areas.

The forested part of urban and peri-urban forests itself is a very important component, as it is the source of a number of key ecosystem services, such as protecting drinking water sources, sequestering carbon, preventing land degradation and providing outdoor recreation. For urban and peri-urban forestry to be truly successful, it must aim to sustainably manage forest resources and continuously provide ecosystem services for present and future generations. It should also optimise benefits to local communities while minimising potential negative aspects that may limit recreational use of urban and peri-urban forests, such as exposure to allergens and perceived risk of crime.

Б. Current urban and peri-urban forest area indicators

While it is recognised that urban and peri-urban forests (UUFs) are an important source of ecosystem services, surprisingly little is known about their extent.

To date, few countries have attempted a comprehensive assessment of their PPG resources. At the local level, many city authorities do not have a full understanding of their SFP resources, and when inventories do exist, they mostly only include trees owned and managed by the state. This is gradually changing as more and more cities and megacities are attempting a more comprehensive inventory of their urban forests. This shows that they realise the importance of having up-to-date information on SFP resources as a basis for planning and sustainable management. This is not an easy task due to the diversity of SFP structures and ownership. However, it is important to note that the level of involvement of national governments varies; for example, national authorities in the Russian Federation, the Caucasus and Central Asia have traditionally been more involved in the management of SFPs. Although "forest ecosystems", which are part of urban forests, are often included in national forest inventories, it remains difficult to get a complete picture of this important component of SFM. For example, there may even be problems in defining the boundaries of urban and peri-urban areas. From the available data, a picture emerges of a small but very important resource that faces its own specific challenges due to different ownership, intensive use and fragmentation. Urban forest areas are often fragmented and small, which can undermine their ecological viability; their management can be complicated by the diversity of public and private owners (including municipal governments).

B. Potential for sustainable urban and peri-urban forestry Urban and peri-urban forests are critical to urban areas and urban communities. They provide a wide range of ecosystem services and benefits that are increasingly recognised and validated through research.

Sustainable urban and peri-urban forestry contributes to climate change mitigation, adaptation and disaster risk reduction SFPs provide essential regulating ecosystem services for climate change mitigation and adaptation. In fact, GPLs can be considered as vital infrastructure, i.e. an asset necessary for the functioning of society and the economy; for example, urban trees reduce the local ambient air temperature by as much as 8 degrees Celsius. This helps urban communities reduce the health impacts of temperature extremes and adapt to projections of worsening of these temperature extremes in the face of climate change. Trees planted near buildings also sequester carbon while reducing greenhouse gas emissions by reducing energy use (and costs) for air conditioning. GPLs can also reduce land degradation and provide critical infrastructure for disaster management. For example, GPLs contribute to disaster risk reduction by helping to stabilise slopes to prevent landslides. Another very important function of GPLs is that they significantly limit stormwater runoff and pollution by intercepting and reducing rainfall intensity, as well as infiltrating and absorbing stormwater and reducing nutrient loading. For example, tree canopy can significantly detain stormwater runoff, thereby alleviating stress on urban drainage systems. The economic benefits of GPGs fulfilling these functions are substantial, with a recent national study in the United States commissioned by the Arbor Day Foundation showing that the environmental benefits of urban trees in the country are valued at $73 billion per year, of which $65 billion is generated by urban trees. Of that, $65 billion is attributable to carbon sequestration. Of this, $65 billion is attributable to carbon sequestration by urban trees and $3 billion is attributable to their contribution to carbon management. Of this, $65 billion is attributable to carbon sequestration by urban trees and $3 billion to their contribution to stormwater management. While countries such as the United States have made progress at the local and national levels in terms of justifying investments in GPGs, research on the associated costs and benefits in much of the UNECE region is limited.

Sustainable urban and peri-urban forestry contributes significantly to improving our health and well-being. Research shows a concrete contribution to improved physical, mental and social health, as well as cognitive development. People who live in greener urban areas and/or have easy access to public green spaces have better mental and physical health and are more likely to engage in social interactions in their neighbourhoods.

During the COVID-19 pandemic, urban green spaces that remained accessible became much-needed 'islands of escape' for urban dwellers. Studies from around the world show that people have become significantly more appreciative of urban green spaces, including local forests, and use them for recreational purposes, in light of the global pandemic, scientists and policymakers called for rethinking existing concepts and transforming cities to respond to the reality of COVID-19 and to be able to respond to possible future pandemics by building more resilient, inclusive and sustainable cities. Trees in local streets and public gardens demonstrated their value during the COVID-19 pandemic by becoming much-needed greenery near residences.

Moreover, studies have also shown that specific components of GPGs (e.g. street trees versus park trees) have their own specific health impacts. For example, trees in schoolyards can benefit children's health and cognitive development, community gardens can promote social cohesion, and suburban forests provide a wide range of benefits, including for mental health. Trees are often featured in studies on the health benefits of urban nature. For example, a Toronto study found that when an urban neighbourhood has an average of 10 more trees, there is an improvement in health perceptions comparable to a CAD 10,000 increase in annual personal income, leading to increased life expectancy. Increasing urban forests and green spaces can also improve health and reduce deaths from air pollution. It is estimated that this would prevent nearly 43,000 deaths in European cities each year. It would also have a significant economic impact through reduced health care costs. SFPs can also have beneficial effects on health due to the role they play in food production and can even contribute to local food security, more sustainable local food systems and improved nutrition, for example through food forests.

Sustainable urban and peri-urban forestry can help conserve biodiversity and promote ecosystem restoration, and biodiversity levels in cities can be very high, partly as a result of the presence of non-native species in gardens and parks, but also because cities are often located at ecosystem interfaces and represent a wide range of habitats. Among green spaces, urban parks often have the highest levels of biodiversity. A study of urban and peri-urban parks found that they are home to about 50 per cent of all bird species found in the region, as well as more than 60 per cent of all amphibian species. A link between biodiversity and health benefits was found, with GPLs also important for urban dwellers, maintaining a connection with plants, animals and natural processes. This may help to increase awareness and appreciation of the value of forests and forest policies among urban and peri-urban populations, including policies traditionally more rural orientated.

Sustainable urban and peri-urban forestry contributes to greening and regeneration, as nature-based solutions that help respond to societal challenges, SFPs can be part of cost-effective strategies to combat climate change. Moreover, GPLs tend to be a source of several benefits at once, making them an attractive tool for addressing many urban challenges. These benefits include important economic benefits. For example, the US urban forestry sector contributes $64 billion to the US economy through annual sales and employment. The urban forestry sector in the United States contributes $64 billion to the economy through annual sales and employment, with approximately half a million jobs created as a result of the activities of private sector authorities and organisations. In addition, recent studies have calculated that the GPL accounts for approximately $31.5 billion of the total value of property assets in the country. In addition, GPLs account for approximately $31.5 billion in the total value of real estate property assets in the United States. In addition, PPGs are often a critical means of protecting urban drinking water resources, which are highly valuable in both monetary and non-monetary terms.

The current emphasis on urban greening and tree planting will also lead to increased economic activity and entrepreneurship and contribute to the creation of new green jobs around the world. For example, a study conducted in Sweden, which has a population of just over 10 million, found that around €1.8 billion is spent annually on managing urban green spaces. This represents an important opportunity for green investment and job creation during periods of economic recovery, including after the COVID-19 pandemic.

Enhancing the impact of sustainable urban and peri-urban forestry in realising the full potential of SFM needs to consider the following aspects:

- Urban and peri-urban forests at the doorstep of all urban dwellers The multiple benefits of sustainable urban and peri-urban forestry should be enjoyed by all urban dwellers, regardless of age, gender, income, education and cultural background. Ecological equity in terms of fair and equitable distribution of benefits should be part of any SFM programme as stipulated in SDG 11.7.

Research has clearly shown that people benefit optimally when they have easy and direct access to SFPs, i.e. they can see the trees from their home window, have a decent tree canopy in their neighbourhood and are no more than a five-minute walk from the nearest public green space. More diverse and resilient urban and peri-urban forests are urban and peri-urban forests that are diverse in their species composition, more resilient to the effects of climate change, pest infestations and disease outbreaks. Diversity also means a wide range of urban and peri-urban forestry components, from quiet urban forests to green schoolyards and community gardens, from crowded urban parks to clutter-free cemeteries. Each can have multiple uses and be a source of diverse experiences and benefits.

Tree planting is good and sustainable management is even better, but it requires long-term planning and calls for action to combat climate change Tree planting is receiving increasing public and political attention, including in urban areas, and often on a massive scale. This is a good thing, as increased tree cover can help address climate change and support efforts to maintain planetary boundaries while ensuring sustainable development. However, tree planting in urban and suburban areas must be linked to long-term, adaptive management of SFM and will only make sense if there is a significant increase in tree establishment. Sufficient resources (including financial) and capacity must be available for this. The benefits of urban trees will increase as they reach full maturity.

There is an urgent need for predictable, long-term funding and resources, and sustainable management of urban and peri-urban forests depends on long-term planning. Without predictable long-term funding and resources, it is more difficult for urban authorities to plan, commit to and effectively implement longer-term SFM plans. SFM plans that are not based on realistic budgets may not achieve their objectives if sufficient funds are not eventually available. Unrealistic budgets may also cause poor performance if the resources available are ultimately greater than those envisaged in ambitious plans and targets. As such, municipal budgets can be one of the most predictable sources of funding for urban forests.

A full assessment of the benefits of SFM can justify budget increases, and better SFM planning can improve the efficient use of available resources. National and subnational funds and programmes can also be predictable sources and help leverage funding from other sources, including increased allocations to urban forests from municipal budgets.

A key element is to organise the management of SFPs serve local communities, therefore it is very important to involve them in organising the management of these spaces. This can help to ensure that areas are properly prepared and maintained, helping to conserve these spaces while building stronger relationships between people, trees, communities and forests. Organisational management also incorporates an important longer term perspective as it promotes a culture of understanding, interaction and partnership between generations. This can help ensure long-term resident support for SFM policies and programmes, as well as for rural forest policies and afforestation efforts in general. A range of cultural and other characteristics of local communities, including indigenous peoples, need to be taken into account in the organisation of governance.

Specific strategies, planning and management plans for SFM is not easy. Cities are very dynamic with constant change, and trees and forests usually take a long time to reach maturity; even if fast-growing tree species are used to get quick results, the

next generation of trees must be thought of. In order to reap their ecosystem benefits, green spaces such as forests, trees and associated vegetation in and around cities should be placed at the centre of urban planning. In particular, SFMU programmes need a longer-term vision developed with local communities to ensure they are focused and set policy direction. Clear goals, objectives and performance indicators should be defined in the planning process based on a shared vision. The development of a SFM Master Plan for the city can help to clearly articulate these measures and ensure that sufficient resources are allocated, these plans should be properly aligned with other municipal policies and programmes Sustainable urban and peri-urban forestry that is based on sound information and reflects best practices The planning, establishment and management of SFM should be based on sound evidence and reliable, up-to-date information. This should include information about the GPG resource and the local community in which the forest is located. The application of modern practices can enhance efforts to ensure sustainable management, through knowledge sharing and peer learning, as well as the existence of clear guidelines and standards to provide direction and guidance on forest management practices and appropriate and equitable access to green spaces. This requires supporting and expanding research, education, training and knowledge transfer on SFM. Tracking and demonstrating success, as well as close monitoring of SFM programmes and activities is often lacking today . Ideally, city governments, urban and peri-urban forest owners, communities and other stakeholders should establish reliable baselines and then track the impact of their SFM programme. This includes not only the development of the SFM resource, but also changes in the provision of the various ecosystem services and benefits they provide, as well as local community perceptions and participation. This kind of success monitoring can be a good basis for comparative analyses between cities, and 15
also to inform citizens about the benefits of GPGs, based on the rapid growth in the use of geospatial and other tools that can be used to measure effectiveness, the emergence of specialised companies and other organisations that can support these efforts.

Using sustainable urban and peri-urban forestry to strengthen interactions at the urban-rural interface Cities often have a strong impact on their surrounding areas. Given that much of SFP includes land on the periphery of cities, this opens up opportunities for better planning and management to ensure integration at the urban-rural interface. This can create new opportunities for more sustainable land use and agricultural activities, carbon sequestration, protection of drinking water sources, and improved management of wildfire risk in urban and peri-urban areas. Improving the interconnectedness of green spaces (green structure) and land use at the urban-rural interface will provide a more holistic view of our food systems, including sustainable production at local and regional levels, positively impact food security and biodiversity, and help change systems that are not utilising their full potential. Strengthening partnerships and co-operation requires "horizontal" integration, for example between different municipal departments and other stakeholders. But this should not only be handled by the city government and not only by one particular department in the municipal administration. It also requires "vertical" integration through the coordination of local, regional and national policies, legislation and programmes. A wide range of authorities, landowners, interest groups, businesses, communities and demographic groups need to be involved. This highlights the need for collaborative approaches that take into account the specific needs, skills, mandates and resources of these different partners, build synergies between them and mobilise them. Feasibility study on the feasibility of sustainable urban and peri-urban forestry. It has become evident that SFM is of vital importance to urban populations, and a growing body of research confirms this.

The benefits of investing in trees can be five or six times the investment costs. However, not everyone is aware of this. With many competing and pressing interests to consider in urban and suburban decision-making, it is important to make a strong case in favour of SFMT, such as the need to address key issues such as climate change and public health threats. A more compelling feasibility study is needed to support these efforts 16

the feasibility of developing SFM. Benefit-cost ratios for SFM, as well as evidence of non-monetary and policy benefits, can provide compelling evidence that this area deserves to be a policy priority and investment. The contribution of SFM to the green economy and its potential should also be highlighted

All of these aspects of enhancing the impact of SFM requires attention. Addressing these issues will require new multi-stakeholder partnerships, with a focus on local and regional actors. However, international organisations can play an important role in enhancing the implementation and impact of SFM by working with authorities and various stakeholders at different levels and fostering a culture of cooperation, coordination and integration. This is also in line with the integrated nature of SFM. This may include efforts to support the sustainable management of all types of forests by strengthening national capacities and monitoring systems. Addressing the above priorities will advance efforts to develop and implement SFM in the near and long term, thereby benefiting and strengthening urban and peri-urban communities. Realising global and national policies and goals at the local level through the development of sustainable urban and peri-urban forestry The importance and contribution of urban and peri-urban forests is clearly reflected in the global goals, these include:

- United Nations Sustainable Development Goals, in particular SDG 11;
- the call of the United Nations Forum on Forests to focus on forests and trees in urban settings;
- international processes on sustainable forest management ;
- Numerous afforestation, reforestation and tree planting campaigns

- to address climate change, biodiversity loss and degradation of the landscape.

National goals and policies often reflect global goals, although they are nationally oriented. The SFMO provides an important framework for achieving national and global goals through local action, with scope for significant strategic expansion of the SFMO to facilitate further progress.

Coordination of sustainable urban and peri-urban forestry with other sectors and SFM policies contributes to the development of a wide range of other sectors and policy implementation in different areas. By integrating policies and programmes, important synergies can be achieved. These include urban planning, public health, public education, climate change action, land use, forestry in general (including rural areas), agricultural policy and economic development. It is often the case that the lack of policy coordination and harmonisation makes it impossible to achieve such important synergies. Elements that can enhance coordination and impact include sound baseline data and monitoring, clear plans and targets, effective coordination mechanisms and strong political support. Greater involvement and cooperation of national and regional authorities and policymakers in strengthening governance and cooperation for sustainable urban and peri-urban forestry In many countries, SFPs are managed by local governments, but there is a need to expand governance. This includes leadership at regional and national levels, policy frameworks and support mechanisms, and better alignment with international policies and agreements. National governments can advance efforts to make SFM a priority. For example, by developing specific national policies, programmes and funding mechanisms for SFM, governments can foster a culture of cooperation at different levels. In collaboration with local stakeholders, innovative ways to promote SFM should be identified, for example by exploring co-management opportunities.

Mobilising and diversifying funding sources for sustainable urban and peri-urban forestry is a nature-based solution that supplies communities with essential goods and services.

However, its development requires predictable and reliable financing to enable the development and implementation of long-term plans. The contribution of SFM to climate change mitigation, air pollution reduction, public health, and even food security and sustainable food systems can justify leveraging existing and new public and private sector funds. Feasibility studies on the feasibility of developing SFM can help in obtaining and enhancing access to sources of finance. Careful planning, proper monitoring and reliable public funding can also help mobilise other sources of finance. Successful examples of innovative financing can also be disseminated and replicated among city, subnational and national governments.

Good examples of successful SFM exist in the UNECE region and around the world. In order to foster a culture of mutual learning, it is important to share and discuss these examples, existing models and experiences. Due to differences in local conditions, approaches cannot always be fully replicated, but there are often some key elements in programmes that can serve as a stimulus and a basis for action. There is an emerging demand for guidance and tools to support practitioners, and such knowledge products can be developed based on knowledge sharing among experts and good practices.

Building a culture of regional and cross-border co-operation involves countries with very different contexts, challenges and opportunities. However, countries in the region also face common challenges such as urbanisation, climate change, health, biodiversity loss and unsustainable food systems. They all share the same urgent task of developing resilient, healthy and economically competitive urban areas. Regional and transboundary cooperation can take many forms. It includes cooperation across administrative, environmental and other geographical boundaries at the international, national and subnational levels. This type of cooperation can often be actively supported through joint research and planning, specialised management mechanisms and political, technical and financial support at different administrative levels (city, national, regional, international). It can also include co-operation on thematic issues, including across immediate boundaries. Co-operation can often take place at the formal level, but informal co-operation, including through networks of experts, can also play an important role. Examples include the Informal Network of Experts on Sustainable Urban Forestry and the European Forum on Urban Forestry Assessments, monitoring and benchmarking across the region As part of their efforts to plant and care for SFM, cities and countries will benefit from regional assessments, monitoring and benchmarking. This will help to assess the situation of SFM in the region (e.g. in terms of the PPG resource and the benefits they provide) and track progress over time. National and international organisations can help coordinate these efforts by linking them to existing data collection and monitoring programmes.

Encouraging the use of international standards and guidelines, various guidelines and norms related to UGPLH have recently emerged, such as the WHO Guidelines for Facilitating the

access to public green spaces in Europe and tree canopy level targets set by cities. A recent example of more comprehensive guidance is the "3-30-300 rule" for SFM. Efforts to develop, disseminate and adopt such guidelines, as well as the development and application of standards for sustainable urban forest management, can contribute to the expansion of SFM as a nature-based solution.

Promoting awareness of the importance of sustainable urban and peri-urban forestry

There is an opportunity to communicate the benefits of SFM to a wider public to educate children, schools, local communities and businesses, as well as to increase participation and ownership of this nature-based solution. Questions such as "How do urban trees benefit us?" and "How can I get involved in organising the management of my local SFP?" can help raise awareness of the importance of urban trees and forests. More importantly, they can help leverage public and private sector funds to harness this nature-based sustainable solution for the benefit of future generations. One of the more effective development of the transition to new, clean, safe, health-friendly and inclusive mobility and transport is provided by the Transport, Environment and Health Pan-European Programme on Transport, Environment and Health (TEEP).

Transport is one of the largest economic sectors in the European Region, and travel and mobility are essential components of modern life, providing access to services, goods and activities. At the same time, transport can cause significant health and well-being burdens and even damage the region's economies due to: pollutant and greenhouse gas emissions, noise pollution; traffic congestion; injuries; fragmentation of space, society and biodiversity; socio-economic inequalities; land acquisition and reduced opportunities for physical activity. Transport, health and the environment are inextricably linked. THE PEP - the Transport, Environment and Health Pan-European Programme - helps to take into account the links between these three sectors.

THE PEP is the first and only international programme to integrate environmental and health considerations into transport, mobility and urban planning strategies. Since the establishment of the HSESAP, the region has seen positive developments towards healthier, cleaner and more sustainable transport and mobility; however, a number of challenges remain, namely:

- Each year in the WHO European Region, more than 500,000 people die prematurely due to air pollution. Emissions from transport account for a significant share of pollution.
- Transport accounts for about a quarter of energy-related greenhouse gas emissions.
- Every year, more than 110,000 people die on the roads in the UNECE and WHO pan-European region. On average, this means that one person dies every five minutes. Road traffic injuries are the number one cause of death worldwide among young people aged 5-29 years.
- At least 20 per cent of the population in the UNECE and WHO pan-European region lives in areas where road traffic noise is considered harmful to health. In urban areas in most countries this figure exceeds 50 per cent.
- In the WHO European Region alone, lack of physical activity is estimated to be responsible for about 1 million deaths per year and obesity for another million.

This is why the HSESAP works to support countries in finding the best balance between the needs of transport and mobility, human health and well-being, and environmental quality.

The HSESAP activities aim to achieve healthy, clean and sustainable transport and mobility in the pan-European region in order to fulfil the objectives that:

- Make urban, suburban and rural environments healthier, safer, more accessible and better connected by transport;

- Ensure social equity, inclusive mobility and the highest level of health and well-being for all;
- Better integrate gender perspectives into transport, health and environmental strategies;
- achieve the goals of the main international agreements - the Paris Agreement on Climate Change and the 2030 Agenda for Sustainable Development.

In its work, OPTOSOS solves current problems by:

- cross-sectoral co-operation and promoting a better understanding of the relationship between transport, health and the environment;
- providing member States of the UNECE European region and WHO with an intergovernmental intersectoral platform for policy development and stimulating the involvement of the health and environment sectors in transport and urban planning;
- providing scientific evidence on the benefits of healthy and sustainable transport;
- developing strategic and practical tools for implementing green, healthy and inclusive mobility;
- providing capacity-building support for integrated and cross-sectoral strategic action in transport, health, environment and urban planning The UNECE and WHO European Region or "pan-European Region" refers to the European regions of UNECE and WHO combined. The two organisations share a majority of member States. Stakeholders in the European Region, home to 17% of the world's population, the 56 States of the UNECE and WHO European Region cooperate in the framework of the HSESAP, involving national, intergovernmental organisations and local authorities and all stakeholders.

OPTOSOS serves Member States and works with them through:

- Ministries and national bodies dealing with transport, health, environment and spatial planning;
- city and local authorities;
- transport and urban planning specialists, transport engineers;
- health care workers;
- environmentalists;
- Stakeholders from business and industry, working with

on creating environmentally friendly and safe mobility;

- representatives of the scientific community;
- non-governmental organisations;
- the general public - with a focus on vulnerable groups, older people, children and young people.

More efficient development through a shift to new, clean, safe, healthy and inclusive mobility and transport How HSSEAP works HSSEAP is a three-part pan-European policy framework that brings together the transport, health and environment sectors on an equal footing. It is jointly operated by the UNECE and

the WHO Regional Office for Europe. The highest decision-making body of THE PEP is the High-Level Meeting on Transport, Environment and Health, which is convened at ministerial level every 5-6 years.
All Member States are encouraged to actively support the HSESAP delivery mechanisms such as Partnerships, Relay and the Academy to implement the HSESAP work programme. To this end, Member States nominate national focal points representing the health, environment and transport sectors.
The scope covers a wide range of policy and action areas, from political relations and policy-making to the design and implementation of cooperation programmes.
Working together in the framework of the HSESAP, Member States are contributing to the 2030 Agenda on several fronts, accelerating the achievement of numerous goals and targets, including those related to health, energy efficiency, climate and environmental protection, quality of urban life and equality. The first ever Pan-European Cycling Master Plan was approved, a historic milestone and a key part of the Vienna Declaration, along with recommendations on green and healthy sustainable transport, conclusions on sustainable urban mobility and spatial planning, recommendations on eco-driving, as well as a comprehensive work programme of the HSESAP based on:

- Child-Friendly Mobility Partnership of the HSESAP and youth to ensure that the views of future generations are incorporated into the work of the HSESAP;
- The HSESAP Partnership on Sustainable Mobility in the Tourism Sector to exchange information on good practices and develop related guidelines and tools;
- The active mobility partnership of the HSESAP to promote the implementation of the new Pan-European Cycling Master Plan, to integrate pedestrian traffic into the new Pan-European Active Mobility Master Plan, to develop the Trans-European Bicycle Network (TEB) and to establish a pan-European competence centre for active mobility. With the approval of the Pan-European Cycling Master Plan, countries have given further impetus to the transformation towards clean, safe, health-friendly and inclusive transport and mobility in the pan-European region.

The Master Plan calls for:

- recognise the bicycle as an equal mode of transport;
- significantly expand cycling in each country to achieve a doubling of cycling in the region by 2030;
- Allocate additional space for pedestrian and cycling traffic;
- expand and improve cycling infrastructure in each country;
- Significantly improve cyclist and pedestrian safety to reduce fatalities;
- Develop a national cycling policy supported by cycling plans, strategies and programmes;
- Integrate cycling into public health policy,
- land use, urban, regional and transport infrastructure planning.

Recommendations on Cleaner and Health Friendly Sustainable Transport - "More efficient further development", in response to the events and challenges during the COVID-19 pandemic, the Steering Committee of the Pan-European Programme on Transport, Environment and Health decided to establish a Task Force to develop Recommendations for Member States on more efficient further development and the transition to cleaner and health-friendly sustainable transport.

The present study Recommendations for Cleaner and Healthier Sustainable Transport - "More Efficient further development" outlines the findings of the Task Force and highlights seven key recommendations that Member States should follow in order to develop their transport systems in a more sustainable manner.

Member States of the ECE European Region and WHO have developed the Transport, Environment and Health Pan-European Programme. THE PEP provides cross-sectoral and intergovernmental policy mechanisms that promote mobility and transport strategies that take into account environmental and health concerns. Over the years, the HSESAP has developed various implementation mechanisms to support the activities of Member States, to assist Member States in integrating transport, health, quality of life and environmental objectives into urban and spatial planning policies. The Guide contains many references to case studies, best practices and city-based examples from across the Eurasian region and beyond. A wide range of thematic areas are covered, including the future of sustainable urban mobility; spatial planning as a function of sustainable urban mobility and accessibility; public transport planning as a basis for sustainable urban mobility; active mobility and how it contributes to improving health and the environment and the potential of Intelligent Transport Systems in the urban context.

The present Handbook presents a methodology for sustainable urban transport planning and provides a short list of key ideas and recommendations that will serve as a substantive contribution to the Fifth High-level Meeting on Transport, Environment and Health.

The HSESAP Partnerships bring together partners from Member States, intergovernmental and non-governmental organisations with common interests in cooperation on specific issues to develop common strategies and plans, achieve visible results and implement specific projects. HSESAP Partnerships also provide an opportunity to share best practices, build capacity and provide mutual support for the implementation of HSESAP at national and pan-European level. The HSESAP Academy links science, policy and practice and provides a platform for key stakeholders, including policy makers, civil servants, practitioners and academics, to build capacity to integrate transport, environment and health into urban and spatial planning.

As a platform for creating and sharing knowledge and expertise , the HSSE Academy facilitates the implementation of HSSE and makes an important contribution to the fulfilment of various regional and global commitments. The range of activities undertaken by the HSSPSPS Academy includes close co-operation with the HSSPS Partnerships. Better development through the transition to new, cleaner, safer, HSSPSS-friendly and inclusive mobility and transport The HSSPSS Toolkit has produced a series of user-friendly tools, guides and information materials that provide an overview of the most pressing transport-related health and environmental challenges in the pan-European region, and present solution mechanisms and opportunities for action to assess and address these challenges.

Health Economic Assessment Tool for Walking and Cycling (HEAT)

HEAT is an easy-to-use web-based tool for estimating the economic value of the impact of regular walking or cycling on mortality and answers the following questions: If X people walk or cycle a distance equal to Y on most days, what is the economic value of the health benefits that result:

- reduction in mortality attributable to their physical activity;
- how much air pollution or accidents affect these results;
- What are the implications in terms of carbon emissions;

The Health Economic Assessment Tool for Walking and Cycling (HEAT) and National Transport, Health and Environmental Action Plans (NTHAPs), which cover different areas and provide an integrated and cross-sectoral way to plan and implement transport, health and environmental actions at the national level. The step-by-step guide for policy-makers and planners helps Member States to identify: key goals, objectives, priority actions, coordination mechanisms, roles and responsibilities; timelines and budgets; and implementation, monitoring and evaluation recommendations for developing sustainable and health-friendly transport in the country.

Developing national action plans for transport, health and the environment: a step-by-step guide for policy makers and planners Plans for the future are mapped The Vienna Declaration details the priorities for strengthening the commitment to co-operation to realise the new vision of the HSESAP:

- environmentally friendly, safe, favourable to health;
- inclusive mobility and transport for the happiness and prosperity of all;

Other areas of work include:

- Developing a comprehensive pan-European transport, environment and health strategy to transform mobility towards zero-emission, health-promoting active mobility and safe and efficient transport (including legal options) over the next decade;
- Increasing walking and cycling in each country, ensuring the safety of cyclists and pedestrians, and integrating active mobility into health policies, as foreseen in the Pan-European Master Plan to promote cycling;
- Enhancing co-operation on implementation and stimulating joint activities of Member States and international organisations
- Addressing inequalities related to transport and urban sprawl, promoting inclusive and equitable transport systems across the pan-European region;
- Developing a communication strategy to raise awareness of the opportunities and benefits of sustainable and healthy transport and to communicate the results.

CHAPTER 2

## 2 Systems principles and requirements for a low-carbon model of development health in natural resource management.

In view of the urgent need for action to combat climate change, the world is rapidly moving towards a low-carbon development model. Countries around the world have experienced widespread flooding, drought and heat waves in recent years. Climate change is affecting the spread of infectious diseases, exposing populations to the risks of new diseases and epidemics. Mitigating the effects of global warming requires energy, transport and digital transition. At the same time, climate change is creating acute shortages of fresh water and food. However, the deployment of low-carbon technologies will also require huge amounts of critical raw materials. Therefore, the only way to mitigate and adapt to climate change is through a fundamental change in our approach to managing natural wealth.

Given the unprecedented challenges we face in the future, it is clear that the current model of natural resource use, which is based on a fragmented and linear approach, needs to be reconsidered. A new paradigm of integrated sustainable management of natural resources that promotes resource efficiency and a transition to a circular economy is of particular relevance. The UN Economic Commission for Europe (ECE) has been taking action to address these challenges since the adoption of the 2030 Agenda for Sustainable Development in 2015. Among other things, it has developed the UN Resource Classification Framework (UNRC), a unified system for classifying and accounting for resources based on social, environmental and economic feasibility, technical feasibility and the degree of reliability of resource valuation. It is encouraging to note that the UNFC is now widely adopted by a wide range of stakeholders, including governments, industries, the financial sector, academia and civil society.

In 2017, ECE member States decided to expand the scope of the UNFC, transforming the classification system into a dynamic resource management tool that helps countries, organisations and companies respond to sustainable development challenges. The Expert Group on Resource Governance (EGER) was tasked to develop the United Nations Resource Management System (UN-RMS), a voluntary global standard for integrated and sustainable resource management through public-private partnerships and civil society. If properly managed resource extraction, processing, use and reuse can provide favourable outcomes for both 27
society, and for the environment. The expansion of the UNFC into a full-fledged management system, UNSAS, has created a dynamic set of tools that link investment principles to sustainable development goals, which helps users transform their activities to build a self-repairing and responsible natural resource management model and contribute to improved livelihoods. This study outlines the UNCSD Principles and Requirements and offers recommendations for transforming a model of natural resource use and reuse for the benefit of present and future generations, which builds on the fundamental principles and

requirements for assessing the sustainability of resource management. In the future, the toolkit is expected to be further expanded and specialised tools will gradually be added to the system to address a variety of issues related to sustainable resource management, such as regulatory modernisation, environmental stewardship, social inclusion, value addition, innovation, circularity and capacity building. They will incorporate standardised methodologies and approaches to achieve common sustainable development goals.

Principles and requirements of the Resource Governance Framework Integrated Resource Governance System is designed to support the implementation of the 2030 Agenda for Sustainable Development, sustainable development requires resources, but their extraction, processing and consumption must be consistent with the principles of sustainable development, based on a voluntary global standard for integrated resource governance in accordance with the principles of sustainable development. This standard applies equally to all resources.

UNSAS has been developed based on the concepts outlined in the following documents:

- "Transforming our world's natural resources: fundamental change

United Nations Resource Classification Framework?";

- "Concept and Structure of the UN Resource Management System."
- "Application of the UN Resource Classification Framework to commercial valuation - an update";
- "Concept Note on the UN Resource Management System: objectives, requirements, key features and the way forward".

A summary of the UNSAS concepts is presented in the European document

UN Economic Commission for UNU (ECE) "UN Resource Management System: Overview of Concepts, Objectives and Requirements".

It also provides definitions of basic terms. The UNSAS submission has the following structure:

(i) Fundamental principles of sustainable resource management; (ii) Requirements;

(iii) A conceptual description of the UNSAS tools, to be completed in subsequent phases of UNSAS development.

A. Purpose of the UNSAS

The goal of UNCSD is to ensure integrated management of natural resources in accordance with the principles of sustainable development for present and future generations. The adoption of the 2030 Agenda for Sustainable Development heralded a new era of global development, with the integration of social, environmental and economic goals as a major challenge.

To fulfil the multidimensional objectives of sustainable development, natural resources must be extracted and used in an optimal and responsible manner. However, we currently face many obstacles to the sustainable use of resources. Among them are economic obstacles such as market volatility, the need to promote responsible investment, to combat the effects of excess profits and to ensure that no one is forgotten. There is a need to make a proper assessment and offer a satisfactory explanation of the social impacts for all the targets outlined in the commitments from the UN climate change conferences. This work has to be done in a context of geopolitical conflicts and high uncertainty. It should be recognised that some of the challenges mentioned above are specific to the economy and the industrial sector as a whole, but the primary role in sustainable resource management is played by the state, combined with the active participation of industry and the responsibility of the financial sector. If properly managed, the extraction, processing, use and reuse of resources will yield favourable results for both society and the environment, contributing to the equitable distribution of benefits, poverty reduction and the elimination of conflicts.

As it happens, resource management decisions are made in the context of individual projects or sectors, usually by a single government agency and companies working in the relevant sector - mining, oil and gas, renewable energy, nuclear power, human resources, groundwater and geological resources. This fragmented approach has significant disadvantages, as it does not allow the whole picture to be seen, the full range of interdisciplinary knowledge to be utilised and the diversity of perspectives to be taken into account in decision-making. The limitations of fragmented management approaches are becoming increasingly apparent. They lack integrated analyses, leading to suboptimal decision-making and risk of serious damage to natural capital. The world needs to rethink resource planning and management practices by moving away from isolated processes towards more integrated approaches.

UNCSD embodies the essential concept of integrated resource management, where complexity, different scales and competing interests are taken into account and provide a common basis for informed decision-making. The process of sustainable resource management begins with an understanding of the state of the world's natural capital and natural resources, including the effort required to develop and utilise them, and an understanding of how these resources relate to the current and future needs of society. Natural capital is the world's stock of natural assets. It includes various elements such as water resources, geological structures, minerals, biodiversity, soil and the ozone layer. Natural capital is characterised by properties such as environmental sustainability and ecosystem health and integrity.

Natural resources are the part of natural capital that is used to produce goods and provide services through economic activity, can be considered minerals, petroleum, nuclear fuel, reservoirs, man-made resources, and renewable energy sources such as geothermal, solar, wind and water power and biofuels. When natural resources are utilised for the benefit of society, net natural capital can increase rather than deplete. Sustainable resource management is defined as a set of policies, strategies, regulations, investments, operations and opportunities in public sector, public-private and civil society partnerships that are implemented in an equitable and transparent, ecologically and socio-economically appropriate and technically feasible manner, which in turn determine which resources are developed, when and how they are developed, extracted, consumed, reused and recycled by the public at large. UNCSD-based sustainable resource management is designed to optimise sustainable benefits for stakeholders in the human-planet-prosperity triad. The approach emphasises cross-sectoral linkages and the minimisation of potential negative impacts, and is: (a) a global and voluntary resource management system for use by the public sector, industry, investors and civil society, and to promote the principles of sustainable development, applied by ;

(b) An innovative integrated resource management system for natural resources to support the development of policies and regulations for sustainable management, contributing to the implementation of the Sustainable Development Goals (c) An extensive information base and methodology for resource management;

d) A holistic system for managing the life cycle of resources, including their extraction, storage, transport and consumption (use and reuse);

e) A framework of sustainable development principles to apply to resource sector finance;

f) A system that allows local and indigenous people to evaluate and analyse projects for compliance with stated environmental, social and economic objectives;

g) A mechanism to take into account the long-term commercial and regulatory aspects of projects;

h) a set of conditions that allow the industry to utilise integrative dynamic capabilities;

i) A toolkit designed to assist in ensuring that projects comply with applicable regulations;

j) a tool for sustainability reporting and financial reporting.

B. UNSAS users and intended uses The main users of UNSAS are governmental and regional authorities, industry, investment actors and civil society, including academia, non-profit organisations, indigenous peoples and the general public

Each stakeholder group will use UNSAS for its own purposes. As UNSAS is a principles-based system, requirements must be fulfilled in order for it to be applied in accordance with the requirements, some requirements are satisfied by compliance with other existing standards and guidelines, which are currently incorporated by reference into the detailed UNSAS manual and will be described at a later date. Where existing documents do not provide guidance on fulfilment of requirements, the text will be developed within UNSAS.

Main users of UNSAS and its intended uses

A. Governments/regional bodies

a) Meeting climate change targets

b) Development of regional and national energy and commodity programmes for sustainable development

c) (d) Planning, including the development of fiscal policies, to ensure security of supply and demand, including assessing global stocks and flows and ensuring access to resources

(e) Developing the necessary laws and regulations (f) Assessing global and national risks and opportunities

g) maintenance of national data registers

h) revenue management

i) development of international standards in addition to existing ones, necessary to meet the complex challenges of the future

j) supporting the development of the global market

k) Improving resource management efficiency and maximising the benefits of resources at the point of extraction

l) development of tangible and intangible infrastructure

m) addressing social issues

(n) Land-use management

o) addressing labour issues

p) addressing environmental issues

q) implementation of labour protection, safety and environmental protection measures

(d) Facilitating partnerships and conflict resolution

s) Improving education and research

t) mitigation and management of climate change

u) disaster management

v) Determination of disclosure requirements

B. Industrial sector

a) Strategic planning, including resource portfolio, supply chain and production chain management

b) Ensuring harmonisation of the interests of different actors

c) support for capital investment decisions

d) Strengthening social and environmental controls

e) increased sustainability

f stress testing

g) operational management

h) servicing of financial obligations

i) capacity expansion and deployment

j) partnership building

k) assistance in research and development

l) assistance in merger and acquisition transactions

m) Evaluating business proposals, including risks and opportunities

(n) Ensuring a return on investment

o) managing opportunities and risks at the portfolio level

p) managing projects, corporate risks and opportunities

q) managing disclosure requirements

C. Investors

a) support for investment analysis and investment decision-making
b) improving equity participation policies and practices
c) Determining the requirements for disclosure of information by investees (d) Developing requirements for self-reporting of information
D. Academia, non-profit organisations, indigenous people and the general public
a) modelling resource flows at different spatial and temporal scales
b) (c) Assistance in the development of technologies from a systems approach (d) Interdisciplinary capacity-building
(e) Supporting sustainable development
(f) Education and training (g) Gender equality and diversity (h) Respect for the traditional rights of indigenous people (i) Promotion of futurological research (j) Improved communication among stakeholders (k) Establishment of international centres of excellence for sustainable resource management (ICES-SRM)
B. In addition, references to existing compliance manuals will be included in the UNCSD and new documentation will be developed where existing manuals are not available. A preliminary list of desired outcomes is provided below: (a) Resource security, i.e., ensuring the availability of resources for sustainable development;
b) Addressing the negative externalities of resource extraction and utilisation, such as pollution, waste, tailings, and so on;
c) eliminating the risk of unfair or irresponsible behaviour, i.e. avoiding the promotion of actions that exacerbate negative externalities and unjustified profits, including excess profits;
d) Providing affordable, equitable services that are consistent with the principles of sustainable development;
e) equitable distribution of benefits to all stakeholders and alignment of incentives that promote sustainable development.
When referring to the UNDMS for analyses, reporting and resource management planning, it is recommended that the fundamental principles be used as a first level checklist and the UNDMS requirements as a detailed checklist. Definitions provide a condensed form of the language, concepts and terms needed to define the UNSAS. This list serves only as a starting point; future versions of this document will include more terms. The following definitions are provisional and may be adjusted according to the needs of stakeholders. These definitions also need to be aligned with the glossary of commonly used terms and similar definitions used in international initiatives.
- A resource is the total quantity of products that are produced and/or consumed by a project from a given date and estimated at the project milestone(s). A resource has environmental, social and economic value and may be renewable (e.g. solar, wind, groundwater) or non-renewable.
Resources may be intended for primary use (e.g. minerals, hydrocarbons, renewable energy, groundwater, pore space for CO2 storage) and may be derived from or after primary use as secondary resources (e.g. anthropogenic resources,

residues and tailings from mining, processing or refining waste, construction waste).

- Governance is the activity of controlling resources, using resources or disposing of resources in an efficient manner, taking into account the needs of present and future generations.
- A system is a set of definitions, principles and procedures, organised schemes or methods under which resources are managed for environmental, social and economic benefits.

The UNCSD framework will include the underlying principles and requirements for managing resources for sustainable development. The system will also include tools for analysis and decision-making.

A. Fundamental Principles of Sustainable Resource Management To ensure the integrity of sustainable resource management, i.e., taking into account multiple variables, temporal and spatial scales and life cycles, such management should be guided by principles.

Thc Principlcs provide a guideline for dctermining the overall direction of sustainable resource management.

The fundamental principles of sustainable resource management are listed below:

1) the rights and responsibilities of States in resource management;
2) responsibility to the planet;
3) integrated resource management;
4) social engagement;
5) service-orientation in the use and reuse of resources;
6) integrated resource recovery;
7) Creating added value;
8) closed-loop principle;
9) health and safety;
10) innovations;
11) transparency;
12) Continuous strengthening of core competences and capabilities.

On the basis of such underlying principles, lower level requirements are established.

Principle 1. Rights and Responsibilities of States in Resource Management States (governments) have rights and legal and regulatory responsibilities with respect to resources within their territories.The 2030 Agenda for Sustainable Development, adopted by all UN Member States, is a common plan of action to ensure peace and prosperity for people and the planet today and in the future. The centrepiece of the The 2030 Agenda is the 17 SDGs: urging all countries to take action to manage resources sustainably.

A State has sovereign rights over all resources within its territory. It has independent legislation and full rights to the sustainable management and use of resources. States are encouraged to apply

The principles of good governance envisaged in UNCSD are voluntary. States (governments) play a major role in the production and consumption of resources. In weighing the costs and benefits of various activities, States usually take a long-term perspective. They set resource policies through various legal instruments, statutes and laws, and strengthen the roles and capacities of resource management agencies such as ministries, regulatory bodies, geological surveys and universities.

Principle 2. Responsibility to the planet

The primary goal of sustainable resource management is to ensure the sustainable well-being of the Earth, its inhabitants and the environment. The principle of environmental limits to sustainable development is recognised in the Brundtland Report (1987) and is reflected in Agenda 21, the Rio Declaration, the Millennium Development Goals and the Sustainable Development Goals . The Brundtland Report states that "the concept of sustainable development does imply certain limits to the exploitation of natural resources, but these limits are relative rather than absolute and are related to the current level of technology and social organisation, as well as to the capacity of the biosphere to compensate for the effects of human activities. At the very least, sustainable development should not jeopardise the natural systems on which life on earth depends: the atmosphere, water resources, soil and living beings".

Sustainable development is defined as development that meets the needs of the present without compromising the ability of future generations to meet their own needs.

Sustainable development also means considering the balance of costs and benefits for society and the planet. The production and consumption of resources can have negative consequences. Therefore, a sustainable trade-off between advantages and disadvantages must be found.

The Paris Agreement states that "climate change is a common concern of humankind". Its overarching goal is to enhance the global response to climate change by keeping the increase in global average temperature below 2 °C above pre-industrial levels in the current century and working to limit the temperature increase to 1.5 °C.

The primary responsibility for the continued well-being of the planet also lies with the Equator Principles-a system adopted by financial institutions to assess and manage environmental and social risks.

Principle 3: Integrated resource management

Sustainable resource management is undertaken through public sector, public-private and civil society partnerships in an integrated and indivisible manner, consistent with its social, environmental and economic viability and systems, and taking into account the principle of the full life cycle. The Brundtland Report (1987) emphasises the need for an integrated approach to natural resource management. The report states: "Until recently, our planet has been a vast world in which human states have different legal structures, so the term "state" is used in a broad sense and, accordingly, in this document the term "state" and "government" are used interchangeably.The International Commission on Environment and Development published a report entitled "Our Common Future". This document is also known as the Brundtland Report, after the name of the Commission's Chairperson, Ms Gro Harlem Brundtland. It sets out the guiding principles of sustainable development as it is currently interpreted activities and their consequences have been clearly delineated within States, sectors (energy, agriculture, trade) and broader fields of endeavour (environment, economy, social relations). [...] However, sustainable and long-term development is not an unchanging state of harmony, but rather a dynamic process in which the scale of resource exploitation, the direction of investment, the vector of technological development and institutional changes are aligned with current and future needs. [...] However, most of the institutions dealing with these issues tend to be independent and unrelated agencies; they have relatively narrow profiles and their decision-making processes are closed. The agencies responsible for natural resource management and environmental protection are organisationally separate from the agencies dealing with economic issues". Many of the environmental and development challenges we face stem from this separation of responsibilities. Sustainable development requires overcoming this isolation. The 2030 Agenda emphasises the need for an approach based on the interface between the natural and social sciences, and between the research community and policy-makers.

The 2030 Agenda states that the SDGs "are integrated and indivisible and balance all three dimensions of sustainable development: economic, social and environmental". The interlinked and integrated nature of the SDGs is critical to ensure the timely realisation of the goals of the 2030 Agenda. The need for effective partnerships between the public sector, public-private associations and civil society is envisaged in SDG 17.

The Brundtland report states that "problems cannot be solved by individual siloed agencies and fragmented strategies. They are interconnected within a complex system of causes and effects". Natural resources are consumed by socio-economic systems directly or as a function for the purpose of producing other resources, for general production and consumption purposes, or for the built environment. Systems thinking suggests that researchers and practitioners should assume a broader understanding of interrelationships, but can focus on individual critical interrelationships between separate layers. Focusing on individual resources, economic sectors or different types of environmental or human impacts as isolated elements will not advance progress in improving resource use and, more broadly, the realisation of international agreements and SDGs.

Addressing issues in one area without considering other areas may even lead to negative consequences. A systems approach is crucial for maximising benefits across sectors and mitigating the negative impacts of natural resource use. A systems approach to the design and implementation of environmental policy addresses many global challenges; it is no longer optional, as it is now the only possible way to transform society to achieve global sustainability. Resource life cycle management is based on a systems approach. Life-cycle analysis is a method for assessing environmental impacts that covers all stages of a product's existence, from raw material extraction to material processing, production, delivery, use, repair and maintenance, and disposal or recycling (cradle-to-cradle concept).

Principle 4. Social engagement

Sustainable resource management must ensure a sufficient level of social engagement. Social inclusion is necessary to ensure that all stakeholders involved in the sustainable development of natural resources for the benefit of all present and future generations interact with each other. Stakeholders, including governments, industry, customers, employees, suppliers, investors and civil society, must build trust and work together to develop responsible practices in the areas of human rights, labour, environment and anti-corruption. Respect for the human rights and interests, cultural sensitivities, customs and values of workers and associations affected by resource extraction is an integral part of sustainable resource management. This is emphasised in the United Nations Guiding Principles on Business and Human Rights. Such an approach should contribute to improved social performance and socio-economic and institutional development. The involvement of key stakeholders in resource management is necessary to address sustainable development challenges in advance. It should also take into account opportunities and produce transparent, independent reports on progress and performance, and be independently verified.

Sustainable resource management can have complex social impacts related to displacement, land rights, cultural heritage, indigenous peoples, gender equality, employment, public health, occupational health and safety, sexual exploitation and abuse, and other issues. Resource projects should apply human rights-based social safeguards, inclusive dialogue and risk management principles to ensure that projects benefit the poor, no one is forgotten and human rights are respected. Infrastructure planning processes should also include inclusive, participatory, transparent and regular stakeholder consultations.

According to the United Nations Declaration on the Rights of Indigenous Peoples, sustainable resource management should be based on free, prior and informed consent. The above views are supported by several targets in the SDG framework, such as SDG targets 1.4 and 16.7.

Principle 5: Service orientation in resource use and reuseResources are extracted primarily as a service to society. Removing the dependence of economic activity and human well-being on the amount of natural resources used and the degree of environmental impact is essential for the transition to a sustainable future. Removing this dependence can bring significant social and environmental benefits, including compensation for past environmental damage, while supporting economic growth and human well-being.

Service orientation is one of the main principles to eliminate this dependency. Service orientation should be applied to both the use and reuse of resources. By applying such a service model, the industrial sector will be able to create long-term benefits for both shareholders and society.

Principle 6. Integrated resource recovery

Sustainable resource management promotes the creation and maintenance of a knowledge base and systems for integrated resource recovery at all stages of operations. One of the basic tenets of resource management should be the concept of integrated resource recovery, i.e. the idea that environmental disturbance should be minimised by extracting all possible beneficial elements and prioritising them from a full life-cycle perspective. This principle can be extended to all stages of the life cycle in which tangible and intangible beneficial elements are extracted and utilised. Integrated resource recovery is also one of the main principles that contribute to eliminating the correlation between the amount of resources used and development.

Principle 7. Creating added value

Sustainable resource management should promote and facilitate the creation of added value throughout the life cycle. Value addition is defined as any economic, environmental or social benefit from downstream processing of resources and downstream production. The purpose of value addition is to increase the gross domestic product (GDP) associated directly with processing and production, as well as to reduce unemployment and achieve other benefits, including from multiple supplier industries such as engineering, design, eco-technology and equipment supply. Reporting should be done along the entire value chain, including increasing the share of local content in the local, regional or national economy. Sustainable resource management requires linkages of upstream stages to industrial goods production and the service sector; downstream stages to beneficiation, refining and distilling, industrial and consumer goods production and the service sector; and horizontal linkages to infrastructure (electricity, logistics, communications, water) and to skills and technology development. Careful assessment of the potential for added value creation is required and the results of the assessment should inform resource management, particularly in terms of social, environmental and economic viability. Potential social and environmental challenges can be turned into opportunities when the opportunities for value addition are viewed through a full life cycle lens.Private sector participation and investment are critical to integrated and sustainable resource development and resource efficiency, and play a critical role in value addition. In resource management, opportunities for mutually beneficial co-operation between government, the private sector, civil society, local communities and other stakeholders should be carefully explored.

Principle 8. Closed loop principle

Sustainable resource management promotes the establishment and maintenance of a knowledge base and systems for responsible development, use, reuse, recycling and waste minimisation at all stages of operations. The circular economy is a systematic approach to industrial processes and economic activities that maximises the utility of a resource for as long as possible.

The most important considerations in implementing the closed-loop principle are the reduction and rethinking of resource use, the pursuit of renewability and reusability of resources and the durability, substitutability, repairability and upgradability of value-added products. Disposal of residues as waste should be the last and least favoured option.

Sustainable resource utilisation requires sustainable management of renewable resources. It should aim to recycle non-renewable resources so that they can be reused, resulting in a circular economy in which waste is minimised. A by-product of one process becomes a raw material for another process. In a circular economy, the efficient use of resources throughout their life cycle, from extraction to production, consumption and utilisation, recycling and reuse, is crucial. The circular economy also plays a key role in eliminating the dependence of development on the amount of resources used.

The Brundtland report states that "all countries should anticipate and prevent the emergence of these pollution problems, for example by strictly enforcing emission standards that reflect likely long-term impacts, promoting low-waste technologies, and taking timely action on the impacts of new products, technologies and wastes."

Sustainable resource management should aim to conserve all resources through responsible production, consumption, reuse and recycling of all products, packaging and materials, without incinerating them as far as possible, and without burying them in soil, discharging them into water or the atmosphere, which threaten the environment and human health. This requirement is also relevant to achieving the SDGs. Principle 9: Health and safety at work

Sustainable resource management promotes the establishment and maintenance of a knowledge base and systems to continuously improve health and safety performance with the ultimate goal of zero harm, within reasonably achievable limits. Ensuring maximum safety for workers and local communities is a requirement of international labour standards on occupational safety and health10 and other international conventions. Resource management can only be effective and feasible if the basic concept of safety is given the highest priority at all stages of the life cycle.

Principle 10. Innovation

Sustainable resource management promotes the creation and maintenance of a knowledge base and systems that foster innovation towards hybrid technologies and diversification of extraction and utilisation. Bringing together different research areas, technology developers and industry is becoming a reality. Hybrid technologies, diversification and smart approaches are being utilised to break the deadlock and turn the results of scientific research into lasting value. This principle is recognised in the 2030 Agenda, which calls for "achieving productivity gains in the economy through diversification, technological upgrading and innovation, including by focusing on high-value-added and labour-intensive sectors".

Principle 11. Transparency

Sustainable resource management ensures that the public understands the distribution of revenues and costs - this stimulates public debate on which to base informed choices about sustainable development options. Openness and reliability of information enables more effective policy making and promotes a social licence to operate. The need to avoid corruption from the contracting and licensing stages to the procurement of goods and services makes transparency in the provision of information for public debate and the identification of realistic sustainable development options particularly important.

To reduce the risk of corruption and to ensure the proper use of revenues, many governments, public and private organisations

improve governance processes and increase transparency in the sector. Ultimately, information on who controls and benefits from resources is used as a key tool to fight corruption and counter illicit financial flows in all sectors of the economy.

Public understanding of the distribution of revenues and costs stimulates public debate on which to base informed choices about sustainable development options. This requires the disclosure of accurate and verifiable information at all stages of the value chain.

The proper utilisation of natural wealth should be a critical factor in sustained economic growth that contributes to sustainable development and poverty reduction. However, its mismanagement can have negative economic and social consequences.

Principle 12: Continuous strengthening of core competences and capabilities

Sustainable resource management ensures that the core competencies and capabilities of organisations and personnel required for interdisciplinary research, development, demonstration, deployment and operation are continuously strengthened. The integrated and indivisible management of resources requires an interdisciplinary approach to problem solving and working in teams composed of experts from different backgrounds. This approach goes beyond what the traditional education system offers and requires continuous improvement of competencies and capabilities.

B. Requirements

The UNCSD principles are accompanied by the following requirements that should be taken into account. Some requirements may not apply to individual resource sectors. The decision to apply UNSAS to a particular resource sector for integrated resource management should be made on a case-by-case basis.

1. Rights and responsibilities of States in resource governance (a) National policy and strategy: supporting the implementation of sustainable resource governance in line with the 2030 Agenda;

b) Regulatory compliance: establishment of regulatory bodies responsible for sustainable resource management;

c) Coordination: coordination with the various authorities responsible for regulating sustainable resource management;

d) Technical service provision: provision of technical services required for sustainable resource management;

e) Compliance with international obligations and international co-operation agreements.

2. Responsibility to the planet

a) (b) Strategic environmental assessment: Strategic environmental assessment (SEA) is a systematic process for assessing the environmental impacts of a proposed policy, plan or programme that examines cumulative impacts and gives due consideration to them, along with economic and social considerations, at the earliest stage of decision-making;

c) Climate change related activities: all activities are in line with nationally determined contributions (NDCs), the conceptual vision of investors and companies, and climate change policies;

d) Resource and energy efficiency: actions to reduce the amount of resources and energy used to extract resources;

e) a measure of GHG emission intensity : expressed in g CO2 eq/MJ;

f) water use and management: how to optimise water abstraction, wastewater discharge to the environment and water management in accordance with the country's legislation;

g) land use and management: measures aimed at minimising negative impacts on land or optimally managing such negative impacts;

h) proper management of all wastes and effluents;

i) biodiversity conservation and enhancement activities: all activities to conserve and enhance biodiversity in a given area;

j) Preparation of periodic reports on sustainable development issues for various purposes.

3. Integrated resource management

a) Information platform, data interoperability, dashboard: the availability of prompt, accurate and complete information about an area or project on which to base decisions;

b) Estimating resources and determining the level of confidence in the UNFC estimates;

c) Opportunity and risk management: identifying, assessing and prioritising opportunities and risks, followed by the coordinated and cost-effective application of resources to minimise, monitor and control the likelihood or degree of impact of adverse events, including resource-related conflicts, and to maximise the realisation of opportunities;

d) productivity: ensuring that the necessary measures are taken to improve the efficiency of extraction. A productivity indicator is usually calculated as the ratio of total output to unit or total costs in the extraction process, i.e. output per unit of cost, usually over a specified period of time;

e) Counteracting illicit financial flows, erosion of

43

tax base and profit shifting (TPT): illicit capital flight. Internal taxation MFATs are possible because multinational enterprises exploit existing gaps and inconsistencies between tax systems in different countries affect all countries. The higher reliance of developing countries on corporate income tax means that they are disproportionately affected by MFNTs;

f) sustainable investment principles: a set of company performance standards that socially responsible investors use to select potential investment targets;

g) Artisanal and small-scale mining (ASM): if there is ASM in the area, it should be integrated into development programmes;

h) competent and qualified assessments: all criteria necessary to ensure the quality of the data and information provided;

i) Establishment of cash reserves for decommissioning, including the preparation of plans for closure and decommissioning of the plant from the time of its commissioning. Such plans are subject to regular updates.

4. Social engagement

a) Human rights protocols to prevent child and forced labour and protect workers' rights;

b) Indigenous peoples: in accordance with the UN Declaration on the Rights of Indigenous Peoples;

c) "stakeholder capitalism": a focus on satisfying the interests of stakeholders such as customers, suppliers, employees, shareholders and local communities;

d) communication and outreach activities.

5. Service orientation in the utilisation and reuse of resources

a) A service model of resource utilisation and reuse is a business model in which customers pay for a value-added product or service, such as heat, light or mobility, rather than for resources. Environmental life cycle, waste management, recycling, etc. can be part of a long-term service contract.

6. Integrated resource recovery

a) Management of by-products and co-products: maximising the benefits of all by-products and co-products;

b) Making the most of land plots/maximising their value: optimising land use by taking land plots out of inefficient use.

7. Creating added value

a) Interdisciplinary approach: identifying opportunities to diversify activities to support different sectors of the economy;

b) Feasibility studies: detailed studies that look at resource and energy efficiency, performance and analyse all possible outcomes;

c) Assessing and publicising opportunities associated with previous, subsequent and parallel processes;

d) management of all links between previous, subsequent and parallel processes in resource management;

e) Supply chain optimisation to ensure optimal supply chain performance;

f) Life Cycle Assessment: a methodology for assessing the impact on the environment relating to all stages of the life cycle of a resource's use.

8. Closed loop principle

a) Waste hierarchy model: The 'waste hierarchy' organises waste management options in order of their environmental optimality. The model prioritises waste prevention from the outset;

b) Closed-loop design: designing to minimise expected waste and pollution, to conserve the products and materials used and to restore natural ecosystems;

c) anthropogenic resource management: utilisation of residues as secondary resources.

9. Occupational health and safety

a) Crisis management, emergency response: emergency preparedness measures that anticipate likely emergencies and plan in advance for key elements of the response, including innovative monitoring systems and automated feedback management systems;

b) safety protocols: a system of protective measures to mitigate existing or unregulated risks;

c) standards for the protection of worker and public health: compliance with international and national standards and regulations to protect workers and the public;

d) Tailings and residue management: ensuring the safety of tailings and residues and critically assessing the implications of different options for the utilisation of residues, mainly anthropogenic resources.

10. Innovations

a) Models of innovation in the form of a combination of hybrid technologies and approaches applicable to different technologies;

b) create-evaluate-learn: a method for quickly obtaining feedback on the usefulness of a new product or service;

c) minimum viable product (MVP) development: A prototype that is evaluated solely for internal quality; (d) Innovation accounting: a quantitative approach to see if innovation is bearing fruit and providing valuable experience.

11. Transparency

a) Transparency and traceability of the supply chain: to ensure supply chain transparency, companies need to know what is happening in previous, subsequent and parallel stages and share this information internally and externally;

b) due diligence: conducting an investigation, audit or review to confirm facts or clarify details;

c) Governments should analyse and report on the links between companies' previous, subsequent and parallel processes, as well as their supply chain due diligence processes;

d) data quality: evidence of accuracy and validity, legality and validity, reliability and consistency, timeliness and relevance, completeness and comprehensiveness, availability and accessibility, degree of detail and uniqueness;

e) assessments carried out by competent authorities and qualified professionals.

12. Continuous reinforcement of core competencies and capabilities (a) Institutional strengthening (ICGO-ESD): building institutions with a long-term mission to create sustainable value and change the world for the better;

(b) Vocational retraining: preparing workers for project completion and equitable transitions.

C. SURON instruments

The UNCSD will consist of several tools to promote integrated natural resource management in line with the principles of sustainable development. They will incorporate standardised methodologies and approaches to achieve UNCSD objectives. A conceptual description of the starter toolkit is presented in a standardised form to reflect UNCSD requirements Users of UNCSD may include government, industry, the financial sector, civil society and academia. In analysing, reporting and planning resource management based on specific requirements, UNSAS users are encouraged to follow the structure presented below. Depending on the specific purpose of the analysis, reporting or planning to be carried out using UNSAS, the details may vary. The procedure may be performed for public administration, company management or for the preparation of published reports. The following list is not exhaustive and may be adjusted as necessary.

1. References to regulatory documents

a) The 2030 Agenda for Sustainable Development;

b) Paris Agreement on Climate Change;

c) Regional visions, strategies and requirements (e.g. European Green Deal, European Union Principles for the Sustainability of Raw Materials; African Union Agenda 2063;

Africa's Mining Vision Programme);

d) National concepts, policies and strategies;

e) UN policy brief "Transforming Extractive Industries for Sustainable Development";

f) UN instruments and conventions relevant to this requirement;

g) key links to public health and wellbeing.

2. Terms and definitions

3. Integration with all UNCSD principles

a) Transformation;

b) opportunities to adapt to local priorities and needs;

c) verification, feedback and audit mechanisms.

4. Scope and context
a) Organisation and conditions for the implementation of its activities;
b) stakeholders;
c) substantiation of claim;
d) optimisation;
i) desired results;
ii) The link to resources as a public good;
e) Conceptual vision and leadership:
i) Commitment;
ii) Policy;
iii) Creating value for stakeholders in the long term;
iv) roles and responsibilities.
5. Compliance with the Sustainable Development Goals
a) On the demand side:
i) balanced and integrated resource management;
ii) The value chain to the point of delivery;
iii) compliance and outcome measurement parameters;
b) on the supply side:
i) description of resource development modes;
ii) relevance to the sustainability of supply and value chains;
c) Efficiency:
i) stakeholder satisfaction indicators;
47
ii) key performance indicators;
iii) monitoring, measuring, analysing and evaluating;
iv) internal audit;
v) management analysis.
6. Planning
a) General;
b) short-term;
c) medium-term;
d) long-term;
e) critical control points/ dashboard indicators.
7. Support
a) Human/institutional resources;
b) competences;
c) awareness;
d) information interaction;
e) information.
8. Operating activities
a) Controls;
b) risk assessment;

c) risk management.

9. Improvement

a) Corrective Action;

b) continuous improvement.

Conceptual description of tools UNCSD proposes a range of tools for sustainable resource management based on principles and requirements. These will include standardised methodologies and approaches to achieving the objectives, and a brief description of the individual tools is provided. These tools will be further developed based on case studies in different countries.

Other tools will be added to the RMS as needed.

1. Clean Energy Index

Combating the global climate crisis and implementing sustainable resource management have become a major priority of our time. Managing resources in accordance with the principles of sustainable development serves the interests of present and future generations. Sustainable resource management will require coherence with the SDGs such as poverty eradication, climate change and affordable energy.

The energy of the future must be low-carbon. The energy transition to a low-carbon economy offers opportunities primarily related to the development of renewable energy and conventional sources with reduced CO2 emissions.

Global energy markets are making the transition from hydrocarbon energy to sources with reduced CO2 emissions. The United States Environmental Investigation Agency predicts that the share of renewable energy sources will soon double, while the share of natural gas relative to total consumption will remain at the same level but grow by 35 per cent in absolute terms. The fuel and energy sector needs to invest aggressively in clean energy. Between 2008 and 2017, only between 0.5 per cent and 4 per cent of oil and gas companies' investments were in renewable energy, mainly to reduce operating costs and develop green, clean technologies for the conventional energy sector. Renewable energy is an important additional source of energy that can, at low cost, meet the growing global demand for energy supply. The Environmental Investigation Agency predicts that onshore renewable energy generation will increase tenfold by 2050, while offshore energy will grow forty three times and solar 17 times.

Renewable energy development involves the extraction of critical raw materials. Their critical importance stems from a strong dependence on low-carbon energy and limited reserves. For example, experts estimate that lithium extraction needs to increase 42-fold for the further development of renewable energy. At the same time, most lithium is extracted from brine. Consumption of cobalt, nickel and graphite is also expected to increase by 20 times. At the same time, exploration and extraction of rare earth elements are associated with CO2 emissions. In order to compare the carbon footprint of different types of energy it is necessary to consider the full life cycle.

It is therefore required to view energy as a holistic process of resource extraction from different low-carbon sources, including exploration and extraction of critical materials and waste management.

Understanding the full life cycle impacts can have a positive impact on cost reduction in the process of generating electricity from different sources. Consequently, an objective comparison of the carbon footprint and efficiency of different types of energy based on a clean energy index should be made.

This tool estimates the carbon footprint of energy from different sources throughout the entire production cycle, including exploration, extraction and waste management. An objective comparison of the carbon footprint and efficiency of different types of energy based on their net energy indices will also serve to achieve a balance between different types of energy. This tool will help to develop an unbiased approach to achieving the SDGs.

The Clean Energy Index will be used by a variety of stakeholders, including governments and businesses. This UNCSD tool will be the starting point for assessing and comparing all types of energy. The Clean Energy Index will play a role in building a circular economy and in integrated resource management.

2. Service orientation in the use and reuse of resources To achieve the goals of the 2030 Agenda, an uninterrupted supply of resources is required. Current resource consumption patterns are highly imbalanced, with high-income countries consuming more than 25 tonnes of resources per person per year. At the same time, annual consumption in the least developed countries is below 2.5 tonnes per capita. Increasing production is not enough to meet the demand for resources. Uncontrolled increases in extraction would have serious environmental consequences and leave a large carbon footprint. Resource efficiency needs to be dramatically improved. Existing commodity models have been developed for linear economies. They are not suitable for a cyclical economy. An alternative to the commodity model is the service model, which takes into account the products, tools and technologies that suppliers provide to users as a service.

All industries around the world, including retail, journalism, manufacturing, media, transport and enterprise software, are currently being transformed by the service model.

Today, many large companies derive most of their revenues from the sale of services rather than raw materials or products. Commerce is moving to a subscription model that allows companies to forecast their revenue.The focus has now shifted from commodities to consumers and outcomes. A service-oriented industry will not focus on producing more goods, but on using as few resources as possible to achieve a certain outcome. The focus will be on resource efficiency, which means efficient production with minimal impact on the environment and climate. Industry and consumers become true partners and develop together. Consumer loyalty will become widespread and strengthen the social contract on natural resources. It will not be difficult for a "commodity" industry to turn into a "service" industry. Along with many other sectors, changes are also taking place in the manufacturing industry.

Instead of focusing on products, inventory and promotion, this industry has focused on the audience, its customers.

The reorientation towards services will contribute to the development of a circular economy. There will be a shift from inefficient use of resources to maximising resource efficiency and eliminating the dependence of development on the amount of resources used. The potential benefit to the industry is the elimination of unpredictable market volatility, which regularly goes through phases of ups and downs. Even if complete control over unpredictable factors is not possible for complex supply chains, at least it will be possible to improve forecasting accuracy and preparedness for market fluctuations. Resource market stability will benefit governments, which will have greater planning capabilities in a stable economy. This transformation will generally contribute to a more equitable distribution of benefits among all stakeholders in society and strengthen the foundations of the social contract for natural resources. The UNCSD tool provides stakeholders with options, checklists and guidance on how to make the transition.The transition can take place in phases. Integrated resource recovery, value addition and closed-loop approaches are incorporated into the tool.

3. Resource supply system

Most of the resources needed by society are extracted from thousands of individual projects (mines, oil fields, wind farms, etc.), which are usually fairly well understood individually. However, there is a lack of holistic understanding of the functioning of the totality of these projects, which form a dynamic and complex adaptive system consisting of hundreds of interconnected and interdependent elements. Such systems usually respond to change in a non-linear and unpredictable manner. The Resource System Tool provides a holistic conceptual understanding of the system, including its degree of complexity, for further research.

The Resource Supply System tool can serve as the basis for analysing the resource supply system. It will include the actions required to supply products while being a small part of the economic system of the human world. The tool will have several basic components: the source, the physical system (extraction, transport, processing), the financial and economic elements, and the conditions of the activities (legal requirements, regulation, etc.). It will include modules on needs, agents, sources, physical systems, financial and other socio-economic issues.

In its structure, the tool can be seen as a normalised representation of the project's drivers, resources and flow of operations. Each block can consist of many, often hundreds, of agents or activities linked together in a network that forms a dynamic adaptive complex system. In order to simplify and make the management of this complex system more efficient, a system based on blockchain technology has been developed.

4. Blockchain system and machine learning/artificial intelligence model for resource management

The old resource management system chronically failed to address one of the most important challenges of the transition to a cyclical economy related to illicit financial flows, including corruption and tax evasion.

Collectively, these phenomena cause ongoing and significant economic damage annually to many countries supplying critical and other resources to other countries. With distributed ledger technology, a blockchain-based tool will provide an "in-built" solution while providing end-to-end, continuous traceability and transparency of material and cash flows.

If all extracted resources are accurately tagged (tokenised) using blockchain technology, starting with recovered and reused secondary resources, which always take precedence over primary resources, the unique nature of each resource unit, whether it is a single resource or a combination of multiple resources, will essentially make each resource unit unique and therefore "irreplaceable".

With blockchain, zero waste will become a programmed outcome of the circular economy as well as one of the ethical pillars of sustainability. Through the functionality of distributed ledger technology, blockchain adoption will address a range of challenges in linear supply and value chains that lead to illicit flows of funds, such as loss of data integrity, lack of transparency and traceability, and confusing or inefficient governance.

A significant advantage of blockchain is the use of smart contracts, where "smart" now essentially means automation: a contract can be embedded in the system, with the terms of the contract available in a transparent and verifiable form. When the conditions are fulfilled, the transaction is carried out automatically and a new block is added to the chain to record the fulfilment. It also becomes much more difficult to falsify or tamper with records, and tracking instances of falsification or tampering becomes easier. In case of any change in transactions as a result of such intervention, a new block is generated and recorded as part of the chain.

The tool will be developed based on:

a) preliminary specifications for the various instruments included in UNCSD;

b) existing systems (such as various tools for food supply chains and customer service);

The structure of a blockchain-based cross-industry supply chain process for tracking, recording, translating and potentially transferring critical data and analytics to all relevant parties will be clarified. A tool for resource management based on blockchain technology and machine learning/artificial intelligence will be developed: blockchain-based tokenisation identifies transparent and traceable flows of materials and cash as fungible objects in the circular economy, contributing to several key objectives such as reducing or completely eliminating illicit flows of both resources and cash. The use of blockchain combined with machine learning and artificial intelligence to implement smart contracts in UNCSD-supported supply and value chains is becoming standard procedure to avoid avoid avoidable losses and unproductive costs by better matching supply with resource requirements (especially critical raw materials) in a sustainable, financially transparent and fair manner.

5. Critical Raw Materials Dashboard Energy transitions are highly dependent on the availability of critical raw materials. Critical raw materials are dependent on geographical aspects, sustainability issues of production and utilisation, and supply chain complexity.

To properly manage critical raw materials, stakeholders from governments, industries, financial institutions, academia and civil society need up-to-date information on the availability, extraction, utilisation and reuse of critical raw materials. In the age of digitalisation, there is no shortage of data. However, the biggest challenge is to extract information from the data set that can be useful for decision-making.

Collecting data on critical raw materials and harmonising them based on UNFC standards helps to meet this challenge. However, UNFC-based data should be considered in conjunction with other production information, especially social and environmental aspects. Particular attention should be paid to supply chain information and data on the utilisation and reuse of other inputs.

CHAPTER 3

## 3 Ensuring carbon neutrality through technology-based interactions of screening for the prevention of noncommunicable diseases

The compromise agreements at the UN on climate change (COP 26) reflected the wide range of interests, contradictions and political will that we see today. Together with my team of experts, I attended COP 26. to meet with activists, diplomats and heads of state from the UNECE region and beyond, and to find common ground on a range of topics important to achieving the goals of the Paris Agreement and the 2030 Agenda for Sustainable Development. This included issues related to sustainable energy. Energy is critical to maintaining peace, co-operation, sustainability and quality of life in our region. The experts found clear pathways for policy makers towards a zero-carbon energy system.

Improved energy efficiency, renewable energy, highly efficient fossil fuel combustion technologies with carbon capture, utilisation and storage, nuclear power, hydrogen, integrated and sustainable management of natural resources are all part of the solution to achieve carbon neutrality. However, only bold, immediate and sustainable action can decarbonise energy in time to avoid a climate catastrophe, which defines international cooperation and is essential to support all countries in the UNECE region in building sustainable energy systems and accelerating the energy transition towards carbon neutrality. UNECE continues to offer its member States a platform to engage in exclusive and transparent dialogue, share best practices and learn from each other, to jointly achieve the energy goals of the Sustainable Development Goals.

Inaction is a political choice that will lead to more serious and possibly insurmountable problems in the future. Political decisions need to be made now to prepare society and build the necessary infrastructure and make the best use of our natural resources. The magnitude and complexity of these challenges are becoming more evident every day, as is preventing catastrophic climate change and achieving the goal of limiting global warming to 1.5°C.

This study calls for ambitious and bold action by government, the private sector and regulators. The development of these technologies requires a new regulatory framework to support immediate commercialisation. Policy frameworks should also include legally binding commitments to increased international technology transfer, harmonised standards and definitions for green hydrogen, energy efficiency and energy conservation. All solutions should be evaluated against existing and upcoming net zero carbon and climate neutrality targets, with all energy infrastructure built to be zero-energy. The integration of innovative energy technologies along with the transformation of energy markets and downstream industries is a challenge and an opportunity.

The investment required to achieve a low-carbon economy will pay off financially and avoid the incalculable costs of economic, social and human disruption from climate catastrophe.

Approximately 80 per cent of primary energy in the UNECE region currently comes from fossil fuels. While different countries will support different technologies in different ways, we need to deliver sustainable energy to address climate change and ensure quality of life at the global level. In short, inaction is not a viable option.

All should be supported in taking action to accelerate the transformation and sharing of best practices in urban and rural development, especially cities, industry, buildings and transport, while achieving the goals of the 2030 Agenda for Sustainable Development and those of the Paris Agreement.

This study builds on the recommendations of the Sustainable Energy Pathway Project and the UNECE Carbon Neutrality Project and is based on a series of technology briefs that directly support the implementation of the Carbon Neutrality Project.

The main objectives of this study are as follows:

- Informing policymakers about the range of options and solutions for achieving carbon neutrality
- Supporting the efforts of all countries to achieve carbon neutrality and attracting investment in green infrastructure projects - Building the capacity of economies in the UNECE region to achieve common goals
- Key findings from climate model-based problem solving show that current national actions and international climate targets set in the Paris Agreement and COP 26 do not achieve carbon neutrality and limit global warming to 1.5-2°C.
- This mission is feasible because governments have achievable pathways to develop and build carbon-neutral energy systems through technology synergies.
- Technology interactions, since carbon neutral energy systems consist of:

I) diversification of primary and final energy supplies;

II) accelerated phase-out of traditional fossil fuels;

III) electrification of all sectors through renewable energy and nuclear power;

IV) widespread deployment of low- and zero-carbon technologies (including CCUS, hydrogen and next-generation nuclear power, and energy storage solutions).

- In the UNECE region, there is a need to increase:

I) technology transfer and implementation;

II) institutional capacity to plan and implement an ambitious transformation of energy systems;

III) participation and acceptance by all stakeholders to create secure, affordable and carbon-neutral energy systems.

- Immediate action must start now to maximise the use of all low and zero carbon technologies to achieve carbon neutrality by 2050.

-Governments need to:

(I) Raise awareness of the benefits of all low- and zero-carbon technologies;

(II) Develop a policy framework in support of carbon neutrality; (III) Create a level playing field for financing an equitable transition to carbon-neutral energy systems consistent with the needs of Member States.

- UNECE's role, coordinated international co-operation will be essential to achieve carbon-neutral energy systems. UNECE provides a much needed exclusive and neutral platform for developing rules, standards and norms for systemic changes in lifestyles and infrastructure.

Supportive policies, incentives and regulatory frameworks encourage regional and subregional technical cooperation in the energy, industry, construction and transport sectors for projects of common interest and public-private partnerships. The future carbon-neutral energy system has clear pathways to achieve carbon-neutral energy systems by combining existing and emerging technologies into integrated energy systems. All low and zero carbon technologies have a role to play in interconnected systems where no energy system will exist in isolation. Innovation and digitalisation enable energy systems to be efficient, sustainable and capable of providing a net zero-emission region.

As the recent report of the Intergovernmental Panel on Climate Change (IPCC) confirms, it is clear that human influence is relevant to warming the atmosphere, ocean and land. It is now or never if we are to limit global warming to 1.5°C; this will not be possible without immediate and deep cuts in emissions across all sectors. Climate change is causing extreme weather events and subsequent social and economic disruption in all regions of the world. At the same time, sustainable energy systems are crucial for quality of life and underpin the realisation of the 2030 Agenda for Sustainable Development. Climate models show that current carbon reduction policies and Nationally Determined Contributions (NDCs) fall short of what is required to achieve the goal of limiting global warming by 1.5-2°C. There is a mismatch between the energy and climate targets agreed by countries in line with the Paris Agreement targets and the progress already actually being made. We have little time left to limit the effects of climate change. Inaction is a political choice that could lead to more serious, potentially insurmountable consequences in the future. Complex global energy systems underpin every economy. On the supply side, then, national energy systems are not isolated, but are part of optimised interconnected intra- and inter-regional systems.

These systems are characterised by the availability of natural resources and technologies that can affect sustainable growth. Namely, a changing technological landscape driven by low-cost technologies, as well as environmental and geopolitical challenges that significantly influence the structure and policy options of the energy system. Once energy systems begin to change, it will take industrial users and downstream consumers considerable time to adapt their operations to the new energy systems.

Clean and low-cost energy technologies are advancing rapidly, but most are still in the early stages of deployment. While technological options exist for most nations, prohibitive costs, regulatory barriers and social pressures prevent large-scale deployment. There are innovative ways to produce low- and zero-carbon energy, including renewable energy technologies, hydrogen, fossil fuels, carbon capture, utilisation and storage (CCUS) and nuclear power. The multiplicity of choices also requires an integrated approach to selecting the optimal mix of technologies. On the demand side, there has also been some decarbonisation through system efficiency, electrification of the energy system and digitalisation. Innovative measures in industry, transport and construction are playing a key role.

The necessary momentum towards carbon neutrality amidst increasingly urgent calls for action, high-level energy convened the first global energy meeting on global energy, and for the UN Framework Convention on Climate Change, which held its 26th Conference of the Parties (COP 26), which called for accelerated technology development, deployment and diffusion, and policy approval for the transition to low-emission energy systems, including through the rapid deployment and generation of clean energy, as well as the development and deployment of clean energy technologies. This report presents an analysis based on modelling results and explores different ways in which policymakers can achieve zero carbon through technology collaboration and implementation of the 2030 Agenda. It should be noted that the modelling undertaken for this report assumes that all technologies will achieve decarbonisation on time and in full. If technology development and deployment is delayed in any way, or if a technology is removed from the agenda, the projection for achieving carbon neutrality will need to be revised.

The changing landscape of energy technologies affects energy systems, ways to achieve carbon neutrality are compatible with national interests. must urgently finalise their current pathways and adapt their energy systems in line with the objectives of the Paris Agreement. The transformation of energy systems must start now and cannot be done in isolation.

Carbon neutrality means achieving zero carbon emissions to limit global warming to 2°C (aiming for 1.5°C) in line with the Paris Agreement. Carbon neutrality requires careful balancing of actual carbon emissions with carbon removal through natural sinks, engineered carbon utilisation technologies and the elimination of carbon emissions. Under the Paris Agreement, carbon neutrality is defined as achieving a balance between anthropogenic emissions from sources and removals by sinks of greenhouse gas emissions in the second half of this century.In the context of this project, carbon neutrality refers to achieving net zero carbon emissions that limit global warming to 1.5-2° C by balancing reported carbon emissions (mainly carbon dioxide and methane) with carbon removal through natural sinks or engineered carbon utilisation technologies.

Carbon neutrality is not an end result. It is an integral part of the journey towards stabilising greenhouse gas concentrations in the climate. However, as a stand-alone goal, carbon neutrality policies alone will not be sufficient to limit global warming. If carbon neutrality is achieved too late, net negative carbon emissions will be needed to eliminate the excess. It is hoped that achieving carbon neutrality in the future will allow carbon emissions to be managed over time and will need to be periodically reviewed and issues such as historical emissions addressed.

Sustainable energy systems based on the three pillars of energy security, quality of life and environmental sustainability will protect society from future risks. Energy security refers to providing the energy needed for economic development; quality of life refers to ensuring affordable energy available to all at all times; and environmental sustainability refers to limiting the impact of energy systems on climate, ecosystem and health. A rapid transition to sustainable energy requires careful decision-making to balance all three pillars to fulfil the widely recognised 2030 Agenda for Sustainable Development.

Sustainable energy and carbon neutrality frameworks are needed to analyse technology interactions. Modelling and expert commentary assume that the rate of economic development in each UNECE member state will be maintained and each country will have its own energy preferences and transition pathways based on natural resource endowment, technological and infrastructure basis, cultural heritage, historical pattern of economic development and regulatory framework. The commitment to ensure access to affordable, reliable, sustainable and modern energy for all is included in the UN Sustainable Development Goals (SDGs). This approach embraces the SDGs and emphasises the interlinkages between the different aspects of sustainable energy and the trade-offs between the three pillars.

Finding a balance between the three pillars is a complex social, political, economic and technological challenge. The dialogue within the UNECE Committee on Sustainable Energy will be an important step for countries to identify trade-offs and synergies for energy security, quality of life and environmental sustainability. While there are no simple answers, there is an urgent need to balance these competing but interrelated interests, how carbon neutrality is achieved, why innovative technologies are needed, reaching consensus on the energy transition to carbon neutrality is a complex issue. Policy choices affect existing and new energy technologies and economic growth, and depend on the availability of national energy resources. Increasingly tight timeframes mean that ideal pathways to carbon neutrality are becoming less and less feasible without harming society. As each country has unique circumstances, there is a need to ensure equal access to resources to achieve carbon neutrality.

The ability to adapt to such a complex transition is vital to developing consensus-building mechanisms among stakeholders to ensure timely and rapid decision-making. Rapid transition can disrupt societies if policymakers do not utilise all available options. Even undesirable options may be required.

Carbon neutrality is achieved through a combination of low and zero carbon technologies and changes in social behaviour. Energy demand will be driven by economic activity, lifestyle changes and energy efficiency, low carbon fuels, smart technologies and electrification of all sectors and supports an integrated approach to energy technologies to represent the interests of all member countries and maximise synergies between different energy sources, fossil fuels currently dominate energy supply due to outdated infrastructure, ease of transport, storage, infrastructure and density Existing and emerging low and no-carbon alternatives need to be utilised to support sustainable development. Sustainable innovative solutions such as CCUS, hydrogen and next generation nuclear power must be scaled up to match the cost and technical competitiveness of conventional technologies through innovative advances, economies of scale and closer alignment with market demand. An analysis based on modelling results is presented and an expanded set of available technical options is shown to support policy development and international energy cooperation.

Solutions and technologies analysed include energy efficiency, renewables, fossil fuels, nuclear and hydrogen, as well as carbon sequestration approaches such as CCUS, BECCS and direct air capture.

Policy makers should use Life Cycle Assessment (LCA) studies to validate their approach. LCA compares technologies on the basis of lifetime environmental impact, from those with the smallest carbon footprint to those that require significant carbon capture and storage to be carbon neutral. It is almost certain that all low- and zero-carbon technologies will be required in the transition period. For example, policymakers can transition to a hydrogen economy at the rate that electrolysers are utilising low-carbon wind and solar power as well as nuclear power. They can also share investments using hydrogen from natural gas with CCUS to accelerate hydrogen ecosystem infrastructure. Battery storage and improved management of distributed resources can stabilise and optimise electricity on the grid. Fossil fuels with CCUS and nuclear as controllable energy sources can act as baseload and provide flexibility for intermittent renewables such as wind and solar, and ensure the reliability of the energy system.

To achieve a carbon-neutral energy system in the region, all currently available low- and zero-carbon technologies for energy supply must be rapidly deployed, and the efficiency of the system must be improved. This includes transforming energy supply by installing CCUS technologies in fossil-fuelled plants, scaling up renewable energy projects, deploying nuclear power, launching large-scale sustainable hydrogen projects, and deploying all other technologies discussed in this review. In addition, national grids and interconnections must be strengthened and expanded in accordance with the combination of energy supply and transnational balancing requirements. An expanded set of technologies is needed to achieve carbon neutrality by 2050 and realise the 2030 Agenda. All energy technologies have disadvantages that can be minimised if used together and strategically.

Carbon neutrality will ultimately require significant changes in how the economy works, potentially leading to many unintended consequences. Any rapid implementation of change requires coordination of technology development, commercialisation and public acceptance 1. "Readiness levels" is a commonly used metric to describe what needs to be addressed during change implementation. Energy infrastructure built now must meet zero energy requirements to avoid asset issues. All infrastructure scale assets have a useful life of more than 30 years. Consequently, any assets built now must meet national emissions targets or be easily retrofitted in the future. Given the timeframe and nature of this transition, modelling shows that a very large scale CCUS system is required over many years. It acts as a last resort if the transition is delayed. Which in turn allows for the continuation of key industries such as cement, steel and chemicals that are difficult to reduce, and even if carbon neutrality is achieved, further reductions in greenhouse gas emissions may be required. As the rate required for decarbonisation is now very high, CCUS can extend the life of non-compliant infrastructure, limit excessive energy transition costs and avoid social disruption. Energy efficiency and optimisation will be the foundation of all energy policies. It is an essential element of managing energy demand in a zero-emissions world by 2050. Which in turn will require the rapid deployment of efficiency measures and the creation of optimal demand for buildings, industry and transport. Policy measures will involve significant investment and training to fulfil the monumental task.Policy should encourage, not delay, change in the energy system. Modelling from the Pathways to Sustainable Energy project has shown that progress has been too slow, and to achieve carbon neutrality towards the 1.5-2°C target, UNECE countries must either further reduce or sequester at least 90 Gt of carbon dioxide by 2050 in the 'middle of the road' socio-economic projection. 90 Gt-equivalent to current global CO2 emissions over four years. Policies should be implemented to reduce and optimise energy demand, decarbonise energy supply and introduce engineered and natural carbon removal technologies

Life Cycle Assessment studies show that there is no completely carbon neutral energy solution. All technologies require materials and high-temperature processes that result in greenhouse gas emissions. Renewable energy solutions require steel, cement and silicon. Electric vehicles and grids in batteries require rare earth metals. Hydrogen can enter the atmosphere and have negative impacts. Investments in energy could mean increased emissions today, reducing emissions in the future. The modelling does not require this change to be factored into the outlook, energy models and greenhouse gas (GHG) emissions models of the economy as it is modelled using historical trends;

1 UNECE Technology Interoperability: Technology Readiness Levels (TRLs) are a method for assessing the maturity of a technology. Commercial Readiness Levels (CRLs) are a method to assess various indicators that affect commercial and market conditions beyond just the level of technological maturity. Social Readiness Levels (SRLs) are a method to assess the extent to which new ideas and innovations resonate with individuals and groups, as well as whether they will be integrated into society and decisions regarding their application in the form of regulatory and

financial treatment.
2 Pathways to Sustainable Energy, the reference scenario allows us to analyse the likelihood of achieving specific goals in the world on its current trajectory. This is a vital part of all research. An analysis of specific indicators based on the outcome of the reference scenario may suggest that a long-term performance goal (LPG), such as a 25 per cent reduction in energy intensity by 2050, is more likely to be achieved given our current assumptions about the pace of economic development and the emerging linkages between energy and economic development. The results of the baseline scenario may also suggest that specific LPG is unlikely to be achieved under the current set of assumptions and interconnections. The baseline scenario for the Pathways project is the overall socio-economic pathway representing the 'Middle of the Road' pathway.
Modelling and analysis of energy technologies:
-Wind power is a renewable energy source that uses turbines to convert wind on land and sea into electricity.
-Solar power is a renewable energy source that uses sunlight through photovoltaic cells (PV) or a set of mirrors and lenses to concentrate a large area of sunlight onto recipients to generate electricity (concentrated solar power).
-Hydropower is a renewable energy source that encompasses a wide range of technologies that harness the forces of the natural water cycle.
-Geothermal energy is a renewable energy source derived from heat within the Earth's crust. It can be used to generate electricity or used as a direct heat source.
-Biomass is a renewable energy source made from biological feedstocks that include solid biomass, wastewater biomass, forest residues, algae and agricultural residues.
-Nuclear power plants convert nuclear energy into useful energy, conventional nuclear power plants produce heat to drive a turbine to generate electricity. Nuclear power plants can provide heat for urban district heating and industrial processes.
-Natural gas is a fossil fuel typically burned to produce the heat needed to run a steam turbine. It also has other applications in heat, cooking, industry, transport. -Coal is a solid fossil fuel usually burned to run a steam turbine to generate electricity and heat.
-Carbon Capture, Utilisation and Storage (CCUS) is the process of capturing carbon dioxide (CO2) emissions from fossil energy production and industrial processes for storage deep underground or reuse. This technology can be combined with coal, natural gas and biomass.
-Hydrogen is a bulk chemical substance that is currently used mainly in oil refining and the production of ammonia (for fertiliser) and methanol. In the future, hydrogen could be used as an energy carrier and energy storage medium.
-Electricity and the process of turning an energy system into an electrical system through electrification is seen as key to the rapid deployment of renewable energy.Electricity storage is the capture of energy for later use and includes

lithium-ion batteries, controllable hydrogen assets and hydro storage power plants. Future long-term energy storage may include developments in mechanical, thermal, electrochemical and chemical storage.
Energy efficiency aims to use less energy to provide the same useful output to meet the required energy needs.
Scenario modelling: a tool for informed decision-making and the interplay of technologies is crucial for energy system transformation. Interconnection is key to balancing energy supply and demand with economic viability and sustainability. Technology chains link energy supply from resource extraction, conversion, storage, transmission and distribution to the provision of energy services. Quantitative modelling of these chains helps identify the combination of technologies that shape supply and investment schedules at the lowest cost while meeting energy security and climate goals. Scenario modelling allows policymakers to see the implications of climate policy on emissions, energy costs, security of supply, storage and fixed supply requirements versus variable supply . Policy makers can use modelling to identify technology and performance gaps and decide which technologies to support by understanding investment costs, lead times, and including all their benefits and risks. Early engagement of policy makers in modelling is needed to ensure awareness, flexibility and agility, with the aim of developing policies to achieve carbon neutrality by 2050. Policy agility and flexibility will be needed to change pathways if the technologies currently being developed do not meet expectations. Trade-offs will need to be made between different technology options, costs, pathways, energy security and environmental protection. Modelling necessarily entails many assumptions about various future events. These include intertemporal dynamics, technology availability and performance, socio-political preferences, constraints and boundaries. These assumptions will shape the conclusions as model developers generate scenarios. Future scenarios are based on transparent assumptions about future events affecting all relevant aspects of the energy system. Analysts and planners face difficulties in quantifying parameters and variables, especially when different stakeholders have different perspectives on problems, dynamics or desired outcomes. These assumptions aim to take into account various factors, such as the levels of technical, commercial and social readiness of different technologies, but they may not fully reflect uncertainties about the pathways to deployment, and such technologies may not be available in a timely manner and at expected prices.
For the purposes of this project, a modelling methodology for medium and long-term energy system planning, energy policy analysis and scenario development, the MESSAGE3 model, was applied. This model uses lowest system cost to optimise energy systems under different technology and policy scenarios to achieve carbon neutrality by 2050. Policy makers may wish to use additional criteria reflecting local and national conditions, capabilities and objectives of their energy system. This may include favouring local resources, maximising energy security, social

welfare and intergenerational equity.

3 The IIASA MESSAGE model provides a flexible framework for a comprehensive assessment of major energy challenges and is widely used to develop energy scenarios and identify socio-economic and technological strategies to respond to these challenges. The modelling framework and its results serve as the basis for major international assessments and scenario studies such as the Intergovernmental Panel on Climate Change (IPCC), the World Energy Council (WEC), the German Advisory Board on Global Change (WBGU) and, most recently, the Global Energy Assessment (GEA).

The scenarios modelled in the context of this project represent energy system transformation, technology interactions and climate change mitigation in a geopolitically stable world. A common mistake is to use scenarios for analyses for which they are not intended. Thus, major geopolitical shocks require not only separate scenarios and sensitivity tests, but also a significant revision of the energy system model. Carbon neutrality scenarios explore plausible internally consistent development trajectories to 2050. The modelling uses a simplified representation of real energy systems. This modelling combines geographical areas, economic sectors and technologies to form judgements about required future technologies, lifestyle changes and socio-political acceptance. Naturally, quantification involves making assumptions under uncertainty. Because the future is unknown, modelling should not be an isolated project but an ongoing process based on the emergence of new ideas.

Conventional management of UNECE energy systems, will not bring about the changes required. Given the longevity of existing energy infrastructure and the lack of time to achieve carbon neutrality, the role of "guaranteeing the future" is becoming increasingly important and relevant. The limitations of the critical raw materials required for the energy transition add uncertainty and complexity to the judgements that need to be made. The carbon neutrality scenario modelled for this publication sets out a potential pathway to achieving carbon neutrality by 2050, using an 'average' socio-economic perspective to determine energy demand. The model starts from existing UNECE energy systems and considers the cost of different energy technologies and implementation timelines to estimate the technologies and capacity needed to supply energy at the lowest system costs to support the underlying assumptions of economic growth. When constraints are imposed, such as greenhouse gas emissions consistent with zero emissions by 2050, the energy supply mix will change to achieve a zero-carbon scenario. The model also details investments in energy infrastructure and trade from resource extraction to distribution.

The model takes into account economies of scale. Energy costs and technology development time are based on estimates of technology experts.

The calculated "cost" includes an adjustment for the return on investment for the presentation of the investment case and consists of an assessment of 'cost learning'

through efficiency improvements, optimisation and economies of scale. The model considers energy demand, technology and infrastructure to achieve zero emissions using low and zero carbon technologies alongside existing energy technologies.
Scenario Definitions, Reference Scenario (REF), this scenario is developed from a set of baseline assumptions based on historical trends and current policies. It describes an assessment of the world as it is today. The baseline scenario allows us to analyse the likelihood of the world achieving certain targets on its current trajectory. Future emissions are determined by the relative economics of a portfolio of current and future supply alternatives, as well as the pace of technological learning and innovation and assumptions with trends underlying the baseline scenario. Throughout the publication, the results of the carbon neutrality scenarios are compared to the baseline scenario.
Carbon Neutrality (CN) Scenario. The Carbon Neutrality Scenario sets a binding carbon neutrality limit by 2050 and aims to limit the global temperature increase to less than 1.5°C. This scenario assesses the feasibility of achieving zero carbon emissions by 2050 under the technology, innovation and infrastructure assumptions of the baseline scenario. Fossil fuel-based supply options become economically less attractive. Renewable and nuclear energy are largely replacing fossil fuels. Given the portfolio of future supply options, innovation and technology uptake rates in the baseline scenario, the carbon neutral scenario minimises the deployment of these technologies. Demand management side effects mitigate supply pressures. Carbon Neutral Innovation Scenario (CNI). A carbon neutral future differs markedly from the baseline scenario and fair technology assumptions. The Carbon Neutral Innovation Scenario focuses on the potential benefits of innovation and deployment policies that accelerate market uptake of innovative technologies. These include:

- Carbon Capture, Utilisation and Storage (CCUS) using decarbonised fossil fuels using captured CO2 recycled in the cyclic carbon economy or stored, and using direct capture of CO2 from the atmosphere.
- Nuclear power with large-scale reactor designs and the new Small Modular Reactors (SMRs), as well as additional energy services beyond electricity, such as the transition to synthetic fuels, technologies and industrial processes.
- Hydrogen with a role as a synthetic fuel and hydrogen as a fuel for direct and indirect end-use.

Carbon neutrality at a glance is far from being achieved Carbon neutrality produces 39% of global CO2 emissions and has historically had high emissions, including countries with the highest levels of economic development in the world.
Despite positive commitments by countries, the region remains heavily dependent on fossil fuels. And still, fossil fuels account for more than 80 per cent of energy supply. Although sustainable energy capacity is growing rapidly, the rate of growth is insufficient. In the baseline scenario, Western Europe and North America will account for more than 75 % of total UNECE CO2 emissions in 2050. The

electricity and transport sectors account for more than 60 % of UNECE emissions due to continued dependence on fossil fuels.

Progress towards carbon neutrality and economic development differs across subregions, hence highly developed subregions should not only strive to meet individual targets, but also need to support countries for which achieving carbon neutrality is more challenging . Richer countries should also aim to be carbon negative to offset historical emissions.

CO2 emissions by sector, carbon neutrality requires emission reductions in all countries and in all sectors. Sectoral emissions from industry, buildings and transport must be significantly reduced. Some sectors contribute more than others. Large sectors such as electricity generation, transport and industrial processes contribute most to CO2 emissions. This is due to their heavy reliance on fossil fuels. In a carbon neutral scenario, transformed fossil fuels, electricity infrastructure and land use contribute to offsetting CO2 emissions, combined with significant emission reductions in other sectors.

Methane emissions matter. Immediately after emission, methane (CH4) is 120 times more powerful than carbon dioxide (CO2) in polluting the climate. Like CO2, methane levels in the atmosphere are currently at record highs. It is the second most abundant anthropogenic greenhouse gas after CO2. Methane's high global warming potential means that its leakage into the atmosphere must be minimised. With a leakage rate of around 3-4 per cent, the advantage of replacing coal with gas is likely to disappear. Enhanced monitoring and reporting would provide more robust mechanisms to address this issue. The oil and gas sector has an important role to play in methane regulation and wider decarbonisation of the energy system. Reducing fossil fuel extraction will help reduce CO2 and CH4 emissions.

Agriculture, forestry and other land uses (AFOLU) continue to be major sources of methane emissions. Reduced coal, oil and gas production, reduces emissions from the supply and recovery of liquids and solids in a carbon neutral scenario. Waste emissions are also significantly reduced through more substantial methane control.

CO2 emissions will need to be significantly reduced in all sectors and in all regions by utilising all low and zero carbon technologies. No sector of the economy can be ignored and no technology option can be excluded. Action will need to be taken to tackle the massive challenge ahead. While decarbonisation of energy supply is critical to achieving carbon neutrality, and is just one of many sectors where action needs to be taken now. More efficient land use, natural carbon sinks and carbon capture technologies require sufficient support and investment. Industrial processes and end uses, including transport and buildings, reduce CO2 emissions.A carbon neutral future is achievable with the right policies, incentives and technology synergies. Scaling it at unprecedented speeds will require different kinds of technologies. The necessary technologies already exist, and many are economically viable with the addition of an appropriate regulatory framework. Nevertheless,

carbon neutrality will be challenging but imaginable.
4 Efficiency is defined in terms of economics, price and demand elasticity, lifestyle changes, intensity (MJ/GDP) and engineering efficiency. It does not refer to thermodynamics. Energy efficiency refers to the price-driven reduction in energy demand resulting from additional system costs compared to the baseline scenario. This includes both technological and behavioural indicators at a high level of aggregation, which are modelled through an iterative link between the energy system and the top-down macroeconomic model for each region.

Overall, replacing the supply chain and developing low and zero carbon technologies is not enough to achieve carbon neutrality. Energy system transformation for prioritisation must include end-use infrastructure such as electric vehicles, charging infrastructure, heat pumps, fuel cells, storage systems.All regions reducing demand through large-scale investments in lower energy intensity and higher energy efficiency infrastructure significantly reduce the continued use of fossil fuels.

Subregions are starting to implement CCUS and hydrogen infrastructure, scaling up renewable and nuclear energy, and implementing infrastructure for giant power generation. Technology, commercial and social readiness levels, which are presented in the information technology summaries, readiness levels are based on the United Nations Framework Classification of Resources (UNFC), a universally acceptable and internationally applicable framework for the sustainable management of all energy and mineral resources. Policy makers can use this framework to assess where to focus investments and which technologies to focus on.

The investments required for low- and zero-carbon technologies require a significant shift in the allocation of investments in future energy systems. The modelling shows that investments in fossil fuel extraction are diverted to other sectors of the energy system. Investment in renewable energy quadruples and investment in energy efficiency grows to account for a quarter of total energy investment. Nuclear, CCUS and hydrogen are also seeing significant investment growth.

All regions must redirect resources now before it is too late. Significant investments in energy efficiency and transmission, distribution and storage benefit all stakeholders. Consumers can benefit from lower energy costs with more energy efficient homes. Energy suppliers and industries can also reduce energy production costs with modernised transmission and storage.Policy makers and the financial world should develop an investment framework for all low-carbon energy projects. Governments should support development projects with an appropriate risk-sharing structure and facilitate access to affordable finance to accelerate the deployment of innovative technologies. Coherent policies and market mechanisms are needed to provide favourable investment signals and attract private finance to high capital cost projects. Policymakers should be empowered and rewarded for making strong investment decisions.

Investments in clean energy infrastructure in subregions How much will the transition to net zero emissions cost? The cost of transitioning to carbon-neutral energy systems is much lower than anticipated. The cost of inaction is much higher, as vulnerable energy systems are exposed to the environmental, economic and social impacts of climate change.

Energy investment as a percentage of GDP (gross domestic product) decreases slightly from 1.24% in 2020 to 1.05% by 2050 in the baseline scenario. To achieve carbon neutrality, the share of energy investment must increase to 2.05% from 2025. This is a modest increase, but it will rise if procrastination persists. Failure to act is likely to make climate compatibility more costly and burdensome for future generations. Raising awareness of investment benefits is thus essential to overcome fears of socio-political acceptance.

Final energy costs as a share of GDP can show marginal values at each stage of the energy supply chain, as they include operating, maintenance and fuel costs. The Baseline Scenario foresees a moderate increase from 6.2% in 2020 to 8.0% by 2050. In the Carbon Neutral Scenario, investments in energy and energy services increase to 15.2% of GDP.

Energy systems of the future: region based, rapid transition from fossil fuels to low- and zero-carbon technologies is vital to achieving zero emissions. According to the analysis, the use of traditional fossil fuels will decline as technologies such as solar, wind, nuclear, hydrogen and CCUS develop. The practical realisation of any rapid pathway to carbon neutrality will depend on infrastructure capacity and access to natural resources.

The sustainability of the energy system can be improved in several ways through energy efficiency, diversification of energy supply and an interconnected infrastructure of all low- and no-carbon technologies. In addition, technology development and investment strategies should be part of broader climate policies. Low and zero carbon solutions must be prioritised and built at scale to ensure that carbon neutrality goals are met. If we continue with business as usual, the world is on a path to average global temperatures that are 4-6$^0$C above pre-industrial levels. These levels are considered catastrophic and existential threats to humanity that must be urgently addressed.

Final energy consumption specifies the energy carriers used to deliver it to the final consumer. In the context of this project and modelling, this includes:

- Electricity is used for lighting, appliances and various electrical equipment. It is also used in electric heating, for heat pumps and for cooling buildings. It facilitates the electrification of industrial processes such as electric furnaces and electric transport.
- Solar energy is used to heat buildings and industry.
- Geothermal energy is used in buildings and industry for heating.
- Heat is district heating, including block heating and heat from industrial

cogeneration.

- Hydrogen fuels vehicles such as fuel cell vehicles, providing process heat in industrial processes such as steel and ammonia production. Hydrogen powers fuel cells that generate heat and electricity in buildings and industry.
- Gas is used for cooking and heating in buildings, for heat in industrial processes and low carbon fuel for transport.
- Liquids include both fossil and synthesised renewable fuels. This provides light and heavy fuels and bio-liquids such as ethanol and methanol. Liquids are used for heating/cooling and cooking in buildings, process heat and raw materials in industry.
- Biomass is used for heating in the residential and commercial sectors and in industry.
- Coal is used for combustion in boilers and cooking cookers in buildings, as well as for process heat and raw materials in industries such as steel and cement.

The transition from the current energy end-use mix to a carbon-neutral end-use mix requires structural change. A carbon-neutral final energy supply requires an increase in energy intensity, a shift from traditional fuels to low- and no-carbon fuels, and deep electrification.

Energy efficiency is a simple solution that can significantly reduce energy demand and improve the carbon intensity of the final energy system. Improved energy efficiency is required in industry, transport and construction, and effective action-oriented campaigns are needed to unlock this potential.

The efficiency of the system goes beyond optimising energy consumption. Improving material efficiency and recycling has become important for raw material production in a cyclical economy. To increase resilience to external shocks, improving recycling and recovery capabilities towards full cycling can reduce emissions, availability and cost of raw materials.

System-wide digitalisation can address gaps at the system level while opening up new opportunities. Digital technologies can unlock huge potential through demand-side flexibility, which can be a key tool for balancing the energy system and cost-effectively achieving net zero emissions.

Widespread innovation of low- and zero-carbon technologies is reducing the carbon intensity of energy systems. Along with efforts to improve energy efficiency and digitalisation, a shift from conventional energy sources to low-carbon fuels such as natural gas, biofuels and biomass will be required. The next generation of low- and zero-carbon fuels, such as hydrogen and synthetic fuels, are expected to be scaled up and fully commercialised.

Sustainable hydrogen from renewable energy sources and nuclear power through electrolysis, natural gas, coal and biomass with CCUS can decarbonise hard-to-reach sectors such as long-distance transport or energy-intensive industries. Hydrogen is expected to play an increasingly important role in a carbon-neutral energy system from 2040.

The largest reductions in $CO_2$ emissions require increased electrification of the final energy system. Energy supply is reduced by 35 per cent in the Carbon Neutral Scenario as fossil fuels are displaced by renewables, nuclear power and energy efficiency. Energy demand also requires electrification across all sectors, including industry, buildings and transport. The holistic interdependence of inter-sectoral and regional electricity supply systems will phase out carbon-intensive fuels and significantly reduce carbon emissions. The effect of doubling electricity demand will have the opposite effect. Electrification still implies a doubling of electricity demand. This will require the installation of more transmission cables to increase capacity and efficiency. The reliability of the electricity system will become even more important as it risks becoming a single point of failure, affecting every aspect of life. Electricity generation capacity growth must outpace demand growth to avoid blackouts and excessive energy prices when demand exceeds supply and there will increasingly be a balance between short-term supply and demand. The lack of technology for electricity storage significantly reduces the ability to cope with changes in energy supply over a longer period.

Significant structural changes must take place. The future electricity generation system will have to partly include decentralised and intelligent systems and require CCUS to mitigate $CO_2$ emissions from coal, gas and biomass power plants.

Conventional coal cannot remain a widespread source of electricity generation, the emission intensity of coal-fired generation is incompatible with environmental goals, thus should be

Consider efforts to rapidly invest in and deploy carbon capture, utilisation and storage (CCUS) and high-efficiency low-emission retrofit technologies (HELE) for existing coal-fired power plants, especially where there are no viable alternatives.

Renewables, nuclear and gas with CCUS will be the main elements of the future energy system. It is expected that for every GW of fossil fuel burning capacity phased out, 2.6 GW of low-carbon capacity will be built, of which 75 per cent will be intermittent renewables. The implementation of distributed renewable energy generation projects will reduce grid losses and minimise power flows. New ways to compensate for the use of highly variable energy sources will be required. New forms of energy storage (electrical, mechanical, thermal, chemical) should be developed to reduce the need for backup fossil fuel sources. The concept of baseload energy will be replaced by uninterruptible energy, meaning that supplies cannot be cut off for critical applications.

Whether the carbon neutrality scenarios reflect 'coal phase-out efforts', coal use is dramatically reduced in all modelled carbon neutrality scenarios. The modelling takes into account technology costs and lead times to optimise how carbon neutrality is achieved. The use of coal with CCUS may well be 'economically' optimal in some countries, given additional modelling conditions such as energy security, availability of CCUS facilities and policy preferences. For example, coal is used together with CCUS to produce hydrogen in modelling cases where natural gas or renewables are not viable in some modelled scenarios, the goal is to achieve carbon neutrality using different technologies (CO2 and CH4 emissions are either captured or offset to meet the emissions target)

Carbon neutrality requires an unprecedented reduction in energy intensity of 2.5 per cent annually until 2050. The increase in energy intensity will be associated with economic restructuring and extensive reallocation of resources in the energy system. Phasing out fossil fuels will reduce primary energy production through integrated and intelligent design that meets demand through clean electrification, smart digital technologies, efficient buildings and infrastructure, and a circular economy approach to water, waste and materials. This is embedded in a whole system approach to structural change in technology, lifestyles and the economy.

Primary energy offers provide efficiency gains. Energy efficiency and energy intensity improvements occur entirely within these chains. Converting primary energy into electricity generation, refining and synthetic fuel production, can be more efficient. In addition, energy transmission and distribution, as well as end-use sectors including buildings, transport and industry, are key players in achieving carbon neutrality.

Coal, oil and natural gas in the overall energy supply will need to be significantly reduced. To achieve carbon neutrality by 2050, renewable energy supply will grow fastest, followed by nuclear power. All technological solutions leading to carbon neutrality must be supported. For example, flexible policy incentives to increase access to onshore and offshore sites for wind and solar power plants, permits for new nuclear power plants, and permits to finance geological CCUS. The success of policies to promote renewable energy must be considered to kick-start the transition to alternative energy sources, CCUS, small modular nuclear reactors, and new energy storage systems. Energy systems will become dependent on access to critical raw materials. Current and future energy systems require vast quantities of raw materials, including critical raw materials, so the principles and requirements of the UN Resource Management System (UNRMS), which emphasises resources as a service, value addition, cyclicality and innovation, should be applied.

Innovative solutions for carbon-neutral energy systems they will be the basis for carbon-neutral energy systems. The world started thinking about the transformation of energy systems more than half a century ago. Non-energy industries started this transformation much later. Typically, technology cycles span more than 100 years. Policy makers should expect and be open to a range of innovations over the next decades. Adoption of all low and zero carbon technologies will contribute to achieving carbon neutrality. To make this a reality, technology transfer and deployment must be scaled up, institutional capacity must be expanded, and support for secure, affordable and carbon-neutral energy systems must be secured.

An overview of the properties and potential of three innovative low- and zero-carbon technologies: new generation nuclear power, CCUS and hydrogen - to achieve carbon neutrality. Next generation nuclear power is an important source of low-carbon electricity and heat that contributes to achieving carbon neutrality. Along with current proven commercial reactor designs, many new nuclear reactor technologies are being developed that could open new markets, improved load control, high-temperature heat for industrial processes, combined heat and power, and electrolysis for hydrogen production. Countries that choose to use nuclear power can play an important role in decarbonising energy systems, a review of nuclear power technologies reflects the potential role of nuclear power in achieving the goal of zero emissions and has led some countries to seek all potential low-carbon energy services provided by nuclear power, nuclear power can be selected as it can play an important role in their energy mix as a viable decarbonisation option. Other countries have chosen not to use nuclear energy for various reasons, some because of their natural resources and others because of their safety and waste concerns. However, society is increasingly aware of the risk of not meeting climate targets. The drive to decarbonise energy systems, along with higher energy prices and better safety measures, is changing people's attitudes towards nuclear power.

This will create new markets for the penetration of current large-scale reactors and next-generation nuclear power technologies. Policy support is needed to reduce the financial risks and high capital costs associated with the completion of large-scale nuclear power plants and to accelerate the development and deployment of small modular reactors (SMRs). Nuclear SMR technology can provide a range of energy services, including electricity, cogeneration of heat and power, and high-temperature heat for industry. The model assumes capital cost assumptions per unit of rated capacity ($/kW) similar to large reactors, but with much shorter construction periods.

Large-size NPPs are presented with the ability to operate in two modes:

- base load mode with a high power factor of 95% and low flexibility
- flexible mode with a power factor of 75 per cent and the same flexibility as gas-fired combined cycle power plants. From an energy security perspective, extending the lifetime of existing reactors that can continue to operate safely can significantly alleviate the use and dependence on fossil fuels and energy costs without the financial risks and long-term commitments associated with new energy projects.

Small Modular Reactors (SMRs) are modelled within an innovative carbon neutral scenario. They include the possibility of flexible control of the power system. In addition, they provide low-temperature district heating (DH) in the mode of cogeneration and produce high-temperature process heat for use in industry, replacing fossil fuels. In the future, SMRs will combine high-temperature heat with other processes to increase hydrogen production, while SMRs will have shorter construction times due to modularity and small reactors.

Nuclear power is suitable for producing significant amounts of low-carbon energy using small areas of land. Nuclear power has been shown to be low carbon from an environmental life cycle perspective, but also has a number of co-benefits. It results in low land occupancy and life-cycle transformation due to the high energy density of fuel cells, which minimises the extraction area per kW, and the relatively low occupancy of power plants, it is suitable for providing significant amounts of low-carbon baseload and uninterrupted demand. Micro reactors and small modular reactors are widely used in the innovative scenario. These innovative designs benefit from standardised factory design and economies of scale. In this scenario, the modelling indicates a moderate increase in nuclear power capacity in the energy supply from renewable energy sources such as offshore wind power. There is also a significant reduction in installed capacity as nuclear power is more efficient at providing baseload power than variable renewables and reduces the requirement for large-scale electricity storage.

Carbon capture, utilisation and storage, carbon capture, utilisation and storage (CCUS) technology is needed to mitigate climate change. However, public perception and acceptance of CCUS remains low Ideally CCUS should be avoided, but practically it cannot be ruled out as an option, as it is one of the few utilisation methods that removes atmospheric carbon in significant quantities. If society cannot convert quickly enough, it is potentially the last technology.

CCUS can pave the way to carbon neutrality and meet emissions targets while mitigating the social and economic disadvantages of a rapid phase-out of fossil fuels. It is also important for energy-intensive industries that cannot easily decarbonise. Today, most CCUS is financed by enhanced oil recovery (EOR). In the future, the amount of CO2 that needs to be captured will be enormous - at least 2.2 billion tonnes per year. CCUS needs to be funded as a CO2 utilisation technology, for example in saline aquifers or as a solution for a circular carbon economy. This requires an environmental taxation approach to finance CCUS.

In this innovative scenario, carbon capture technologies are typically installed at point sources such as fossil fuel power plants and polluting industries. As fossil fuels are phased out, the number of suitable sources decreases, with further development of biomass energy with carbon capture and storage (BECCS) and direct air carbon capture and storage (DAC).

A point source CCUS system will not cover all emissions. Increasing the fraction of CO2 captured increases capital and operating costs in power plants and industry. There are also emissions from the use of fossil fuels in transport that have not been decarbonised. Achieving full carbon neutrality therefore means that all fossil fuel power stations with CCUS installed and all transport emissions must be aligned with negative emissions opportunities such as BECCS or DAC. DAC must be fully compatible with other CCUS technologies. Increasing DAC is a robust solution for carbon sequestration because it provides truly permanent storage, unlike most land uses, and is not dependent on natural resources, unlike BECCS and land use.

Carbon capture is necessary to achieve carbon neutrality, low carbon energy technologies and lifestyle changes are insufficient to limit global warming to well below 1.5-2 °C compared to pre-industrial levels. Society therefore realises that CO2 capture and storage will be a necessity. CO2 needs to be actively removed from the atmosphere. Various options are being explored, including accelerated implementation of CCUS and DAC. Although some scientists believe that the ability to remove CO2 from the air will reduce the relevance of an energy system based on non-fossil fuels, and it is important to note that without the implementation of all CCUS technologies, the UNECE region will not be able to achieve carbon neutrality and the goals of the Paris Agreement.

DAC sees exponential growth in the innovative carbon neutrality scenario due to faster technology learning and market penetration. It requires energy inputs and comes with costs. DAC costs money and unlike CCUS in power plants, there is no source of revenue to cover the cost. While DAC provides a higher and longer-term fossil fuel presence in the energy system, it has numerous invaluable indirect social impacts on the feasibility and ease of transitioning to carbon-free energy, reducing the need for variable renewable energy generation, electricity storage and nuclear power.

The broader sustainable energy system aims to keep fossil fuels in the ground. However, fundamental transformational change in energy systems takes time. Many critical sectors of the economy are difficult to decarbonise. By modernising fossil fuel plants with carbon capture and underground carbon storage technologies, we can mitigate the impact of the fossil fuel industry. In 2050, fossil fuels will account for a smaller share of the total energy mix. Outside the energy system, significant industries that are difficult to decarbonise, such as cement, steel and chemicals, will need fossil fuels, albeit in much smaller quantities and will be transformed by measures to limit CO2 emissions.

In the carbon neutrality scenario, CCUS plays an important role. In the priority scenario for carbon neutrality, CCUS means that natural gas use remains constant while oil and coal use declines, but not to the low levels seen in other carbon neutrality scenarios. In this scenario, the UNECE region needs to install about three billion tonnes/year of CCUS capacity by 2050.

CCUS is a last resort that adds flexibility for residual and hard-to-reach industries such as cement, steel and chemicals. It should not be seen as a way to preserve the use of fossil fuels. The cost of wind and solar energy has fallen dramatically over the last decade, making them cheaper than fossil fuels. However, not all activities, including energy-intensive industries, can be easily decarbonised. CCUS has struggled with cost overruns and disappointing results in test centres and needs strong policy support.

Hydrogen is an innovative solution to achieve carbon neutrality and decarbonisation in sectors where emissions are difficult to tackle. Sustainable hydrogen has been proposed as the basis for a modern, decarbonised and energy efficient society. Hydrogen is already used as a chemical feedstock; for example, ammonia is used in fertilisers or hydrocarbons used for plastics. In the future, hydrogen can be used as an energy carrier and energy storage. It has extensive, viable applications in various sectors that need to be decarbonised, such as transport, industry, power generation and building heating. However, it has drawbacks due to which its implementation is not easy. It is difficult to transport, difficult to store in large quantities, poses an explosion hazard and has an indirect global warming potential (GWP) if allowed to escape into the atmosphere. The economics of production depend on the price of the resources needed to produce hydrogen, like natural gas, coal electricity from renewable sources and nuclear power.

The Carbon Neutral Innovation Scenario models a potential hydrogen-based economy. This includes hydrogen electrolysis using solid oxide electrolysers that can run on the high-temperature heat of nuclear power. In addition, the hydrogen-to-fuel pathway is modelled, including the conversion of hydrogen into methane, into methanol and other liquid fuels. This suggests that hydrogen can be used to produce liquid synthetic fuels that can, for example, replace petrol used in various sectors. This scenario shows an increase in the use of hydrogen by citizens to heat buildings and power vehicles, suggesting increased government support and incentives.

Hydrogen can contribute to the decarbonisation of hard-to-reach sectors, such as energy-intensive industries that use high temperatures in their processes or long-distance transport. These are examples of critical economic activities where end-use electrification is only partially possible or such technologies do not yet exist. Consequently, a rapid transition to a "hydrogen ecosystem" is consistent with the goals of achieving carbon neutrality by 2050 and the 2030 Agenda for Sustainable Development. This requires a deliberate, rapid and extensive expansion of renewable and low-carbon hydrogen production.

The massive increase in clean, grid-connected hydrogen electrolysers means that low- and zero-carbon power plants are needed to meet increased demand. Certain types of electrolysers, including platinum, iridium and cobalt, require critical feedstocks. Thus, nuclear power, biomass, solar and wind power have greatly increased energy supplies. Hydrogen from fossil fuels with CCUS also plays a significant role, and by 2050 the region will already be dependent on imported hydrogen.

This scenario also highlights the contribution of nuclear power to hydrogen production through electrolysis and steam electrolysis from small modular nuclear reactors.

There is a significant increase in CCUS for hydrogen production from fossil fuels in the innovation scenario. In the chemical industry, hydrogen for chemical products is traditionally obtained from gas, oil and coal. In the presence of CCUS and DAC, coal gasification, natural gas steam conversion and electrolysis are increasing their contribution to hydrogen supply. These proven technologies can be used to create a hydrogen economy, but require deployment of CCUS or another pathway to stop the conversion of carbon to CO2 and emissions into the atmosphere.

To make the hydrogen economy a reality, efforts to decarbonise the energy sector should be intensified. With adequate economic and financial incentives for capital, this modelling scenario shows that hydrogen electrolysis makes a significant contribution to energy systems by enabling cheap and abundant electricity from low-carbon sources such as variable renewables and nuclear power. In the future, energy importing countries will be able to import hydrogen from a wider set of producers. It is envisaged that existing infrastructure such as natural gas transport and distribution can be adapted to facilitate the transition to hydrogen. Government support for research and development and end-user adoption helps create niche markets for hydrogen technologies such as fuel cells.

The challenge of rapidly expanding sustainable hydrogen production means that policy makers must consider all options for sustainable hydrogen production. These include low-carbon sources such as fossil fuels with CCUS, biomass with CCUS, and renewable energy and nuclear power for electrolysis or thermochemical separation of water using high-temperature processes, whether countries can import hydrogen like oil and gas by 2050, where the hydrogen priority model assumes hydrogen imports of 1 EJ per year. This is equivalent to nine million tonnes per year or ninety-four billion cubic metres (bcm). This is relatively small compared to, for example, current European imports of natural gas, which amounted to about 326 billion cubic metres. However, policymakers should be aware that only pipeline transport of hydrogen has been established. Large-scale transport of liquefied or high-pressure hydrogen remains a technical and economic challenge. Large parts of the existing gas infrastructure will be repurposed to integrate hydrogen produced by electrolysis from low-carbon sources (renewable and nuclear) and hydrogen produced from natural gas using CCUS technology into the energy system.

Building sustainable carbon-neutral energy systems in the UNECE region requires the deployment of all low- and zero-carbon technologies in industry, transport and construction.

In order to succeed in this endeavour, it is important:

- Raise awareness and harness the potential of all low and zero carbon technologies to become carbon neutral. This is possible by identifying and sharing approaches that have proven successful (and internally) mobilising stakeholders to ensure widespread and decentralised deployment of proposed solutions. Develop a clear, technology-independent regulatory framework and energy system structure so that all low- and zero-carbon technologies can be deployed in integrated carbon-neutral energy systems, given the considerable uncertainty inherent in any transition. Coherent policies and market mechanisms across the region are needed to ensure favourable investment signals and attract private finance for high capital cost projects.

- Develop financing mechanisms and investment frameworks that enable the deployment of all low and zero carbon technologies. Unlocking both private and public finance will require climate and sustainable finance categorisation based on science and technology neutral methodologies that support the transition to a low-carbon economy.

Decarbonisation of industry is a top priority for achieving carbon neutrality. Energy-intensive industries are among the main sources of greenhouse gas emissions, accounting for about 25 per cent of total global CO2 emissions. Cement, metals, chemicals and petrochemicals are the most significant sources of industrial CO2 emissions, with shares of 27%, 25% and 14% respectively. Policy makers need to ensure that these industries plan for the consequences of energy decarbonisation, as fuel and raw material supplies to these industries are expected to be affected faster than the typical investment cycle of these industries.

Energy-intensive industries are needed to support a low-carbon economy. Among other things, steel and concrete structures are needed to support energy transmission - for wind power, insulation for energy efficiency and lightweight materials for electric vehicles. Oil and natural gas will continue to be needed as fuels and feedstocks for these industries, as decarbonisation of vital processes will remain technically challenging.

Energy efficiency in industry will be crucial to reduce, replace and offset emissions by replacing equipment with more efficient equipment such as the installation of heating control systems and waste heat recovery.

A variety of low and zero carbon technologies will support the industrial processes of the future. This includes deploying technology solutions for carbon neutral industries by encouraging innovation, research and development to accelerate the development and deployment of all low and zero carbon technologies. Industrial energy efficiency, CCUS, hydrogen, nuclear power and heat, and electrification through renewable energy sources are vital to achieving a carbon neutral industrial sector, will have to adapt to a wide range of innovative energy options. These include electricity, biomass, bioliquids, plant and seed oils, plastic waste recycling and hydrogen. This requires the development of circular economy policies. In addition, deployment of CCUS technologies in the cement, chemical and petrochemical sectors will be a crucial factor in achieving carbon neutrality. Funding for projects to reduce methane emissions from coal mines is difficult to obtain and depends on carbon market funding. Any new coal-fired power projects should establish CCUS and fund methane reduction projects at mines that supply coal to the industry.

There is an urgent need to build capacity in infrastructure, power generation and human resources through pilot projects. Projects can focus on hydrogen as an energy source and process agent in industry, improving energy and material efficiency in industrial processes and increasing energy demand flexibility, emphasising the associated benefits of resilience to energy and resource supply and price shocks. Actions will make companies more resilient to a changing environment, while helping overall energy supply costs by preventing /reducing peak load and thereby contributing to the levelling of the electricity grid.

Clusters and the circular carbon economy can stimulate economies across the region. A circular carbon economy based on emissions reduction, carbon capture, reuse and removal, combined with an industry cluster approach, is a means of creating sustainable jobs, green products and industry competitiveness.

Industry should prepare for significant changes in the supply chain. Fossil fuels are the main feedstock for industry. In general, industry requires a basic energy load. Any interruption of supply is likely to be disruptive. Industry can influence energy projects that provide energy supply. Policy makers should prepare to engage with sustainable and innovative low- and zero-carbon technologies to run factories, support high-temperature processes and remove CO2 as a by-product of industrial processes.

The residential and commercial sectors are demanding electrification on a huge scale and at an unprecedented rate. Most people in the UNECE region use natural gas and heat-generated electricity in their homes and businesses. Mass electrification requires a combination of a number of policy decisions, including improving the efficiency of the energy system, installing insulation and smart appliances. Energy efficiency improvements in the building sector can have a direct impact. This includes decarbonisation of buildings using enhanced retrofitting and insulation of existing infrastructure.

Digital approaches can also define efficient, effective and economically transformative solutions. The use of smart appliances, smart meters, leak detection and advanced load management techniques should be implemented to help detect anomalies and optimise energy use while creating sustainable energy systems that can automatically switch energy sources based on price and availability. Educational programmes could also raise awareness of energy and resource consumption measures. These include promoting reduced thermostat settings, encouraging heat pumps and distributing renewable energy production to households, public and commercial buildings.

Hydrogen is expected to become an important source of electricity and heat for homes in many regions by 2050. Deep electrification of the residential sector is required to achieve carbon neutrality. Surging growth will also require renewable energy capacity and modern energy-efficient appliances.

Hydrogen is expected to significantly penetrate the building sector by 2050 under an innovative carbon-neutral scenario. It will be mainly used for home heating as part of a system-wide digital transformation of the energy system. By 2050, natural gas, oil and coal will be excluded from residential and commercial building services. This is due to political support for retrofitting buildings with insulation and improving energy efficiency. Energy efficiency has excellent potential to reduce consumption, help manage load profiles and reduce infrastructure investment. This includes enhanced retrofitting and insulation of existing infrastructure, as well as educational programmes for end users to raise awareness and help reduce thermostat settings. The transport sector will undergo profound structural change. Electric and hydrogen cars, buses, trains and other transport are set to become commonplace in the region. While such an ambitious shift in the transport sector is generating strong momentum, it is important to note that shortages of raw materials such as lithium and cobalt, as well as issues around recyclability and short battery life for electric vehicles, may prevent full electrification of the traditional urban car park.

The current changes are not sufficient. Transport in the region is dominated by liquid petroleum products such as petrol and diesel. In the last 84 years, transport has been modernised by increasing the number of electrified railways and the introduction of electric and hydrogen vehicles. However, to date, they have had little impact.

Adequate policy support is needed for new transport infrastructure to enter the market. Emissions taxes could be considered to incentivise a structural shift towards low-carbon fuels and technologies, with a shift away from diesel cars. Other policy measures include government support for electric charging stations and hydrogen stations, as well as encouraging flexible working hours, car sharing and increased use of public transport. Natural gas vehicles will also need policy support to see modest increases in use along with biofuels such as bioethanol and biodiesel vehicles.

Major technological challenges remain for decarbonising transport. Despite improvements in transport efficiency, lifestyle changes will also be required. All freight transport by road, sea and air continues to cause significant emissions. Rural areas will be more difficult to redevelop than urban areas.

Hydrogen and biomass play a role alongside electricity in decarbonising transport. Reducing oil demand and emissions is an absolute priority. In addition, hydrogen should be promoted for long-distance freight and passenger transport. The use of biofuels for transport purposes should be seen as temporary unless global maize and grain stocks are threatened. Biomass and waste are well suited for use as feedstocks for the production of biogas and advanced biomethane, ready to be injected into the gas distribution network for heavy-duty transport. Electrification of transport will place a significant burden on the public. It requires the public to buy an electric vehicle and adapt to shorter mileage and longer 'refuelling' times. This is particularly difficult in poor and rural areas. Very cold and very hot regions have battery performance issues. Efforts to persuade consumers to buy smaller cars and use less air conditioning will help reduce battery sizes.

Electrification of transport requires a balanced policy stance and brings together two previously unrelated markets that are priced, taxed and regulated separately - fuel and electricity. Electrification of transport will affect the overall price of electricity unless capacity is increased to meet this additional demand. Tax

revenues from fuel will also
will change. Carbon neutrality targets are usually based on a timeframe for achieving zero emissions. However, climate change is determined simply by greenhouse gas emissions. Building electric cars increases CO2 emissions (due to battery production), assuming a similar pattern of vehicle use. Transport-related emissions will only decrease if electricity comes from low-carbon sources. Optimising transport to limit climate change and ensure stable and affordable energy markets will be a challenge.

CHAPTER 4

## 4 Aspects of health-ecological and social systems development environmental climate change

Environmental assessment provides a picture of the progress made in protecting the environment - the foundation of human life and health - while highlighting the many challenges that need to be addressed by society as a whole. There are far fewer successes than failures and setbacks. The assessment therefore provides much food for thought We face a triple planetary crisis of climate change, biodiversity loss and pollution and waste generation, which is being exacerbated in our region. Getting on track to achieve the Sustainable Development Goals requires qualitative changes in both economics and behaviour.

The assessment shows that success is possible with the right tools and political will. For example, in terms of air emissions, nitrogen and sulphur oxide emissions have been reduced in large parts of the region and the use of hydrofluorocarbons has virtually stopped. However, ambient concentrations of fine particulate matter exceed air quality standards throughout the pan-European region, and despite improvements in the western half of the region, greenhouse gas emissions have declined only slightly over time. The stagnation of emissions reflects a failure to control energy consumption or to invest sufficiently in renewable energy - the share of renewables in the energy mix is growing more slowly than the increase in total final energy consumption.

The assessment also clearly shows the existence of outstanding challenges related to environmental topics such as freshwater, waste management and chemicals, biodiversity, environmental monitoring and data availability, and addresses two themes:

a) Greening the economy : working towards sustainable infrastructure ;

b) Applying the principles of the circular economy to sustainable tourism.

Broadly speaking, tourism does not fulfil the principles of the circular economy and infrastructure is not environmentally sustainable. Nevertheless, the assessment indicates how results can be achieved and monitored in working towards sustainable infrastructure and in applying the principles of the circular economy to sustainable tourism.

Policy and technology solutions are available in all areas, for sustainable infrastructure, the assessment recommends to utilise existing tools to promote sustainable infrastructure, strategic environmental assessment and best practice principles for sustainable infrastructure. Economic and financial incentives should be utilised

and create an enabling environment for the life cycle approach and the implementation of circular economy strategies. With regard to sustainable tourism, the assessment emphasises the need for cooperation among different stakeholders, the application of circular economy principles throughout the tourism value chain, access to knowledge, information and finance for small and medium-sized enterprises operating in the tourism sector, and the integration of circular economy principles into tourism-related legislation, policies, plans and strategies. Other areas requiring urgent attention are the promotion of domestic tourism and the use of more sustainable modes of transport. Progress has been made in environmental protection in some areas, but significant shortcomings remain that pose a threat to both human health and the state of the environment in the pan-European region. The following subregions are mentioned throughout the assessment, where possible and appropriate:

1 European Union of 27 member states;

2 Western Europe - Andorra, Israel, Iceland, Liechtenstein, Monaco, Norway, San Marino, Switzerland, United Kingdom;

3 ) Central Asia - Kazakhstan, Kyrgyzstan, Tajikistan, Turkmenistan and Uzbekistan;

4 Eastern Europe - Armenia, Azerbaijan, Belarus, Georgia, Moldova, Russia and Ukraine;

5 South-Eastern Europe - Albania, Bosnia and Herzegovina, North Macedonia, Serbia, Montenegro, Turkey

The assessment covers the trends shown by the arrows in Tables 1-19 indicate an improvement (green, up arrow) or deterioration (red, down arrow) in the situation, rather than an increase or decrease in the value of the indicator.

1. atmospheric air and the ozone layer

Expanding the policy framework for air pollution control, some progress has been made but more efforts are needed.

The health effects of long-term exposure to fine particulate matter (PM) less than 2.5 μm in diameter (PM2.5) decreased by 13 % and nitrogen oxides (NOx) by 54 %. However, the number of premature deaths due to ground-level ozone exposure increased by about 24 per cent during this period, possibly due to higher average temperatures. The phase-out of hydrochlorofluorocarbons as a refrigerant in refrigerators and air-conditioning systems is not yet complete, especially in countries with economies in transition.

Additional technical and organisational measures should be developed to meet target 3.9 of the Sustainable Development Goals, especially for PM2.5 and ground-level ozone. The main responses are to improve and apply best available techniques to prevent emissions of PM, NOx and hydrocarbons from industry and to reduce emissions from traffic (by implementing Euro-6 and Euro-7 measures). All countries should update ambient air quality standards to bring them in line with WHO recommendations. Adequate replenishment of the Multilateral Fund for the Implementation of the Montreal Protocol should be promoted to accelerate the phase-out of hydrochlorofluorocarbons worldwide. *2. Greenhouse gas emissions*

All countries in the pan-European region have made commitments to reduce greenhouse gas (GHG) emissions, but net emissions in the region are still rising. Efforts and achievements are unevenly distributed across the region. Reductions that have largely been achieved in western Europe are offset by increased emissions in the rest of the region. However, some countries still lack firm quantifiable commitments or mechanisms to track progress in their implementation, resulting in significant data gaps. There is a need to strengthen their commitments to nationally determined contributions, to commit to economy-wide absolute emission reduction targets and to report regularly on progress in implementation and achievement of targets.

3. *Decarbonisation*

Decarbonisation is becoming a hot topic across the pan-European region, but action has been lagging, renewable energy has recently increased, but the region is still heavily dependent on fossil fuels, which on average account for about 78% of total final energy consumption.

The increase in the share of renewable energy in the energy mix has been slower than the growth in total final energy consumption in the region. Detrimental subsidies and incentives should be abandoned or reformed and effective positive incentives should be developed to accelerate decarbonisation by shifting investment incentives to renewable energy.

4. Quantity and quality of fresh water

Water quantity in the pan-European region is distributed asymmetrically in space and time, and climate change poses additional challenges affecting human health through various water-related phenomena such as floods, droughts, waterborne diseases and changes in biodiversity in aquatic ecosystems. Anthropogenic pressures, including through hydromorphological changes and barriers, increase the asymmetric distribution of water resources, degrading freshwater quality (see Tables 4 and 5) and aquatic biodiversity, and directly impacting resources through water abstraction. River basins, lakes and aquifers are exposed to multiple stressors. Diffuse pollution and discharges of urban and industrial wastewater remain significant in many places, and persistent organic pollutants are a major public health concern. However, advances in science are providing new solutions and favouring new processes and technologies to combat these negative impacts.

Where freshwater resources and aquatic ecosystems are threatened, the best available technologies should be applied to improve the situation. Some examples of high-readiness solutions include water protection measures and traditional mitigation approaches, as well as measures to protect resources and use water more efficiently, such as digitalisation and precision agriculture, nature-based solutions (NBS) in the creation of water retention basins or in the restoration of coastal zones, and the use of new techniques for environmental flow regimes. The potential of non-conventional water sources needs to be explored.

5. Freshwater - financing for water projects under the international climate agenda is limited and bankable projects are difficult to establish. Technical and managerial shortcomings have a very strong impact on financing patterns, which over the past decade have been constrained by the effects of crises at local and

regional levels.

Economic sustainability of water management must be sought, and innovative financing mechanisms remain in demand in this context. Several financing instruments (e.g. equitable water tariffs, environmental payments, cost recovery mechanisms and incentives) can be used to develop natural and man-made infrastructure, but a clear legal framework is absolutely necessary for success.

6. Integrated water resources management and transboundary water co-operation

The growing challenges in water resources management indicate that fragmented management practices are unlikely to have the desired effect in the long term. Detailed information is important to improve knowledge, and the involvement of public and private actors becomes very important to conduct successful

water policies and good decision-making. Transboundary management of shared rivers, lakes and aquifers remains a challenge

The problem is exacerbated when there is significant water abstraction or retention upstream and downstream countries have no alternative water supply sources. Despite some positive examples, the processes of co-operation and participation in the protection and allocation of water resources, as well as other practical mechanisms in the pan-European region, are not being realised to the extent that they could be. Integrated water management, involving a balance between human needs for water and the availability of water for nature, should be sought. In order to maximise the impact on society, water policy should be more interdisciplinary and transdisciplinary. Therefore, the interconnectedness of water, food, energy and ecosystems necessitates a proactive policy approach to implement short-term projects in the context of a long-term vision for the pan-European region. Water management is more effective at the basin level and requires effective governance to succeed in terms of technology and financing. This integrated approach is even more important for international rivers, lakes and aquifers where floods and droughts can occur. Co-management should focus on environmental protection and benefit-sharing through effective and sustainable transboundary cooperation in the subregions, as envisaged for the protection and use of transboundary watercourses and international lakes.

7. Biodiversity and ecosystems

The condition of ecosystems remains of concern, with no clear positive trend. Only a small proportion of habitats assessed at the European Union level have a good conservation status, and the general picture is likely to be similar in the rest of the region under consideration. The relative proportion of particularly biodiversity-rich primary and intact forests has remained stable at very low levels over the same period . Forest fragmentation remains an important pressure factor. There are significant differences in the percentage of sustainable fish stocks. Fish stocks in the Mediterranean and Black Seas continue to be significantly overfished, while the north-east Atlantic and Baltic Sea show signs of recovery due to better management decisions. In the pan-European region, land acquisition for urban and infrastructure development continues, but the rate of land acquisition has declined in most EEA member countries and even to the contrary in Eastern Europe.

Conditions should be created for medium- and long-term sustainable mobilisation of funds for the conservation of biodiversity and other components of the environment by both accelerating the use of existing regional and global funds and mechanisms and establishing national financial instruments, also removing or reforming subsidies and incentives for products and activities that result in biodiversity loss, and developing effective positive incentives for mainstreaming biodiversity conservation across all sectors of the economy. In addition, Governments should ensure that positive trends in forest areas are maintained and take additional measures to conserve remaining primary and intact forests and their ecological functionality, for example by promoting management standards aimed at maintaining high conservation value forests, preventing forest fragmentation and thus increasing forest connectivity. It is important that there are sufficient areas of natural quality, which should not be limited to protected areas (PAs), to ensure functional biodiversity (biodiversity conservation on a district-by-district basis).

8. Protected areas

The area of protected areas (PAs) in the pan-European region has almost tripled and the total forest area in the ECE region has increased by 33.5 million ha over the last 30 years. The area of terrestrial and marine ORs has increased since 2000 and represents 13.6 per cent and 9.2 per cent, respectively, in the pan-European region. Over the last five years, the area of Marine Protected Areas (MPAs) has increased by 66 per cent and that of terrestrial MPAs by 22 per cent. Despite the increase in the area of terrestrial and marine MPAs, the overall decline in biodiversity continues. An expanded network of protected areas in the region should be consolidated and improved through investments in management effectiveness, ecological representativeness and connectivity, i.e. ensuring that protected areas are linked to each other to facilitate faunal movement and that they represent the diversity of ecosystems in the country. Additional efforts are needed to achieve the target of 10% of coastal and marine areas in the pan-European region to be covered by conservation measures, in particular in Eastern and South-Eastern Europe. Governments in the pan-European region should protect at least 30% of land and sea surface by 2030, in line with the global movement supported by the High Ambition Coalition for Nature and People. In addition, the expansion of protected areas and territories requires transformational approaches to governance and management that go beyond

traditional protected areas and including, for example, other areas that qualify as other effective zonal biodiversity conservation measures or protected areas.

9. Land use and soil

Land use and land use change dynamics in the pan-European region are still largely driven by agriculture. In most affected areas, further reductions in erosion can be achieved through the adoption of conservation agriculture^ Conservation agriculture practices in the pan-European region can also play an important role in carbon sequestration, water management, biodiversity and increasing soil productivity by increasing soil organic carbon (SOC). In Eastern Europe, the average rate of soil erosion has decreased over the last 30 years due to massive cropland retirement and climate change. In the Russian Federation, the total volume of washed away soil and erosion rates have decreased by 56.1 % and 15 %, respectively, over the last 30 years due to widespread retirement of arable land and reduced spring runoff. Despite the reduction in land drainage in most EEA member countries, the practice continues in favour of urban and infrastructure development in the pan-European region, and soil compaction remains a pressing issue.

Better guidance should be provided to farmers on the use of soil conservation practices in areas with degraded (eroded) soils. Policies should also maintain a reasonable balance between soil organic carbon (SOC) storage to increase crop yields and SOC storage for climate change mitigation, in line with initiatives to, for example, increase carbon storage in agricultural soils by 0.4 per cent each year. Measures should also be taken to address the conversion of natural ecosystems to agriculture and the degradation of habitats due to agricultural practices unfavourable to biodiversity, including, for example, better targeting of subsidies and other incentives for sustainable agriculture. In addition, Governments should consistently take measures to further reduce land acquisition and develop and implement policies to combat soil compaction. According to the Food and Agriculture Organization of the United Nations (FAO), conservation agriculture is a system of farming that promotes minimum soil disturbance (i.e. no-tillage), maintenance of permanent land cover and diversification of plant species. It improves biodiversity and natural biological processes above and below the land surface, which contributes to increased water and nutrient use efficiency and improved and sustainable crop production.

10. Protection of the marine environment

Marine pollution from both terrestrial (e.g. nutrients, plastics, chemicals) and marine (e.g. plastics, oil) sources remains a pressing problem in most marine regions. Beach and marine litter, of which plastic litter is a major contributor, is recognised as a serious global threat to coastal and marine ecosystems in most areas, including remote and sparsely populated areas such as the Barents Sea. At the same time, climate-induced changes in coastal and marine ecosystems are occurring with hitherto unseen effects, such as an increase in sea surface temperature of about 0.2 °C per decade in the North Atlantic and 0.5 °C per decade in the Black Sea (since 1981) and an observed acidification of surface waters at a rate of about 0.5 °C per decade in the Black Sea (since 1981).

0.02 pH units per decade in the marine regions surrounding the European Union (and throughout the world's oceans). A holistic cyclic ecosystem approach to the management of coastal waters and marine ecosystems will be essential for the management of coastal waters and marine ecosystems, encompassing different economic sectors and their value chains, taking into account the cumulative effects of multiple pressures, and gradually bringing together social, economic and governance aspects.

This approach is equally applicable to the use of nature-based solutions (NBS) in sustainable infrastructure to enhance coastal resilience and climate change resilience, and the transition to sustainable coastal and marine tourism as part of post-pandemic recovery coronavirus infection (COVID-19).

Fish stocks in the Mediterranean and Black Seas continue to be significantly overfished, while the north-east Atlantic Ocean and the Baltic Sea are showing signs of recovery due to better management decisions. Urgent action should be taken to reduce major pressures in order to halt and reverse the degradation of coastal waters, marine ecosystems and seas. They should also intensify efforts to complete inventories of a range of beach and marine litter components with information on the composition and sources of litter to enable the development of more effective measures, in particular where subregional measures are deemed necessary. Governments should work with the tourism sector along the entire value chain, recognising the high impact of the sector on coastal areas and the land-sea interface for the marine ecosystem.

11. Waste management

Despite the fact that waste prevention is given the highest priority in the waste management hierarchy, the amount of waste generated continues to grow throughout the region. Even where there is a strong political commitment to the development of a circular economy, such as in the European Union and other Western European countries, the amount of waste generated is increasing. Recycling rates vary considerably between countries and are particularly low in Eastern Europe and Central Asia. A recycling rate of more than 45 per cent for municipal waste is recorded in only a few European Union countries and in Switzerland. The situation is improving in all subregions, but slowly. The average volume of waste consisting of waste electrical and electronic equipment (e-waste), which contains both hazardous and valuable components, is stabilising in the region as a whole, but continues to grow rapidly in the economically less developed subregions. Collection and recycling rates of e-waste are extremely low in all subregions; recovery rates also remain low.

Efforts to prevent waste generation during production and consumption, as well as to manage minor and major repairs and refurbishment, including through the use of financial incentives, such as tax breaks, to reduce waste, should be supported. Such waste prevention efforts will improve resource efficiency, also provide public administrations with skilled staff willing to engage with all sectors of society, and continue to improve access to reliable and detailed information to ensure sound management of chemicals and waste, while establishing a resource-oriented pan-European e-waste management partnership with the goals of efficient collection of recyclable raw materials and recyclable materials. The recovery of secondary resources from e-waste is an urgent priority, especially given the rapidly growing amount of e-waste in Eastern Europe, South-Eastern Europe and Central Asia.

12. Chemicals

Chemicals play a vital role in the economy and are essential for the transition to a green economy, but it remains difficult to determine what the full human exposure to hazardous chemicals is. Chemicals and waste management underpins many of the solutions to the current challenges faced by countries in making the transition to a zero-GHG economy.

Should strengthen their waste and chemicals management systems should also endeavour to further promote the comprehensive and harmonised implementation of multilateral

95

environmental agreements (MEAs), including the Protocol on Pollutant Release and Transfer Registers to the Convention on Access to Information, Public Participation in Decision-making and Access to Justice in Environmental Matters

13. Minerals and materials

Minerals are also critical to the transition to a sustainable, zero-GHG economy, particularly those used in electrical and electronic devices and batteries. Global mineral extraction has tripled over the past half century, and it is the extraction and processing of natural resources that is responsible for more than 90 per cent of the loss of biodiversity and water scarcity and about 50 per cent of the impacts of climate change. There is an important and as yet untapped opportunity to reap economic benefits for the pan-European region and reduce its dependence on sources of vital raw materials - the bottlenecks in the transition to a sustainable economy of the future.

They should adopt an approach leading to a "circular" - or resource-efficient - economy and strengthen the management of raw materials, including, for example, through the application of the Resource Classification Framework and the UN Resource Management System. They should introduce clear legal frameworks to assess and minimise the environmental impacts of extractive industries and generally limit the extraction of raw materials and minerals to prevent biodiversity loss, water scarcity and the effects of climate change. 14. Disaster risk reduction

About 65 per cent of the population in the pan-European region is covered by local Disaster Risk Reduction Strategies (DRR). Only 15 countries in the region reported that all their local governments are implementing such strategies under target 13.1 of the Sustainable Development Goals, while 23 countries, which together account for a quarter of the region's population, do not report data on this indicator (see Table 14).

Awareness of potential hazards, including natural hazards, and in particular climate-related hazards, should be raised, especially among poor communities, and regular reporting on the implementation of target 13.1 of the Sustainable Development Goals and the Sendai Framework for Disaster Risk Reduction 2015-

2030 should be enabled.

Local authorities are determined by the country reporting on the relevant Sustainable Development Goal indicator (11.b.2), taking into account the subnational public administrations responsible for developing local DRR strategies.

Funding and public expenditure on environmental protection, for which data are available, revenues from environmental taxes and public expenditure on environmental protection have increased since 2000, closely following the pattern of gross domestic product (GDP) growth.

However, as a percentage of GDP, government spending on the environment (a maximum of about 0.8 per cent) is much lower than revenues from environmental taxes, which means that revenues from environmental taxes are not necessarily channelled into reducing environmental damage. Nevertheless, environmental expenditure by governments is only a fraction of the total environmental expenditure in each country. "Green bonds have become a tool for financing environmentally friendly projects by both the private sector and governments. Despite the negative environmental impacts of fossil fuels, all countries continue to subsidise fossil fuel extraction to varying degrees. The International Monetary Fund (IMF) predicts that these subsidies will continue until at least 2025, with indirect subsidies increasing until then.

Green finance should be encouraged and environmental expenditures should be seen in the broader context of environmental and public finance. Environmental taxes should be used to reduce various types of pollution, and the revenue generated should be primarily used to finance public environmental expenditure.

Governments should only use subsidies when they are really needed, as they always distort markets and increase public sector deficits. Governments should also periodically review subsidised environmental financing in the light of the polluter-pays principle and regularly conduct impact assessment analyses of such financing so that funds can have a real added value. In addition, governments should envisage the use of green bonds, in particular through a range of policy measures, including demonstration issuance, the dissemination of clear guidelines for issuing green bonds and favourable regulatory policies, as additional instruments for environmental financing alongside more traditional ones such as taxes and levies. National environmental policies in the pan-European region should aim at phasing out harmful subsidies and rapidly shifting to greener energy sources.

Investment in sustainable infrastructure is recognised as one of the strategies with the greatest impact on rebuilding on an improved basis after the COVID-19 pandemic. Recently, there has been a general realisation that sustainable development solutions should be included as early as possible in the strategic planning phase. However, most countries in the pan-European region have not yet developed mechanisms to incorporate sustainability considerations (such as climate risk) and externalities (e.g. pollution costs, ecosystem services or biodiversity protection) into cost-benefit analyses of large infrastructure projects, although these analyses are not legally binding in many countries. Access to basic drinking water services is consistently above 90 per cent in all pan-European subregions, with the exception of rural Tajikistan, where it is below 75 per cent. For example, access to sanitation ranges from 82.3 per cent in rural Eastern Europe to 99.5 per cent in urban areas of South-Eastern Europe and Western Europe, with an average of 96.3 per cent. In the pan-European region, full access to electricity is ensured and the countries have at least 83.8 per cent coverage of third-generation telecommunications. The challenges now are to guarantee an increase in sustainable infrastructure using nature-based solutions (NBS), resource efficiency, recycling and reuse in an environmentally responsible, socially inclusive and economically viable approach. It is important to ensure that the needs of all stakeholders are identified and addressed, and that infrastructure is flexible in use, interconnected and able to utilise real-time information to adapt to changing conditions (including climate risks, changes in demand for services and migration dynamics).

A pan-European effort to achieve a common understanding of what sustainable infrastructure means should be engaged and a common strategy to quantify progress across countries should be defined. Governments should utilise existing tools to promote sustainable infrastructure development, including the ECE Protocol on Strategic Environmental Assessment and the UNEP International Best Practice Principles for Sustainable Infrastructure, and allocate additional resources to achieve the institutional and technical capacity needed to plan, design, implement, operate and decommission sustainable infrastructure projects. They should build on the United Nations Environment Assembly resolutions on green and sustainable infrastructure and on nature-based solutions (NBS) to support sustainable development adopted by Member States. Governments should also use economic and financial incentives - in the short and medium term - to support private sector realisation of ROPFs in infrastructure projects, should also promote investment in sustainable infrastructure more broadly.

In addition, Governments should create an enabling environment for a life cycle approach and closed-loop economy strategies consistent with or similar to the Pan-European Strategic Framework for a Green Economy in Sustainable Consumption and Production Patterns or other initiatives such as the European Union taxonomy

A pan-European tourism economy based on closed-loop principles will be more resilient to and better prepared to respond to crises - economic, health and epidemiological or related to the effects of environmental challenges facing the region. This is necessary for sustainable tourism development and the transition to green tourism and can contribute to the achievement of the Sustainable Development Goals (such as Goals 6, 7, 8, 11, 12, 13, 14 and 15). Despite the improved performance of tourism prior to the coronavirus pandemic (COVID-19), there have been growing consequences of its rapid growth, increasingly contributing to environmental crises, biodiversity loss and social problems.

Therefore, after the pandemic, it is necessary to avoid a return to the traditional model by moving towards sustainable tourism. The application of closed-loop principles is the main strategy for the transformation, recovery of the sector and sustainable development in general, and will contribute to the creation of more sustainable societies and economies. However, with the exception of of some selected areas, the application of closed-loop principles in tourism is still in its infancy. Key areas and subsectors of tourism that have strong links to the Sustainable Development Goals and the circular economy are: energy consumption and emissions in transport, hospitality (including refrigeration) and catering; waste management in destinations, hospitality and catering (including food waste and plastics); water use and wastewater management in general; and resource use in civil and industrial construction, interior decoration and domestic premises Opportunities may be most evident in the construction and operation of hotels and restaurants, including waste management. Tourism, if developed sustainably, has the potential for long-term positive impacts beyond the sector itself, through its linkages with other economic activities and direct interactions between producers and consumers.

Challenges in data availability and difficulties in definitions (indicators used in the assessment) remain to be addressed in order to develop indicators for monitoring the application of circular economy principles in tourism. Developing and ensuring the availability of data on the circular economy in the tourism sector is a necessary step to assess the most effective and efficient investments in sustainable tourism and to facilitate large-scale private sector investment and multilateral investment in business models for sustainable tourism.

When planning the transition to closed-loop business models, governments should cooperate with destination, city and regional management organisations. Governments are responsible for key policies on local public services such as transport, solid waste management, water and energy, all of which affect tourism, investment, economic growth and environmental quality. The COVID-19 pandemic vividly illustrated the supply problems arising from fragmented and complex tourism value chains. Therefore, in pursuit of sustainability, governments and tourism businesses must move towards shorter supply chains, shared infrastructure and improved resource efficiency, as well as sustainable consumption and production patterns. Access to cyclical knowledge, information and finance should be facilitated for small and medium-sized enterprises (SMEs) working in the tourism sector, as well as for the promotion of domestic and regional tourism with the expansion of sustainable mobility and climate positive tourism models. Furthermore, Governments should integrate the principles of the circular economy into tourism-related legislation, policies, plans and strategies, especially to achieve the Sustainable Development Goals and the targets of the biodiversity and climate agenda.

Making the transition to a circular economy a priority, with trackable targets and a dedicated budget, is crucial for the sustainability of the sector. Sustainable investment in and financing of the tourism sector should be included in national or local plans. Private and public stakeholders should integrate circular economy principles into their sustainability strategies and set clear targets that can be quantified and monitored. Governments can test the application of circular economy principles in tourism by addressing specific issues such as plastic pollution. Such an approach will help industry stakeholders to better understand and implement the concepts of closed-loop and value chain coordination, and replicate them at a later stage for other topics and operations. This could be achieved through participation in multi-stakeholder voluntary initiatives such as the Global Plastic Tourism Initiative. More generally, Governments should increase responsible travel to natural areas in line with ecotourism principles, thus integrating conservation, communities and sustainable tourism, specific key tourism impact indicators should be selected for inclusion in ECE statistical databases. Indicators demonstrating the extent to which the tourism economy follows a closed-loop model should be aligned with indicators being developed to monitor the sustainability of tourism development and be compatible with the Sustainable Development Goals and climate change targets, as well as in line with the United Nations World Tourism Organization (UNWTO) statistical programme for measuring sustainable tourism indicators.

The environmental governance system in the pan-European region remains partially fragmented in terms of applied policies, institutions, harmonisation of legislation and the participation of 54 countries in MEAs, which is incomplete. The assessment of status and trends, as well as the policy recommendations contained in the thematic chapters of this report, point to the need to strengthen environmental governance and existing policies in the region, and to make adjustments to address significant gaps. Gaps also remain in the implementation of good environmental governance, including with regard to public participation, transparency, responsiveness, efficiency and effectiveness, with implications for the environment and health of the region's population.

Education for Sustainable Development (ESD) equips people with the knowledge and skills to enable them to lead healthy and productive lives in harmony with nature and with concern for social values, gender equality and cultural diversity. Such education also empowers people to play an active role in environmental governance. Countries described progress in ESD Countries have met 78% of the agreed criteria to ensure that policy mechanisms, regulatory frameworks and institutional frameworks promote ESD.

Governments, the private sector, academia and citizens should work together to achieve the Sustainable Development Goals, including in a transboundary context. They should explore new partnerships on topics such as the circular economy, sustainable infrastructure, resource efficiency and waste management.

In addition, Governments in the pan-European region should: (a) consider joining multilateral environmental agreements to which they are not yet parties in order to enhance coherence and harmonisation of policies and legislation;

b) Use the Pan-European Strategic Framework for Green Economy as a basis for committing to circular economy, resource efficiency and sustainable infrastructure development, including by promoting nature-based solutions, with funding to be redirected to these areas to support a just transition and the effectiveness of such investments to be monitored and evaluated;

c) Ensure public participation in action planning and implementation, gender mainstreaming and public access to reliable and timely information to increase the likelihood of successful outcomes;

d) Ensure effective public access to information, public participation in decision-making, protection of environmental defenders and access to justice in environmental matters, as provided, for example, by the Aarhus Convention and its Protocol on Pollutant Release and Transfer Registers;

e) Develop and invest in the capacity and education for sustainable development of responsible authorities, the private sector and civil society to ensure the transition to sustainable development;

(f ) Seek to strengthen science-policy linkages and rapid adoption of innovative solutions, while investing in digitalisation.

Other recommendations in this evaluation provide more detailed information on steps to be taken to improve governance. The availability and accessibility of information and knowledge to help public decision-makers, the private sector, industry and the public make choices to achieve concrete results are improving, but challenges remain, in some sectors more so than others. As this evaluation has shown, this makes it difficult to measure progress towards policy objectives in the pan-European region, including in relation to new policy developments such as the circular economy or sustainable infrastructure. This assessment has identified data gaps across the region in almost all areas, with data available for some countries but missing for others, or lacking recent data. Data for some indicators required for this assessment are not routinely collected, in particular data on emerging strategies, including two conference themes.

Although, according to the final review report on the establishment of a Common Environmental Information System, such national systems have been successfully established in all countries of Europe and Central Asia, these systems differ in form and regularity of updating and in content.

There remain gaps that need to be addressed, including with regard to compliance with all SEIS principles and frameworks, and ensuring that all data streams related to ECE environmental indicators are fully generated and shared. The evaluation for the region identified gaps in monitoring, both in terms of data availability and quality.

The following are some examples:

a) air and climate change: gaps remain in the measurement and analysis of fine particulate matter (PM2.5), and the quality of emissions data varies widely. GHG emission datasets for some countries remain incomplete;

b) noise: noise is not considered in the assessment due to lack of data for the pan-European region. The World Health Organisation (WHO) has identified long-term exposure to noise as an important public health problem and the second leading environmental cause of ill health after air pollution in Western Europe and the European Union;

c) freshwater: the use of geo-information systems needs to be intensified, in particular at the transboundary level, and water statistics need to be improved. Environmental assessment of water quality and determination of hydromorphological loads require knowledge that is not yet available throughout the region. Monitoring of emerging pollutants requires more attention throughout the pan-European region. Monitoring and data are incomplete for the calculation of certain indicators;

d) coastal waters, marine ecosystems and seas: challenges remain in spatial and temporal data coverage, and data gaps remain, for example, on the amount, composition and sources of beach and marine litter in some parts of the region;

e) Biodiversity and ecosystems: data gaps remain for some indicators, including the ECE indicators on "terrestrial protected areas" and "land acquisition", in particular for non-European Union countries. Another problem noted is the comparability of data;

(f ) Land and soil: data gaps were identified for "prevalence of stunting among children under 5 years of age, per cent";

(g) Chemicals and waste: no set of impact-oriented chemical indicators are regularly monitored in the region. In addition, there is a lack of information on the impact of chemicals on the efficiency and economic viability of circular economy models. Gaps remain with regard to capacity and data availability for some indicators, including "total waste generation per capita", "e-waste generation per capita" and "municipal solid waste recycling rate";

(h) Environmental financing: there is a critical lack of quantitative data on environmental financing for the countries of Central Asia and South-Eastern Europe and an urgent need to improve data collection systems; (i) Sustainable infrastructure: significant data gaps were identified both in the proposed social, environmental, institutional, economic and financial indicators and in quantifying the contribution (positive or negative) of infrastructure development on the basis of the following There is a lack of a common definition of the term "sustainable infrastructure", which has implications for quantifying progress in the region;

(j) The circular economy and sustainable tourism: the impact of tourism has long been measured in economic terms, and there is now a need to rethink how success is measured in social and environmental terms, with circular economy indicators playing a key role. There are currently no indicators in the region that provide accurate information on the adoption of circular economy principles and practices in tourism, and for a number of common aspects of circularity, classification definitions vary from State to State, although the UNWTO statistical programme for measuring sustainable tourism indicators should help in this regard. Even basic tourism statistics tend to suffer from a lack of data and are highly context-dependent, while the detailed statistics needed to accurately monitor cyclicality are lacking;

(k) Despite the establishment of CEIS, national systems vary in form, regularity of updates and content. Gaps remain that need to be addressed, including with regard to the full implementation of CEIS in accordance with all its principles and pillars. The gaps identified indicate that countries still need assistance to fully implement the SEIS framework and principles and to fully generate and share all data streams related to ECE environmental indicators and other indicator systems, including indicators on the Sustainable Development Goals.

Governments in the pan-European region should:

a) combine policy and science to develop and implement appropriate standardised pan-European methods and systems for monitoring and information management, including through the application of new technologies, in order to fill data gaps to improve decision-making and ensure the timely availability of information to the public;

b) Utilise the revised ECE Guidelines for the Application of Environmental Indicators, present a set of ECE environmental indicators in line with the SEIS principles and framework and adopt indicators to cover noise and important emerging policy topics;

c) Promote the use of appropriate standardised methods for monitoring air pollutant emissions and the public availability of monitoring data in the pan-European region, as well as increased cooperation and national investment to address monitoring gaps in countries with economies in transition;

d) invest in data collection and information processing, as knowledge plays an important role in water-related decision-making and policy development (e.g. water accounts, ecosystem assessment and related indicators). Continuous improvement of monitoring and communication technologies is a top priority in terms of a water information system for the pan-European region;

e) Increase efforts to supplement inventories of several components of beach and marine litter with information on the composition and sources of litter in order to be able to develop more effective measures. Where subregional monitoring measures are deemed necessary, joint efforts should be made;

(f ) Establish a region-wide scheme for monitoring exposure to chemicals and waste through collaboration between scientists and policymakers to better understand and address the adverse effects of chemicals on human health and the environment;

g) Improve systems for collecting data on environmental financing, such as environmental expenditures, across the region to clarify and report on which actors are spending money on environmental activities, how much they are spending and for what purposes, and who is financing these expenditures;

h) Develop a common definition of the term "sustainable infrastructure" in the pan-European region. This would enable reporting and quantification of progress across countries and subregions;

i) Select a number of specific key tourism impact indicators for inclusion in the ECE statistical databases. Indicators demonstrating the extent to which the tourism economy follows the circular economy model should be aligned with indicators being developed to monitor the sustainability of tourism development (especially the most promising ones) and ensure their compatibility with the Sustainable Development Goals. The development of circular economy indicators could follow the approach adopted in the UNWTO initiative to establish a Statistical Framework Programme for Measuring Tourism Sustainability, and data and statistics should be produced by the various participating data producers according to statistical standards;

j) To assist countries in fully implementing the CEIS basic provisions and principles and ensuring that all data streams related to ECE environmental indicators are fully generated and shared and, where appropriate, apply the updated Recommendations on Enhancing the Effective Use of Electronic Media developed under the auspices of the Aarhus Convention;

k) Strengthen co-operation and interoperability between national and international systems to streamline environmental monitoring and reporting, reduce reporting requirements for countries and improve readability and efficiency - from indicator methodologies to reporting on data flows;

l) Continue the digitalisation of environmental monitoring systems and the use of new technologies to generate more comprehensive, high-quality data to support regular assessments and policy development;

m) Consider the possibility of joint use of pollutant release and transfer registers and SEIS.

Review of the regular environmental assessment, the environmental assessment framework provides an overview of the regular environmental assessment, as well as a mandate for an information study on national reporting and progress on the SEIS, and a review of environmental policy.

The following subregions are mentioned throughout the assessment, where possible and relevant:

a) European Union of 27 member states;

b) Western Europe - Israel, Iceland, Liechtenstein, Norway, UK and Switzerland;

c) Central Asia - Kazakhstan, Kyrgyzstan, Tajikistan, Turkmenistan and Uzbekistan;

d) Eastern Europe - Armenia, Azerbaijan, Belarus, Georgia, Moldova, Russia, Ukraine;

e) South-Eastern Europe - Albania, Bosnia and Herzegovina, Macedonia,

Montenegro, Serbia and Turkey.

A. Regular assessment of environmental conditions

This section opens with past "Environment for Europe" Ministerial Conferences and related pan-European environmental assessments (see figure 2 below). It then presents the mandate for this assessment, explains the choice of topics for the next conference and describes the use of the SEIS as a basis for this assessment.

B. State of Knowledge and the Common Environmental Information System

Access to valid, reliable, comparable and up-to-date data is critical to monitor progress towards policy objectives in the pan-European region and to help policy-makers make informed decisions for the benefit of the region's inhabitants. The COVID-19 pandemic has reinforced the need for relevant, reliable and comparable data across the region. Regular national reporting on the state of the environment and the establishment of SEIS in Europe and Central Asia are important contributions to utilising available data to support policy making

1. environmental reporting

Regular state-of-the-environment reporting in the countries of the pan-European region provides comprehensive, targeted information on environmental conditions, trends and pressures in each country. Such reports provide a strategic vision for policy-making and action. National integrated state of the environment reports, based on a solid evidence base, serve as a source of information and knowledge for decision-makers and the public, and engage readers and influence their behaviour.Most countries in the pan-European region have relevant national legislation, conduct regular environmental analyses and produce integrated national state of the environment reports covering a number of thematic areas, such as energy, transport, health, environment, water, water resources, energy efficiency and energy efficiency. The importance of national reporting on the state of the environment is also confirmed by the Aarhus Convention, which requires each party to the Convention to publish and disseminate, at regular intervals not exceeding three or four years, a national report on the state of the environment, including information on environmental quality and information on environmental loads. As part of the final review of the establishment of SEIS in Europe and Central Asia, ECE member States from the pan-European region were requested to provide information on the regularity and type of reports they produce. The reports vary in terms of regularity, content and form, but they all contribute to the transition towards more sustainable use of resources and environmental protection for human well-being. An overview of the regularity of national integrated state of the environment reports or indicator-based state of the environment reports is provided.

The assessments utilised available data and reports where possible, including the national state of the environment reports mentioned above. Another source of information was the publication "European Environment: State and Prospects for 2030", prepared by EEA using materials from the SDG Global SDG Indicators

Data Platform. Progress in establishing a Common Environmental Information System in Europe and Central Asia. At the Seventh Ministerial Conference "Environment for Europe", Ministers mandated the development of a Common Environmental Information System (CEIS) as the basis for a regular process of environmental assessment across the pan-European region. This mandate was reaffirmed by Ministers at the Eighth "Environment for Europe" Ministerial Conference. Subsequently, the overall Common 107
environmental information system has been successfully established in Europe and Central Asia. All member States have made progress to varying degrees in recent years in establishing a national system and in ensuring the availability and accessibility of environmental information, including for use in regular assessments, such as the seventh pan-European environmental assessment on the availability and accessibility of data flows in national systems, which participated in the final review report on the establishment of SEIS by submitting their self-evaluations According to the final review report on the establishment of SEIS, national systems have made progress in establishing a national environmental information system. The gaps identified indicate that countries still need assistance to fully implement these principles and frameworks and to ensure that all data flows related to ECE environmental indicators are fully generated and shared. The final overview report is based on the assessment framework of the Common Environmental Information System and mainly on the responses provided by 21 member States to the call for reporting sent to all countries in Europe and Central Asia, and is complemented by additional research. Further reviews of the work on the establishment of SEIS in accordance with its principles would help to address shortcomings and thereby support regular assessments and reporting in the region. In addition, the final review report recommends that the work on the establishment of SEIS and the related data streams underlying the environmental indicators be harmonised and aligned with the revised environmental indicators. They should also be aligned with the United Nations Framework for the Development of Environmental Statistics and monitoring and evaluation processes at the regional and global levels, including in the context of the 2030 Agenda and the green and circular economy, in order to enhance their policy relevance. This evaluation also recommends expanding the list of ECE indicators to include other relevant topics, such as "Coastal waters, marine ecosystems and seas".

Based on the country responses received during the final review of the establishment of SEIS, the limitations of cross-country and region-wide comparisons of data streams were assessed for each data stream. Results from the inputs indicated limitations in 44 per cent of cases, partly due to the fact that several countries did not provide references to data streams or time series information. The present assessment confirmed these problems, with noting comparability problems, for example between data under the heading "Land acquisition and conversion data from European Environment Agency member and co-operating countries" and data from other countries in the pan-European region. This incomplete comparability of data from other States is due to, inter alia, the limited availability of reliable remotely sensed data and consistent criteria for their analysis, the degree of consistency of national monitoring efforts and changes in land classification in some member States.

It is therefore recommended to continue to invest in consistent land cover classifications - ideally in line with the Corine land cover system - and monitoring capacity, to harmonise comparable national information for inclusion in SEIS, and to carefully update actual land cover categories with past data to provide reliable trend information. In addition, the final review report recommends further digitalisation of environmental monitoring systems and the use of new technologies to generate more comprehensive, high quality data to support regular assessments and policy development. This was also confirmed during the preparation of the pan-European assessment. Efforts to establish SEIS, including strengthening content, infrastructure or co-operation between competent authorities to ensure data flow, have also contributed to the implementation of the Aarhus Convention, in particular its component on access to information, as noted by the parties during the preparation of the reports on the Aarhus Convention. Parties reported that, despite remaining obstacles (e.g. insufficient interoperability of databases and incomplete and fragmented data resulting in incomplete information), significant progress has been made in ensuring the availability of environmental information in electronic databases that are easily accessible to the public through open telecommunication networks. Numerous effective electronic tools, such as electronic databases, publicly accessible government e-services, websites and information portals, have been further developed in this area and are regularly updated and improved. However, additional steps are needed throughout the region, in particular with regard to pollution and emission registers.

The preparation of the pan-European assessment has identified additional data and knowledge gaps on key environmental issues across the pan-European region. The availability and accessibility of information and knowledge to help public decision-makers, industry and the public make choices to achieve results is improving, but remains challenging, in some sectors more so than others. As this evaluation has shown, this makes it difficult to measure progress towards policy objectives in the pan-European region, including in relation to new policy developments such as the circular economy or sustainable infrastructure. The evaluation for the region identified monitoring gaps, both in terms of data availability and quality.

The following examples can be given:

a) air and climate change: gaps remain, especially in the measurement and analysis of fine particulate matter (PM2.5). The quality of emissions data varies widely. There are also gaps in data availability, as not all countries in Eastern, South-Eastern and Western Europe and Central Asia have submitted emission inventories. GHG emission datasets for some countries in the region remain

incomplete;
b) freshwater: there are gaps in geo-information systems, in particular at the transboundary level, and water statistics need to be improved. Environmental assessment of water quality or determination of hydromorphological loads requires knowledge that is not yet available everywhere in the region, and there are also problems in monitoring new pollutants. Monitoring and data do not provide a complete picture for the calculation of certain indicators;
c) Coastal waters, marine ecosystems and seas: new developments and technologies related to monitoring and data release have not yet been sufficiently applied, and problems remain with spatial and temporal coverage of data. Data gaps were noted, for example, on the amount, composition and sources of beach and marine litter in some parts of the region;
d) (b) Biodiversity and ecosystems: data gaps remain in the production of some indicators, including the ECE indicator on "land acquisition", in particular for non-European Union countries. Another issue noted is data comparability; (e) Chemicals and waste: no set of impact-oriented chemical indicators is regularly monitored in the region. Gaps remain with regard to the availability of data from a number of countries for some indicators, including "total waste generation per capita", "e-waste generation per capita" and "municipal solid waste recycling rate";
(f ) Environmental financing: there is a severe lack of quantitative data on environmental financing for the countries of Central Asia and South-Eastern Europe. This makes it difficult to attempt to assess progress in environmental protection and environmental financing. The lack of reliable data also means that it is not possible to reliably calculate the investment and operating costs of achieving environmental objectives and use them in policy-making. There is an urgent need to improve data collection systems, such as data on environmental expenditure;
(g) Sustainable infrastructure: significant data gaps were identified both in the proposed social, environmental, institutional, economic and financial indicators and in the quantification of the contribution (positive or negative) of infrastructure development and the achievement of the indicators proposed in the assessment. In addition, there is no common definition of sustainable infrastructure in the pan-European region; as a result, there are difficulties in reporting and quantifying progress by country and subregion;
(h) The circular economy and sustainable tourism: the development of indicators for sustainable tourism, not to mention cycle monitoring, is still under development, but the process is hampered by a number of challenges. At present, there are no indicators in ECE member States that provide clear information on the extent to which tourism utilises closed-loop principles. For several common aspects of circularity, classification definitions vary from country to country. Even basic tourism statistics tend to be incomplete and the differing definitions create problems in their utilisation, while the detailed statistics needed for accurate closed-loop monitoring are lacking. Digitalisation offers opportunities for better

and more uniform measurement and monitoring, but depends on the availability of uniform and up-to-date data on the circular economy of tourism.

Accordingly, it is recommended that Governments in the pan-European region: (a) combine policy and science to develop and implement appropriate standardised pan-European monitoring and information management methods and systems, including through the application of new technologies, in order to fill data gaps (including data gaps on the relationship between gender and conservation) to improve decision-making and ensure the timely availability of information to the public;

b) Utilise the revised ECE Manual on the Application of Environmental Indicators, submit a set of environmental indicators to ECE in line with the SEIS principles and framework and adopt indicators to cover important new policy-relevant topics;

c) To assist countries in fully implementing the CEIS framework and principles and ensuring that all data streams related to ECE environmental indicators and other indicator systems, including indicators on the Sustainable Development Goals, are fully generated and shared, and to apply, as appropriate, the updated Recommendations on Enhancing the Effective Use of Electronic Media developed under the auspices of the Aarhus Convention;

d) consider the possibility of synergistic use of pollutant release and transfer registers and the pan-European SEIS;

e) Continue the digitalisation of environmental monitoring systems and the use of new technologies to generate more comprehensive, high-quality data to support regular assessments and policy development.

Environmental policy in the region global, regional and sub-regional policy frameworks in the pan-European region. Policies, as well as their objectives, goals, targets and indicators, all play a role in catalysing country action. Among the most significant global instruments are the MEA, the United Nations Environment Assembly and the 2030 Agenda for Sustainable Development. The "Environment for Europe" ministerial process and the European "Environment and Health" process play a prominent role at the regional level. Key elements at the subregional level include European Union environmental policy and legislation, the European Union accession process and the environmental and sustainable development policies of the Commonwealth of Independent States. Global Framework of Programmes

The 2030 Agenda for Sustainable Development provides a comprehensive framework for sustainable development and integrated environmental policy. The 17 universal Sustainable Development Goals and 169 targets of the 2030 Agenda set policy objectives at all levels with the overall goal of poverty eradication, as well as the economic, social and environmental dimensions of sustainability. The Agenda addresses fundamental issues of governance, institutions, peace and international cooperation. It specifically sets targets for targeted progress on major environmental challenges, including under Goal 6 on water, Goal 7, on energy, Goal 12 on consumption and production patterns, and Goal 13 on climate action, among others, and includes more than 90 environment-related indicators to measure progress in implementing the Agenda. Governments have also identified national targets and indicators.

Sendai Framework for Disaster Risk Reduction 2015-2030

The Sendai Framework for Disaster Risk Reduction 2015-2030 aims to significantly reduce disaster risk and

reduce disaster losses in terms of loss of life, livelihoods and health.

loss of livelihoods and ill health

and the loss of economic, physical, social, cultural and environmental assets of people, businesses, communities and countries. It includes a set of seven global challenges that are indirectly linked to the environment and identifies four priority actions, each with an environmental component, to be implemented at the local, national, regional and global levels.

The Strategic Plan for Biodiversity, including the Aichi Biodiversity Targets, set the global framework for biodiversity action over the past decade. The Plan has five strategic goals, each with three to six targets. The Sustainable Development Goals also include targets and indicators related to biodiversity.Global MEAs, such as the United Nations Framework Convention on Climate Change (UNFCCC) and the Paris Agreement, the Convention on Biological Diversity (CBD), the Convention to Combat Desertification (UNCCD), and MEAs on certain pollutants (such as persistent organic pollutants (POPs), mercury and ozone-depleting substances (ODS)) and wastes also guide environmental policies in the ECE region, along with regional MEAs, including through legally binding limits. through the establishment of legally binding limits. The rapid adoption of global agreements illustrates their political relevance at the international level.

The UN Environment Assembly provides a comprehensive global environmental governance structure, bringing emerging issues to the attention of the world community. It sets global environmental policy priorities and develops new norms of international environmental law. Through its ministerial declarations and resolutions, the Assembly also provides leadership, spearheads intergovernmental action on the environment and contributes to the 2030 Agenda.

At the regional level, the "Environment for Europe" process and its ministerial conferences, organised with the aim of harmonising environmental quality and environmental policies in the pan-European region and ensuring peace, stability and sustainable development in the region, have served as the main framework over the past three decades. The Lucerne Declaration, adopted by the Environment Ministers, defines the political dimension of the "Environment for Europe" process. The Sofia Declaration emphasised the urgent need to further integrate environmental considerations into policies across all sectors if economic growth is to be achieved in line with the principles of sustainable development.

The Nur-Sultan Conference adopted a number of programme commitments, including:

• improving environmental protection and promoting sustainable development; - affirming the importance of involving civil society, including business, women, non-governmental organisations (NGOs) and other groups, in decision-making to improve the environment;

• further implementation of integrated water resources management principles, implementation of the ecosystem approach and integration of ecosystem values into the management accounting system;

• Improving water resources management and strengthening transboundary co-operation;

-continuation of work on completion and implementation of the ten-year framework programmes on sustainable production and consumption. The outcomes of the Nur-Sultan Ministerial Conference were analysed in Batumi, Georgia, including consideration of the final report on the implementation of the Astana Water Action Proposals, the progress report on the establishment of SENS, and the 20-year experience of environmental performance reviews (EPRs).

In addition, participants in the Batumi Conference:

• Endorsed the voluntary Pan-European Strategic Framework for Green Economy and invited ECE member States and other stakeholders to implement it;

• welcomed the Batumi Initiative for a Green Economy (BIG-E), which consists of voluntary commitments to operationalise the Strategic Framework;

• endorsed the voluntary Batumi Clean Air Initiative (BCI) and welcomed initiatives put forward by interested countries and other stakeholders to improve air quality and protect public and ecosystem health. In addition, the conference made commitments to: improve environmental protection, achieve sustainable development, implement the Sustainable Development Goals and ensure access to basic services; strengthen ecosystems and expand ecosystem services as a component of environmental infrastructure, and improve sustainable use of natural resources; lead the transition to a green economy, direct investment and trade to support a green and ecosystem; and support the development of a green and inclusive economy.

Work was undertaken to track the implementation of the commitments made under BIZ-E and BHIP both at the Conference and beyond, in particular through the midterm review conducted by the Committee on Environmental Policy. The evaluation was based on reports on the implementation of each of the three Batumi instruments and MEAs in support of the 2030 Agenda, as well as on activities in support of countries' efforts to green the economy, the establishment of SENS and under the third cycle of EPR24. The evaluation demonstrated the harmonisation and improvement of relevant data flows and the quality of selected environmental indicators, as well as the use of data flows for different purposes. In addition, the evaluation highlighted the progress made in the implementation of voluntary commitments by Member States and organisations participating in BIZ-E and BHIP. It was noted that since 2017, the Sustainable Development Goals and targets had been included in the EPR. The Committee noted with satisfaction the launch of activities to assist countries under review in implementing the recommendations of their EPRs.The Committee noted that countries still needed assistance to fully implement the SEIS framework and principles by 2021 and to generate and disseminate relevant data streams related to ECE environmental indicators on a regular basis. The Committee also recognised the need to allocate sufficient resources to assist Governments, through MEAs, in achieving the Sustainable Development Goals.

The European Environment and Health Process, which was launched in Frankfurt, Germany, following a second conference in Helsinki, Finland, published a comprehensive review of environmental health in Europe, "Caring for Europe's Tomorrow: Public Health and the Environment in the WHO European Region", the third conference, held in London, adopted the Protocol on Water and Health to the ECE Convention on the Protection and Use of Transboundary Watercourses and International Lakes. The fifth conference in Parma, Italy, set clear targets to reduce the adverse effects of environmental hazards on public health in the next decade. At the sixth conference in Ostrava, Czech Republic, Member States committed themselves to developing national action programmes that should take into account the need to accelerate progress on health and the environment and, in particular, on the environment-related health goals and targets of the 2030 Agenda. Other regional processes, other important processes and instruments include the ECE Steering Committee on Education for Sustainable Development, the Transport, Environment and Health Pan-European Programme on Transport, Environment and Health (THE PEP) and the ECE Environmental Performance Review (EPR) programme. THE PEP is a tripartite pan-European framework that brings together the transport, health and environment sectors on an equal footing. It is jointly implemented by ECE and the WHO Regional Office for Europe. The Fifth High-Level Meeting of the HSESAP, where the Vienna Declaration on "Better development through a transition to new, clean, safe, health-friendly and inclusive mobility and transport" was adopted. An important milestone and key component of the Vienna Declaration was the first Pan-European Integrated Cycling Plan. Together, through the work of the HSSPSAP, Member States are pushing forward the 2030 Agenda on several fronts and across a range of goals and targets, including in the areas of health, energy efficiency, climate and environmental protection, quality of urban life and equality and equity. Subregional frameworks, among frameworks below the regional level, European Union policies, including the accession procedure, are one of the most powerful drivers of fundamental change. Subregional environmental agreements also play an important role because of their binding provisions; these include the Alpine Convention, the Framework Convention on the Protection and Sustainable Development of the Carpathians, the

Framework Convention on Environmental Protection for Sustainable Development in Central Asia and a number of regional maritime agreements, such as the Convention for the Protection of the Marine Environment and the Coastal Region of the Mediterranean Sea (Barcelona Convention). At the European Union level, the European Green Deal promotes a holistic approach and defines a road map for achieving climate neutrality by 2050, with sustainability as the new standard for all policies. The programme, while recognising the integrity of the environment and the link to the immediate environment, includes as ambitious directions within and beyond the European Union a biodiversity strategy for 2030, a zero-pollution action plan, a farm-to-table strategy, a sustainable and smart mobility strategy and a transition to a circular economy. Other approaches include the report "Transition in the Tourism Sector "26 prepared with industry and civil society representatives. The new European Union Biodiversity Strategy 2030, which provides an action plan for nature conservation and reversing ecosystem degradation, plays an important role in measuring ecosystem health and halting biodiversity loss in all ecosystems, including marine ecosystems. It will be implemented in parallel with the global process under the Convention on Biological Diversity to develop a post-2020 framework for global biodiversity action.

There have been dramatic socio-economic and political developments in the pan-European region that have exacerbated pressures on the natural environment and led to environmental change, consider four groups of driving forces:

- Urbanisation and population growth in coastal areas
- A more prosperous society with greater resource utilisation - shifts in energy production and use
- an increasingly mobile society (tourism is also considered in detail in this regard).

1. Urbanisation and coastal population growth The region's population has grown slowly, increasing by about 6.5 % (compared to about 38 % globally) from 784.8 million in 2000 to 829.9 million in 2015, and is expected to grow by only 2.7 % year-on-year in 2015, before beginning to decline after 2040. Urbanisation is increasing in the region, with 50-80% of the population projected to live in urban areas by 2050 . Currently, the high concentration of anthropogenic activities within cities is responsible for 70% of global greenhouse gas emissions and increasing air, water and soil pollution, as well as problems caused by noise and traffic congestion. In addition, the effects of rapid and unplanned urbanisation can influence the likelihood of conflict over limited resources. This situation has fuelled the development of sustainable infrastructure and innovative approaches to spatial planning, mobility and energy consumption (e.g. smart cities, smart grids). The concept of sustainable infrastructure is being actively promoted in climate policy to increase resilience to extreme weather events.

The New Urban Agenda promotes the concept of a smart city that harnesses the power of digitalisation, clean energy and technology, and innovative transport technologies, thereby empowering residents to make more environmentally friendly choices.

The population living within 10 kilometres of the coast in the coastal countries of the pan-European region grew by 10% between 2000 and 2015 - faster than the population as a whole - from 133.6 million to 147.7 million. By 2050, 71 % of the world's population is projected to live in coastal zones. Coastal areas with high population densities are characterised by increased urban density due to increased pressure on infrastructure, resulting in increased environmental pressures such as wastewater discharge, sewer overflows and waste generation. Urbanisation of coastal areas leads to urban sprawl, degradation of landscapes, shorelines and habitats, and increased pressure on coastal ecosystems. The impact of these pressures is further exacerbated by the development of tourism, often concentrated in coastal areas and during the summer months, as in the case of the Mediterranean region. Coastal countries are facing increasing challenges in achieving sustainable development and conservation of coastal and marine areas, especially in relation to climate change. Several regions and cities in the pan-European region are experiencing rapid population growth and currently lack the capacity to cope with the growing pressures of these factors.

2. A more prosperous, resource-intensive society As the Organisation for Economic Co-operation and Development (OECD) Global Material Resources Outlook to 2060 report notes, a growing population with higher incomes will drive a significant increase in global demand for goods and services in the coming decades, that technological developments will help decouple the growth in output and material inputs, with the greatest opportunities likely to be in countries with less developed economies. However, the decline in resource intensity may be slower than GDP growth, fuelling a corresponding increase in resource consumption. OECD projections for the period 2011-2060 show material resource use and GDP growing by a factor of 1.5 and 2.5 in Eurasia and 1.8 and 2.5 in Europe, respectively, while material intensity is expected to decline from 0.9 t/dollar to 0.5 t/dollar. The material intensity is expected to decrease from 0.9 tonnes/US$ to 0.5 tonnes/US$. The material intensity is expected to decrease from 0.9 tonnes/US$ in Eurasia and from 0.4 tonnes/US$ to 0.3 tonnes/US$ in Europe. The material intensity is expected to decrease from 0.4 tonnes/US$ to 0.3 tonnes/US$. US$ 0.4 tonnes/US$ to 0.3 tonnes/US$ in Europe. Resource inputs, i.e. the amount of materials extracted from the environment and used to meet the final needs of an economy, and domestic material consumption (DMC), i.e. the amount of materials produced or processed in a country, show that although countries with higher populations use more resources, on a per capita basis, and rich countries stand out as the largest consumers in relative terms Ecological footprint, an indicator that compares the demand for natural resources with the available biomass

In the pan-European region, the national ecological footprint far exceeds the global biocapacity (about 1.7 tonnes per person) in all countries. Prosperity in the region has led to enormous infrastructure development, continued extraction of natural resources, expansion and intensification of agriculture (including in countries outside the region but which are suppliers to the pan-European region), which increases pressure on land. In addition, some 40-60,000 industrial chemicals are traded globally and trade is expected to increase significantly in the future. Chemicals are used, for example, in agriculture, health care and the production of goods such as electronics, textiles, furniture and toys, and a large proportion of them are hazardous; for example, in the European Union, 62 per cent of such substances were classified as hazardous to human health and 35 per cent as hazardous to the environment. The generation of large amounts of waste is also associated with the inefficient use of resources in the environmentally unsustainable consumption and production practices of modern society. In addition to the problems caused by hazardous waste, other waste streams result in wasted materials and energy and exacerbate pressures on the environment, for example through microplastics entering the food chain, with detrimental effects on biodiversity and human health. Single-person housing is an indicator of a more prosperous society, which entails an increase in material and energy consumption per capita. The overall increase in personal wealth is also a major factor in the development of coastal tourism, including the construction of luxury resorts and hotels, other facilities and infrastructure.

3. Shifts in energy production and utilisation

Despite a 25 per cent increase in industrial production between 2000 and 2010 and a 20 per cent increase between 2010 and 2023, the total energy sources have remained virtually unchanged. This indicates an increase in energy efficiency. In parallel, the composition of energy sources is changing, but fossil fuels such as coal, oil and natural gas have only decreased from 84 % in 1990 to 74 % of net energy production, while the share of hydropower, wind and solar energy, biofuels and waste has increased from 5 to 14 %. Figures show a 44% decrease for coal and a 9% decrease for crude oil, but a 21% increase for gas and a 2.4% increase in total fossil fuel consumption. In addition, the relative use of nuclear energy increased by 5 per cent, hydropower by 17 per cent, wind and solar energy by a factor of 11, and biofuels and waste by a factor of two. Energy sources, net of imports and exports, pan-European region, 1990-2023 (in % by source (left axis) and totals in petajoules (right axis))

Changing energy consumption patterns are also leading to a stabilisation of CO2 emissions in the region, albeit with significant geographical

However, the reductions in greenhouse gas emissions needed to keep global temperature rise below 2 °C, let alone 1.5 °C, are still not foreseen.

New trends are expected in electricity consumption. The European Union aims to have at least three million charging stations for electric vehicles by 2030, i.e. three times as many as today. However, this trend will put more pressure on resources, such as lithium for batteries. A new hydrogen fuel cell industry is emerging.

4. An increasingly mobile society

Passenger and freight transport is one of the most significant environmental impacts, with impacts ranging from greenhouse gas emissions to material consumption and pollution to ocean and atmospheric issues. Infrastructure, including transport infrastructure, is growing steadily. For example, the length of motorways continues to grow, albeit at a slower rate than in the past, while road transport continues to grow, and has increased in some countries. Public land transport is growing and rail passenger transport is increasing. However, this trend - along with others - is likely to have been reversed by the effects of the COVID-19 pandemic.

Maritime transport remains the main channel of communication with the world market, with ships transporting around 90% of all goods worldwide. The huge global scale of the maritime transport sector with a focus on the pan-European region and noting the most important and busiest ports and most used shipping routes. The transport of oil and chemicals is predominant in the North Sea, the southern Caspian Sea and inland transport in the Sea of Azov. The Mediterranean Sea is also home to major oil transport routes, with oil shipments via two of the world's six major oil transhipment points, the Suez Canal/SUMED Pipeline and the Turkish Straits, which together accounted for 13.24 per cent of world oil shipping. With the increase in container volumes and ship sizes, there is an increasing need to improve port infrastructure and move to deep water (the Mediterranean region accounted for about 27 % of global international tourism), as well as other trendy coastal tourism destinations. The contribution of tourism to climate change is estimated at 8 %43 , with transport accounting for the majority (75 %) of tourism emissions. The length of the route and the choice of transport mode are key factors in determining tourism transport emissions. Significant increases in transport speed, combined with cheaper transport due to the development of air transport, have been the main factors driving the overconsumption of transport in passenger-kilometres. Aviation has become one of the key drivers of total emissions from the tourism sector. Dynamics of domestic and international tourist arrivals by all types of accommodation. Between 2005 and 2023, the number of tourist arrivals has been growing steadily, except in 2009 due to the economic crisis of 2008, the share of domestic tourist arrivals has consistently exceeded 60 per cent but is gradually declining. There is a slow downward trend in the dynamics of tourism participation of European Union citizens. In other words, the growth of tourism consumption in the European Union is accounted for by a slightly decreasing number of people. Both the benefits and the impacts of tourism are becoming less evenly distributed among the population.

Currently, the environmental impact of tourism is not systematically measured. This inability to measure the effects of impacts affects all indicators relevant to the circular economy. The tourism system includes the elements of accommodation, activities, transport at the destination and transport between outbound markets tourism and destinations. For many closed-loop economy indicators, such as waste recycling and water purification, tourism will not deviate too much from national indicators simply because a country with a 100 per cent circular economy will also become a destination for fully closed-loop tourism. However, the role of tourism is important as long as the country has not yet reached the level of a 100 per cent closed-loop economy. In addition, the greater the resource needs (energy, water, land use, food), the more difficult it will be to achieve full circularity.

At the global level, the authors of several studies show the share of tourism impacts and trends. For example, one article shows projected trends in energy use, water use, land area, food and CO2 emissions between 1900 and 2050. It states that the global tourism system required: 'about 16,700 NJ of energy, 138 KM3 OF fresh water, 62,000 km2 of land and 39.4 Mt of food, which also resulted in the emission of 1.12 Gt of CO2.' Despite efforts to introduce more sustainable forms of tourism, analyses show that total resource consumption in the tourism sector could increase by 92 per cent (water) and 189 per cent (land use) between 2010 and 2050. Consequently, a rapidly growing amount of resources is required to sustain the global tourism system, while the system is simultaneously becoming increasingly vulnerable to disruptions in resource flows". The above figures refer to the global system of domestic and international tourism, but it is likely that tourism in the pan-European region accounts for a share proportional to the share of the number of trips made in the pan-European region in the global number of trips.

The situation is different with regard to climate change. The climate impact of tourism is mainly (75-80 per cent) due to transport from home to destination, with air transport accounting for the largest share, although only about 20-25 per cent of all trips are made by air. An important gap in the measurement of tourism is the measurement of the distances travelled by tourists on each mode of transport. Air transport statistics are more detailed, but only in terms of the number of passengers, not passenger-kilometres. The number of passengers carried per year in the European Union increased between 2009 and 2023 by 52-56%, but in 2020 it fell again to 40% of the 2009 value and 28% of the 2019 level due to the pandemic. If we take the United Nations World Tourism Organisation (UNWTO) definition of a tourist (International Recommendations for Tourism Statistics, thus taking into account holidays, visits to family and friends and business trips involving at least one night's stay, the bulk (over 90%) of air travel is tourism-related. In the case of other modes of transport, tourism accounts for about 10 %. As transport statistics use rather different definitions of the purpose of travel, it is very difficult to identify data that use the UNWTO definition of tourism. The main factors in the development of the tourism system are the level of GDP per capita and the cost and speed of transport. The average number of trips per capita in a country, region or city surprisingly shows a linear relationship with GDP per capita, but with a limit of about five trips per year per capita, the total number of trips varies in proportion to population and differential GDP per capita. However, the choice of destination, as well as modes of transport and travel distances, depend not only on the value of GDP per capita, but also on the cost of travel and journey times using the available transport systems. These selection processes are very complex, as people not only consider the speed and cost of their chosen mode of transport, but also their perceptions of the cost and speed of other modes of transport. In addition, the choice of destination and especially the distance a traveller is willing to travel is highly dependent on the speed and cost of the transport system provided. Therefore, the main factors determining how tourism is shaped and its impact on the degree of cycling are the speed and cost parameters of the entire infrastructure complex (infrastructure, software, marketing, etc.) of road, bus, rail, ferry and air transport, as well as the elements of their interconnection and interdependence.

The range of factors in environmental legislation is wide and sometimes they are quite complex in nature. In the case of infrastructure, the main factors are resource and energy use and emissions of oxides of nitrogen (NOx) and dispersed matter (PM).

Climate policy can also strongly influence the cost and even speed of transport systems. Both maritime transport and air transport are among the sectors where emissions reductions are difficult to achieve, i.e. there are few mitigation options in these sectors and none are implemented on a large scale. In the case of tourism, zero emissions are achievable for buildings, land transport and short line ferries. In the railway sector in particular, there are several national systems that are already almost entirely powered by renewable energy. However, the environmental impact of different modes of transport depends on a number of factors, including passenger numbers by mode, railway electrification and energy production. Electric vehicles have the potential to become zero-emission vehicles as only electricity generation achieves this goal. One potential barrier to a significant spread of electric vehicles is still battery resources, as despite increasing attempts at recycling, the issue of total required battery capacity seriously complicates the challenge of closed-loop resource utilisation, which is not a problem for rail. In general, the highest priority should be given to less frequent journeys with shorter distances, combined with efforts to get more travellers to travel using greener options. In the European Union and partly beyond, tools already exist to compare energy consumption and CO2 and exhaust emissions for planes, cars and trains in the passenger transport sector so that consumers can consciously choose environmentally friendly travel options.

In aviation, the decarbonisation process is still in its infancy. Except for the addition of less than 0.5 % of alternative (bio)fuels, aircraft efficiency improvements are only achieved by conventional methods. The development of advanced waste-based fuels and synthetic electrofuels is currently being intensified in several countries. Electrofuels potentially promise the possibility of achieving zero emissions when flying solely on these fuels. However, the renewable energy costs of producing such fuels are very high. Existing processes operate at an efficiency of around 20 per cent, meaning that without an improvement in this figure, the energy consumption of air tourism will increase by a factor of five. But even with the large-scale efficiency improvements of up to 60 per cent expected by experts54 , an electric-fuelled aviation system could consume about 20 per cent of all renewable energy expected by 2050. Obviously, such a 20-25 % share of renewable energy consumption in the tourism sector alone cannot be acceptable to society. This limitation is significant

an obstacle to aviation growth and an additional argument in favour of a maximum shift in favour of less frequent travel over shorter distances and using more environmentally friendly modes of transport. This will change the geographical structure of tourism in favour of more domestic travel, shorter-distance travel and a lower share of long-distance travel, as well as a greater closed-loop operation of the industry, while ensuring that tourism remains an important economic sector in many countries.

Environmental status, trends and policy responses using the ECE suite of environmental indicators, Sustainable Development Goal indicators and other indicator frameworks as appropriate.

These indicators are selected based on the following criteria:

- political relevance;
- soundness of methodology, preferably based on national sources;

data availability;

- coverage of load, condition and exposure factors.

Consider eight environmental themes:

- atmospheric air and the ozone layer;
- climate change and greenhouse gas emissions;
- fresh water;
- coastal waters, marine ecosystems and seas;
- biodiversity and ecosystems;
- earth and soil;
- chemicals and waste;
- Funding and public expenditures for environmental protection. A. Atmospheric air and the ozone layer

The health effects of long-term exposure to fine particulate matter less than 2.5 μm in diameter (PM2.5) in 41 European countries between 2009 and 2023 were reduced by 13 % and nitrogen oxides (NOx) by 54 %.

However, the number of premature deaths due to ground-level ozone exposure increased by about 24 per cent over this period, possibly due to higher average temperatures. The Montreal Protocol on Substances that Deplete the Ozone Layer has had a positive impact on human health and the environment. The phase-out of hydrochlorofluorocarbons, present as refrigerant in refrigerators and air-conditioning systems, is still pending, especially in countries with economies in

transition.
Over the past decade, emission measurement and air pollution monitoring technologies have been improved through the introduction of newer equipment, advanced portable sensors and networking strategies to increase the efficiency and reduce the cost of operating ground-based monitoring stations, and progress continues. In the pan-European
The region still has gaps in monitoring, especially in the measurement and analysis of fine PM particles. Countries in the region are expanding the policy framework for air pollution control. The assessment and conformity check of the current European Union air quality legislation in 2023, for example, resulted in proposals to strengthen provisions for air quality monitoring, modelling and improvement plans to achieve cleaner air. As a result of the conformity check, the European Union air quality standards will be revised to align more closely with the WHO Air Quality Guidelines, which were updated in 2023.
The Russian Federation is implementing the Clean Air Project, which envisages significant reductions in pollutant emissions in 12 major industrial centres by 2030, as well as radical modernisation of the state system for monitoring air pollution in these cities.Cooperation should be intensified so that non-European Union countries in the region can benefit from the experience of the European Union's Zero Pollution Action Plan. Air pollutant concentrations and air pollution indices are available in real time and are published on maps by various providers, just as the Copernicus European Atmospheric Monitoring Service (http://atmosphere.copernicus.eu) provides continuous satellite data and information on the composition of the atmosphere. The service monitors air pollution, solar energy, GHGs and climate change on a global scale. Governments should develop additional technical and organisational measures to address target 3.9 of the Sustainable Development Goals, especially for fine particulate matter and ground-level ozone. Collecting and analysing data disaggregated by age and sex is a critical step to support policy development. Key measures are to improve and apply best available techniques to prevent emissions of dispersed matter, nitrogen oxides and hydrocarbons from industry, to reduce emissions from road traffic (by implementing measures to Euro-6 and Euro-7 emission standards) and, for example, to apply higher standards for domestic heating appliances.
Governments should facilitate adequate replenishment of the Multilateral Fund for the Implementation of the Montreal Protocol and urge donors to do so in order to accelerate the phase-out of hydrochlorofluorocarbons worldwide.Governments should promote the use of appropriate standardised methods for monitoring air pollutant emissions and the public availability of monitoring data in the pan-European region, and enhance cooperation and national investment to close the gap
Emissions of substances such as sulphur dioxide ($SO_2$), carbon monoxide (CO) and lead (Pb), which were a major problem in the second half of the 20th century, have declined worldwide. However, emissions of other substances such as PM, $NO_x$ and

ammonia (NH3) have increased in many regions. In the last 40-50 years, policy measures to reduce air pollution have been developed at the national level and through successful international cooperation, for example through multilateral environmental agreements, various organisations have committed themselves to the Batumi Clean Air Initiative. For the pan-European region, the Convention on Long-range Transboundary Air Pollution (Air Convention), to which a number of protocols have been signed, has initiated science-based actions to address long-term air pollution problems. The Protocol to Abate Acidification, Eutrophication and Ground-level Ozone, as amended, is the main instrument for setting national emission limits for SO2, NOx, NH3, volatile organic compounds (VOCs) and PM2.5 to be achieved by 2020 and beyond. As black carbon (soot, a short-lived climate pollutant) is a fraction of PM, climate co-benefits are also provided. Other important protocols to the Air Convention are the Protocol on Heavy Metals and the Protocol on Persistent Organic Pollutants. Based on emissions data from the European Pollutant Release and Transfer Register (E-PTR), the EEA has estimated that emissions of air pollutants and GHGs cost society around €277-433 billion (2-3% of EU GDP) in 2022. Of the 11,655 facilities submitting data to the E-PRTR, only 211 large industrial facilities account for 50% of the total cost of damage. Air quality in the pan-European region remains moderate and unhealthy for sensitive populations in many areas, especially in urban and industrial areas, despite some notable reductions in ambient air concentrations, and air pollution is still considered to be the most serious environmental risk to human health, as described in the reference documents on the European Union's Best Available Techniques and their equivalents in the Russian Federation. At present, PM, nitrogen dioxide (NO2) and ground-level ozone (O3) are the substances that most seriously affect human health, even if concentrations do not exceed current established limit values.

3. Status, major trends and recent developments

Over the past decades, air pollution in Europe has generally decreased in the European Union and Western Europe and increased in Central Asia and Eastern Europe, mainly as a result of economic growth. Joint efforts by national and regional authorities have not yet led to the desired results, as some air quality standards are still exceeded, especially in the European Union and Western Europe. urban areas. Long-term human health effects of PM2.5 in 41 European countries were reduced by 13 % and premature mortality was reduced to 417 thousand cases (4.8 million years of life lost). As for NOx, over the same period, its impact on human health was reduced by 54 % and premature mortality was reduced to 55,000 cases (624,000 years of life lost). However, the number of premature deaths due to ground-level ozone exposure increased by an estimated 24 per cent over this period to 20,600 (247,000 years of life lost), possibly due to an increase in average temperatures. In the Russian Federation, the number of cities with high and very high levels of air pollution has decreased by 70 per cent (based on air pollution indices). The Government of the Russian Federation has instructed the authorities of large cities such as Moscow and St. Petersburg to develop a roadmap for setting limits for highly polluting road transport (in line with Euro-3). Other countries in Central Asia and Eastern Europe have seen similar developments in fuel quality. In Uzbekistan, more than 50 per cent of private cars and trucks use cleaner natural gas as fuel.

The Breath is Life global campaign, led by WHO, UNEP and the Climate and Clean Air Coalition, launched in 2022, inviting governments to commit to meeting the WHO Air Quality Guidelines targets in 2030. The campaign aims to halve the number of air pollution-related deaths by 2030 while helping to slow climate change. Through the Coalition, more than 70 States have formed a voluntary partnership with intergovernmental organisations, NGOs, cities and financial and business institutions to reduce emissions of short-lived climate pollutants (black carbon, methane, hydrofluorocarbons and tropospheric ozone).

The WHO Recommendations were revised in 2023 and now propose air quality levels for six pollutants for which the most up-to-date data on health effects are available. Taking action on these so-called classic pollutants - particulate matter (PM), ozone (Oz), nitrogen dioxide (NO2), sulphur dioxide (SO2) and carbon monoxide (CO) - has implications for other harmful pollutants.The second European Union Clean Air Forum discussed the existing differences between the European Union's air quality guidelines and their largely more stringent equivalents adopted by WHO, and ways to address these differences.

The European Union air pollution policy framework comprises three main elements: air quality standards, national emission thresholds for major pollutants and emission limit values for major sources of pollution. A compliance check of the European Union Ambient Air Quality Directive69 in 2019 showed that not all the objectives of the Directive have been achieved and that in some cases there is a significant gap in the achievement of air quality standards, which requires improvements to the current legislation. In specific cases, more stringent emission thresholds in the National Emission Thresholds Directive or more stringent emission limit values in the Industrial Emissions and Mobile Sources Directive may be necessary to fulfil the policy objective of achieving all European Union air quality standards as a first step towards achieving their WHO equivalents in 2030. In 2023, the European Commission adopted an action plan to achieve zero pollution. In 2022, the EEA and the European Commission developed the European Air Quality Index, which, based on monitoring data from over 2000 stations across Europe, provides online information on air quality. The interactive map shows the local air quality situation at station level for five main pollutants: PM2.5, PM10, ground-level ozone, NO2 and SO2.

At the global level, the United Nations General Assembly adopted resolution A/RES/74/212 on International Clean Air Day for Blue Skies. UNEP, in cooperation with the Climate and Clean Air Coalition and WHO, coordinated activities to mark the International Day in order to raise public awareness,

demonstrate the link to the Sustainable Development Goals and promote and catalyse solutions to protect ambient air.
Emissions of air pollutants under the European Monitoring and Evaluation Programme for Long-range Transport of Air Pollutants (EMEP) 43 of 51 Parties to the Air Convention have submitted their emission inventories At the same time, the quality of data is highly variable, which acts as a factor of uncertainty, experts and model developers are working on the challenge of establishing a harmonised methodology for emissions accounting. In the period 2000-2022, the emission trends for major pollutants (SO2, NOx, NH3, non-methane volatile organic compounds, PM10, PM2.5, PMcoarse and black carbon) showed a significant weakening of the relationship with economic growth and a decline in absolute numbers in the western part of the region. Central Asian and Eastern European countries have shown an increase in emissions since 2000, but due to the lack of reliable reporting, these emissions data are often based on expert estimates extrapolated from GDP growth trends.
The largest gap between economic growth and production and emissions of air pollutants in recent decades occurred in the energy and manufacturing sectors. Emissions in the road and off-road transport sector have also declined significantly as a result of stringent emission standards set at the European Union level and, with some delay, in the pan-European region. The agriculture and waste sectors have seen much smaller reductions in emissions. The residential, commercial and institutional sectors did not reduce their emissions much, except for SO2 emissions.
Urban air quality, improvements in air quality monitoring and reporting over the past 15-20 years allow air quality trends to be assessed and reported in a qualitative and statistically reliable manner. For European Union member States, long-term data are available on concentrations of some air pollutants regulated by the European Union Ambient Air Quality Directive. Countries in Central Asia and some countries in Eastern Europe report air quality using a different methodology, in the form of air pollution indices, where three different indicators are used to assess air quality. These indices characterise both short-term air pollution and chronic health and environmental impacts of air pollution. Air quality assessment in Central Asia and Eastern Europe also includes specific pollutants for which hygienic standards are set (more than 700 substances, 160 of which are subject to state regulation). The air quality category established by the set of indicators takes into account the main pollutants for each city assessed against the standards. Assessments for specific pollutants that most affect air pollution levels in cities are regularly published on the Internet.
SO2 concentrations show the largest reduction in the main pollutants in the pan-European region over the last 20 years, with European Union averages showing a 70 per cent reduction at monitoring stations in road traffic and an 85 per cent reduction at monitoring stations in urban and industrial areas.
The decline in SO2 concentrations has slowed down in the last few years. In terms

of NOx concentrations in ambient air in the European Union, an average reduction of 25-35 % over the last 20 years has been observed at all types of plants, with the largest reductions recorded at plants in rural areas. The phasing out of internal combustion engines in cars is expected to accelerate the reduction of NOx concentrations in urban and suburban stations over the next 10 years. Over the last 20 years, annual mean trends for ground-level ozone in Europe have shown no significant change or an increase of about 20 per cent at traffic monitoring stations, with 25 per cent of these sites showing increases of 40 per cent or more, while high ground-level ozone peaks have decreased by about 10 per cent, except at traffic monitoring stations. Increases in average ozone concentrations have been accompanied by reductions in NOx and VOC emissions. Since 2000, annual mean PM10 concentrations in Europe have decreased by 40-50 % at all stations, with the largest decrease at monitoring stations in industrial areas, while the decrease in PM2.5 concentrations was about 30 % (compared to 2008). Regional differences are observed in the seasonal peaks of PM concentrations in areas where firewood is mainly used for domestic heating, e.g. South-Eastern Europe, Eastern Europe and Central Asia.

Consumption of ozone-depleting substances (ECE, response indicator) The phase-out of ozone-depleting substances (ODS) continues, although some limited essential uses, such as for laboratory and firefighting purposes, are still allowed in special cases. Since 2012, ODS consumption figures in the 27 member States of the European Union (production, plus imports, minus exports and destruction) have been negative, declining from 343,000 tonnes of ozone-depleting capacity (ODP) in 1986. In Central Asia and Eastern Europe, ODS consumption decreased from 243 to 34 tonnes between 2014 and 2022, and in the Russian Federation from 684 to 287 tonnes.

To date, ODS emissions have been reduced from 1990 levels by 98 per cent. The obligations of the parties to the Montreal Protocol include phasing out the production and consumption of regulated substances within a specific time frame, reporting data on production, use, imports and exports to the Ozone Secretariat, and establishing a licensing system for imports and exports.

Three possible sources of case studies are suggested. The first is the document Measures to Green the Post-Pandemic recovery, recently published by the Coalition on Environment and Climate Change, which contains interesting case studies under the categories "Transport and mobility, climate measures" - measure 10 (Chisinau), "Transport, air quality, climate measures" - measure 11 (Milan, Amsterdam, Ukraine and Belarus) and "Transport and mobility, air quality, biodiversity measures" - measure 13 (Barcelona (Spain)).

The second and third sources are the City of London Corporation's Air Quality Strategy 2019-2030 and a case study from South East Europe as part of the UNEP report, providing an update on regional air quality policy for the pan-European region.

B. Climate change and greenhouse gas emissions 1. Key findings and recommendations

Despite the GHG emission reduction commitments made by all countries in the pan-European region, net GHG emissions in the region continue to increase.

Efforts and achievements are unevenly distributed across the region. The reductions that have been largely achieved in western Europe are three times smaller than the emissions growth in the rest of the region. National commitments under the Paris Agreement have been reaffirmed by 35 countries in the region that have set more ambitious targets. However, some countries still do not have firm quantifiable commitments or mechanisms to track progress towards their fulfilment, resulting in significant data gaps.

While decarbonisation is becoming a new paradigm for Europe, the gap between words and actions is deepening. Between 2013 and 2023, 29 countries in the pan-European region increased their use of renewable energy, but the region remains heavily dependent on fossil fuels, which account for around 78% of total final energy consumption. The increase in the share of renewable energy in the energy mix has been slower than the growth in total final energy consumption in the region. The estimated share of the population covered by local disaster risk reduction strategies (DRR) in the pan-European region is around 65 %. Only 15 countries in the region reported that all their local governments are implementing DRR strategies under target 13.1 of the Sustainable Development Goals, while 23 countries, which together account for a quarter of the region's population, do not report data on this indicator, should strengthen their commitments to nationally determined contributions under the Paris Agreement, commit to economy-wide absolute emission reduction targets, and regularly report on progress towards achieving absolute emission reductions.

Governments should enable the sustainable mobilisation of funds in the medium and long term for climate action, both by leveraging existing regional and global funds and mechanisms and by establishing national financial instruments, should accelerate decarbonisation by reorienting investment incentives towards renewable energy, should raise awareness of potential hazards, including natural hazards, and in particular climate-related hazards.

As part of global climate action, all countries in the pan-European region have pledged to reduce GHG emissions to prevent global temperatures from rising by more than 1.5 °C, as set out in the Paris Agreement. According to the International Energy Agency (IEA) 2018 data, despite the downward trend in growth rates, global energy consumption could increase by 30 per cent between 2017 and 2040. Energy is expected to remain a major source of anthropogenic GHG emissions. The European Union has defined its decarbonisation strategy with a long-term goal to reduce GHG emissions by 80-95 % below 1990 levels by 2050. In this context, several European Union Member States have already declared their intention to completely phase out the use of hard and lignite coal between 2025 and 2035. Such a goal may prove too ambitious and challenging for countries that are heavily dependent on coal. Countries in the region are in very different situations in terms of fossil fuel reserves and renewable energy potential, technical capacity, energy consumption patterns, infrastructure and labour and capital markets. The decarbonisation process is providing an impetus for the development of new low- and no-carbon technologies, but this does not negate the need to address energy poverty and ensure a just transition. Addressing the impacts of climate change, especially on the most vulnerable communities, requires urgent adaptation programmes that are systemic, multidimensional and transformative. Local adaptation strategies are increasingly being developed across Europe. More than 1,900 local authorities in EEA member and co-operating countries have made adaptation commitments under the Global Covenant of Mayors on Climate and Energy, the next challenge is to implement these strategies.

3. Status, major trends and recent developments

GHG emissions in the pan-European region increased by 1 per cent between 2014 and 2018, while the average carbon footprint per person increased by 0.2 per cent. The European Union's climate action progress report "A leap towards climate neutrality in Europe" states that in 2023 GHG emissions were reduced by 24 % against 1990 levels and that the European Union remains on track to meet its 20 % GHG reduction target. According to the latest IEA80, pandemic COVID-19 led to a 6 per cent overall reduction in global energy-related GHG emissions in 2020, with the maximum reduction recorded in April of that year. However, global emissions were 2%, or 60 million tonnes, higher than in the same month a year earlier. Globally, climate finance has increased significantly, but investment in fossil fuels remains higher.In parallel with the increased uptake of renewable energy, energy consumption is also increasing. Since 2010, the share of modern renewable energy81 in global final energy consumption has remained at around 10 per cent. Including traditional bioenergy use, the share of all renewable energy sources in total final energy consumption will be 18 %.

The IEA report Net Zero by : a Roadmap for the Global Energy Sector83 outlines more than 400 measures that include, starting today, no investment in new fossil fuel projects and no final investment decisions on new coal-fired power plants without carbon capture and storage. This pathway envisages that by 2030, the annual increase in solar photovoltaic power generation will reach 630 GW and wind power generation will reach 390 GW. Together, this is four times the record level achieved in 2020. The roadmap also sets a target of ending sales of new passenger vehicles with internal combustion engines by 2035 and for the global electricity sector to achieve zero emissions by 2040. It outlines a major effort to improve energy efficiency worldwide, resulting in global energy efficiency levels increasing by an average of 4 per cent annually between now and 2030, about three times the average over the past two decades.

While the European Union has set a new target to increase the share of renewables in final energy consumption to at least 32% by 2030, non-European Union members of the Energy Community have not been able to agree on new targets for decarbonisation, renewables and energy efficiency for the period to 2030.

The share of renewable energy in the transport sector in the European Union reached 10.2 per cent in 202084 , in other words, the target of 10 per cent renewable energy in transport by 2020 has been met. Technological development is enabling a shift from fossil-fuelled vehicles to environmentally friendly vehicles. Electric vehicles, combined with renewable energy generation, offer great prospects for decarbonising a large part of road transport. However, electric vehicles account for only 0.2 per cent of the European Union's total vehicle fleet, and if their market share continues to grow at the current rate, it would take about 60 years to replace half of the current passenger car fleet85. At the global level, the share of renewable energy in the transport sector in 2017 was 3.3 per cent, with the majority of this being liquid biofuels, mainly ethanol and biodiesel produced from crops.

The pan-European region attracts tourists from all over the world, and tourism leaves a significant carbon footprint. While the application of circular economy principles to the tourism sector within a country or within an individual resort may reduce this footprint somewhat, the bulk of it is generated by the transport of tourists themselves. Between 2014 and 2023, GHG emissions in the European Union decreased by about 12 Mt of CO2 equivalent, mainly in Germany, but emissions increased in 12 other European Union Member States. High-income countries outside the European Union also achieved emission reductions, with the United Kingdom accounting for 95 per cent of the reductions. In Eastern Europe, the Russian Federation accounted for the lion's share of the increase in GHG emissions, with Ukraine reducing emissions by more than 30 Mt of CO2 equivalent. In South-Eastern Europe and Central Asia, Turkey and Kazakhstan are the main contributors to the increase in GHG emissions, respectively, although data are not available for a number of countries. Share of renewable energy in total energy consumption (Sustainable Development Goal indicator 7.2.1) The share of renewable energy in total final energy consumption is the percentage of final energy consumption derived from renewable resources. Although energy consumption from renewable sources in the pan-European region increased to 1.3 petajoule between 2014 and 2023, their share remained unchanged due to a parallel increase in energy consumption from non-renewable sources.

The share of renewable energy sources (RES) in total energy consumption ranges from 4 % in Eastern Europe and Central Asia to 18 % in the European Union and Western Europe. The average for the whole pan-European region is 13 %. Only Western Europe showed a steady upward trend over the five-year period 2014-2023. To keep global temperature rise within 1.5 °C, the annual increase in the share of renewable energy in primary energy worldwide needs to increase from 0.25 % to 2 %86.Proportion of local governments that have adopted and implemented local disaster risk reduction strategies in line with national disaster risk reduction strategies (Sustainable Development Goal indicator 13.1.3) The Sendai Framework aims to increase the proportion of local governments that adopt and implement local DRR strategies. According to data for Sustainable Development Goal indicator 13.1.3 for the period 2015-2023, 31 countries in the pan-European region reported having such strategies in place, covering 41,850 local communities (see Table 27). More than 600 major cities in the pan-European region (out of 4,360 cities worldwide) are participating in the "Making Cities Resilient" initiative coordinated by the United Nations Office for Disaster Risk Reduction. In addition, 9,919 local communities from 33 countries in the pan-European region are participating in the Global Covenant of Mayors on Climate and Energy initiative. In 2022, around 41% of the EU population lives in municipalities that have signed the Global Covenant of Mayors for Climate and Energy.

Given the large populations of countries with local DRR strategies, it is estimated that 65 % of the population of the pan-European region is covered by such strategies. More than 80 % are covered in Eastern and South-Eastern Europe as well as in Western Europe (85 %), while in Central Asia the coverage is less than 26 %.

Stockholm, the capital of Sweden, plans to phase out fossil fuels by 2040. As explained in the city strategy, "Stockholm aims to completely phase out fossil fuels by 2040 at the latest, eliminating their use within the geographical boundaries of the city. At the same time, the city recognises that it will not be easy to phase out the use of fossil fuels in aviation and international shipping, and that some plastics derived from fossil minerals will still be burned in heating plants in 2040. Nevertheless, climate neutrality or zero net emissions can be achieved by offsetting these residual effects, for example by investing in carbon sinks. Climate neutrality allows the use of fossil fuels, provided that CO2 emissions are offset by measures that sequester carbon or carbon dioxide in some way."

According to the plan, by 2040, the city's energy and heat supply system will completely switch from natural gas to mainly biogas. The district heating company has decided to phase out fossil fuels by 2030. To increase the share of renewable energy in the transport sector from the current 16 per cent to 100 per cent by 2040, the city plans to double the capacity of the public transport system and modernise the infrastructure for pedestrians and cyclists.

The Global Covenant of Mayors is an initiative launched by the European Commission in 2008 to bring together local authorities that have voluntarily committed themselves to the European Union's climate and energy goals. With some 2,000 cities already participating in the initiative, the European Commission launched the Global Covenant of Mayors East initiative. Today, the Global Covenant of Mayors for Climate and Energy represents the largest movement of local authorities willing to go beyond their own national climate and energy goals.

The initiative has 9,919 members from 33 countries in the pan-European region. During the Paris Climate Summit, the European Commission announced the geographical expansion of the Covenant of Mayors for Climate and Energy, opening new regional offices in sub-Saharan Africa, the Americas and in Japan, India, China and South-East Asia.

C. Fresh water

Access to clean freshwater is essential for a life of dignity and economic development. Water is critical for life, nature conservation and biodiversity. In addition, over the coming decade and beyond, there will be deepening interconnections and increasing tensions between water and other sectors of the economy. In the pan-European region, water resources are unevenly distributed in space and time. Climate change poses additional challenges in terms of precipitation patterns and temperature; all future climate change scenarios indicate that hydrological extremes will be longer, more frequent and more intense. Climate change affects human health through many water-related phenomena: floods, heat waves, droughts, waterborne diseases and changes in biodiversity in wetlands and aquatic ecosystems. The impacts of these events are differentiated by gender, with increased vulnerability of the poor, women and children.

Anthropogenic pressures reinforce the asymmetric distribution of water resources, degrading freshwater quality and aquatic biodiversity. In addition, despite increasing efforts to limit emissions at source, diffuse pollution and urban and industrial wastewater discharges remain significant in many places. There is also growing concern about persistent organic pollutants because of their significant adverse effects on public health.

River basins, lakes and aquifers are therefore exposed to numerous stressors that jeopardise their physical, chemical and ecological state and the services they provide. However, advances in science are enabling to develop new solutions and facilitating the emergence of new processes and technologies to combat these negative impacts.

Financing for water projects under the international climate agenda is limited; developing bankable projects is challenging. Over the last decade, the quality and effectiveness of financing models have been significantly reduced due to technical and governance deficiencies and crises at local and regional levels. Growing water management challenges indicate that fragmented management practices are unlikely to have the desired effect in the long term. The involvement of public and private actors is becoming a critical factor in the implementation of successful water policies. With this in mind, one of the main elements of good governance is information. Its granularity is essential to enhance knowledge and link micro- and macro-levels to facilitate informed decision-making. Transboundary management of shared rivers, lakes and aquifers remains a challenge. The problem is exacerbated when upstream countries have significant water abstraction and/or retention and downstream countries have no alternative sources of water supply.

Despite some positive examples, the processes of co-operation and participation in the protection and allocation of water resources, as well as other practical mechanisms in the pan-European region, are not being realised to the extent that they could be.

Recommendations, integrated water management should be sought, involving a balance between human water needs and water availability for nature. In order to maximise the impact on society, including gender- and age-differentiated impacts, water policies should be more inter- and transdisciplinary. Therefore, the interconnectedness of water, food, energy and ecosystems necessitates a proactive policy approach to implement short-term projects in the context of a long-term vision for the pan-European region.

While progress has already been made in various countries to reduce (drinking) water consumption, it is not enough. Where freshwater resources and aquatic ecosystems are threatened, the best available technologies should be applied to improve the situation. In addition to water conservation measures and traditional pollution mitigation approaches, measures for resource protection and more efficient water use are entering the water market and should be put into practice. For example, in irrigated crop production, digitalisation and 'precision' agro-techniques can be applied to reduce water use and agrochemical losses. Nature-based solutions (NBS) can be used in the creation of water retention basins or in the restoration of riparian zones. New methods of environmental flow regime assessment have been developed.

Work is needed to validate the conceptual possibilities of non-conventional water supply sources. These are just some examples of high readiness solutions that can be applied in the pan-European region. Economic sustainability of water management must be pursued and innovative financing mechanisms are still needed in this context. A number of financing instruments can be used to develop natural and man-made infrastructure (e.g. equitable water tariffs, environmental payments, mechanisms for the development of natural and man-made infrastructure).

cost recovery and incentives), but a clear legal framework is absolutely necessary for success. Successful technology and financing activities require good governance. More often than might be expected, effective implementation requires social participation and cultural sensitivity. In addition, water management is more effective at the basin level. This integrated approach is even more important for transboundary rivers, lakes and aquifers where floods and droughts can occur. Joint management should be oriented towards environmental protection and benefit-sharing within the framework of effective and sustainable transboundary co-operation in transboundary basins, as foreseen in the Convention

ECE Convention on the Protection and Use of Transboundary Watercourses and International Lakes (Water Convention). Knowledge plays a crucial role in decision-making and water policy development. Therefore, investments in data collection and information processing (e.g. water accounts, ecosystem assessment and indicators) are needed. Continuous improvement of monitoring and communication technologies is a top priority from a pan-European water information system perspective. From an anthropocentric point of view, the sustainable use of freshwater resources is an ongoing challenge. Drinking water, agriculture, industrial production, energy production, transport and leisure are just some of the human activities that have an impact on water resources. There are systemic and complex non-linear relationships between the main drivers, the pressures acting on freshwater ecosystems, the corresponding impacts on the status and quality of water resources and the linkage to policy objectives. Water strategies therefore aim to move from the sectoral level to a more integrated approach in resource use. Today, the concept of water resources management involves the integration of food, energy and environmental policies, while recognising the central connecting role of water. This paradigm requires improved water governance and scientific knowledge for the development and implementation of effective and efficient water policies, which have an important place at all levels of government, civil society, business and a wide range of stakeholders to advance human rights, gender equality and poverty reduction.

Legislation is the basis of water management systems. Public policy promotes the sustainable use of freshwater resources through command and control measures and measures to reduce pollution at source. The European Union has a comprehensive legal framework for the protection of freshwater resources, ranging from setting mandatory targets for urban wastewater treatment to the conservation of freshwater resources and the protection of aquatic ecosystems. European Union legislation on water management has a significant impact on countries in the pan-European region.

At the same time, nutrient, persistent organic and toxic pollution from diffuse and point sources, as well as hydrological and morphological pressures, continue to occur in the pan-European region, hindering the achievement of water policy objectives. The ecological status of rivers at a higher level is determined by more than one impact factor; therefore, water protection and water allocation processes are more effective at the river basin scale. Attention should be paid to new pollutants; new health concerns require strict limits and further monitoring of surface and groundwater to preserve drinking water quality in the pan-European region.

In addition to existing pressures in freshwater management, climate change is emerging as a key driver for water management. Furthermore, although water resources are not directly mentioned in the Paris Agreement, they are central to most adaptation measures identified in nationally determined contributions and are closely linked to other priority areas. Climate scenarios indicate an increase in peak precipitation intensity in the pan-European region, especially in the mid and high latitudes, where average precipitation levels will also increase. Intense precipitation causes floods and impermeable soils (soil compaction) without green infrastructure favours flash floods. At the same time, water scarcity will worsen at low latitudes and mid-latitudes in continental hinterlands, in particular in the Mediterranean zone.

As recently highlighted, finance is a key aspect to support the implementation of policies and programmes, and "although water is a central element and prerequisite for adaptation, only 5% of all climate finance and just over one-fifth of all climate finance from developed countries to developing countries is allocated to it". The situation appears to be the same across the pan-European region, or even worse in non-European Union countries. The point is that water managers have always had traditional difficulties in dealing with cost recovery. In practice, serious problems do arise. In water-intensive agriculture, for example, it is still necessary to identify appropriate cost recovery measures and exemptions that will be acceptable to society. This is not a reason to stop critically analysing the application of economic incentives for inclusive and responsible water management. The European Union Water Framework Directive (Art. 9) has been a starting point for strengthening economic considerations and cost recovery principles in the water sector. However, it is not clear how exactly cost recovery contributes to achieving sustainable and equitable water use.

In this context, it should be noted that while water resources are always a national issue, they are much more difficult to manage if rivers, lakes or aquifers are shared with other countries. With regard to transboundary waters, assessments often differed from State to State for obvious reasons, but ultimately such waters were a shared resource. In the pan-European region, 52 countries share transboundary rivers, lakes and aquifers, and the Water Convention has therefore been developed to provide the region with a framework, although countries may enter into bilateral or multilateral agreements. International co-operation is essential in times of floods and droughts, when downstream countries are most at risk and depend on decisions made in upstream countries. In general, water allocation mechanisms in transboundary water bodies are mainly considered from a supply-side perspective. However, elements of demand or benefit-sharing analyses can complement supply-oriented solutions and help to ensure integrated water resources management.

The development and implementation of sustainable infrastructure and nature-based solutions (RBFs) in freshwater conservation can bring multiple benefits to society, the economy, the environment and human well-being. Multifunctional ROPFs can meet societal needs and conserve biodiversity while optimising resource use and limiting trade-offs. It should be ensured that the principles of cyclical water economics are prioritised in the tourism and recreation industry. Tourism development that takes into account the optimisation of water resources and the recovery of valuable products has the potential to support all of the Sustainable Development Goals. As one researcher noted, "the linkages and synergies between circular economy methods and the targets of the Sustainable

Development Goals are strongest in the case of Sustainable Development Goal 6 (clean water and sanitation) and Goal 15 (preservation of terrestrial ecosystems)" and these are assessed below. It is important to ensure that the parameters of water services are defined in terms of sectoral needs, namely in terms of food, energy, ecosystems or human dynamics (e.g. tourism). Closed-loop economic techniques for wastewater recycling and reuse, as well as sludge management, are absolutely necessary to achieve Sustainable Development Goal 6 (clean water and sanitation). In order to fully utilise the best practices of the circular economy, infrastructure will need to be upgraded and optimised and innovative infrastructure solutions will need to be developed. One example is toilets equipped with a urine collection device for phosphorus recovery in decentralised systems.

3. Status, main trends and recent developments Renewable freshwater resources in the pan-European region are asymmetrically distributed. The indicator of freshwater abstraction as a share of renewable freshwater resources is characterised by high variability across countries. It is currently a concern in a number of countries; Furthermore, climate change will affect most countries where water supply is already a problem. Therefore, with the exception of the Scandinavian peninsula and some small areas in Central Europe, under pessimistic scenarios, river flows are projected to decrease throughout Europe, but most severely in southern countries. In addition, abnormal heat increases the intensity and number of forest fires, which in turn have a negative impact on aquifer recharge and surface water quality. Recently, more countries have been affected by large forest fires than ever before, including in the northern countries of the pan-European region (e.g., in the Russian Federation, the worst forest fires in Siberia were recorded in 2021; Sweden experienced the worst fire season in its history in 2018).

Freshwater resources and ecosystem biodiversity are still highly relevant in different sub-regions of the pan-European region. Even for a secondary indicator such as "proportion of water bodies with good water quality", in 76% of countries in the pan-European region, more than 60% of water bodies in 2020 were characterised by "good water quality". This indicator has not changed since 2017, suggesting the need to intensify efforts to improve water quality. At the same time, if we apply a more stringent indicator for assessing water quality, say the indicators used in the European Union area, in 2015 only 40% of surface water bodies met the "good ecological status" and 38% met the "good chemical status". A similar picture in the European Union can be seen for the "good chemical status" of groundwater.

In fact, the original European Union policy goal of achieving "good ecological status" for all water bodies has not been met and the deadline has been delayed until 2027 at the most.

Despite these threats, areas of aquatic biodiversity are unevenly distributed across Europe's subregions, and hydromorphological impacts associated with existing or planned water management facilities continue to create environmental pressures. In addition, extreme weather events, in particular floods, can provoke man-made accidents and severe water pollution. The mining industry is an example of how extreme weather events can lead to man-made accidents in several countries in the pan-European region (e.g. Kazakhstan, Romania and Tajikistan). Accidents have potential transboundary impacts, but transnational impacts are often ignored in river basin management plans, despite the fact that the ECE Convention on the Transboundary Effects of Industrial Accidents and the Water Convention require contingency plans and measures to minimise the risk of accidental pollution in transboundary basins. Access to a safe drinking water supply in the pan-European region is on average above 70 per cent, with no significant change in recent years. The highest levels are found in the European Union and Western Europe subregions (98 per cent and 99 per cent, respectively). In the Central Asian subregion, the average is lower but still high (70 per cent).

This may explain why access to drinking water supply systems meeting safety requirements increased by 10 % worldwide between 2000 and 2015, but by no more than 4 % in the pan-European region over the same period. In addition, monitoring of the presence of new contaminants, such as certain animal and human medicines, brominated flame retardants, microplastics and anti-fouling biocidal coatings, needs to be strengthened in the pan-European region. However, more detailed data indicate additional asymmetries at the national level. Countries in the pan-European region are significantly differentiated in terms of sanitation services and wastewater collection and treatment systems. Indeed, on average, 38 per cent of the population, or 344 million people, in the pan-European region are projected to lack access to safe sanitation, with the situation varying across subregions. While the European Union and Western Europe show higher rates (more than 90 per cent), the situation is much worse in Eastern Europe and South-Eastern Europe. In addition, ageing sewerage infrastructure requires serious additional costs. The European Union estimates that the annual investment required to rehabilitate and build new sewerage and wastewater treatment plants is around €25 billion. Summary data for Eastern Europe and Central Asia indicate even higher needs. Finally, non-conventional water sources should be used more extensively; recycling of sewage or domestic wastewater seems to be a common strategy only to save water. In fact, in the European Union, the recycling rate of treated wastewater was less than 3 %. Other non-conventional sources of water in arid zones can be considered (e.g. domestic wastewater, rainwater and atmospheric water harvesting, desalination of low salinity water), but water efficiency measures should be considered first. Further action on the water-energy-food nexus is fraught with risks. The food production sector plays a critical role from a social perspective and deserves special attention. Control of diffuse pollution in agriculture has been slow; over 18 per cent of the groundwater area still has excessive nitrate concentrations. Linking environmental flows to irrigated arable farming practices is an example of how difficult non-excessive trade-offs can be. Excessive groundwater withdrawal weakens the aquifer's ability to mitigate the effects of inter-annual or frequent droughts. Therefore, the best strategy is to utilise smart technologies and more efficient water management systems. The introduction of water-efficient crops, transpiration reduction techniques, precision farming and digitalisation, the use of reservoirs for agricultural purposes and rainwater harvesting for irrigation should be encouraged. However, adaptation techniques should be encouraged to the same extent as emission-reduction techniques, and farmers are eager to adopt these techniques.

Other solutions beyond agriculture are also becoming cost-effective, among which nature-based solutions (NBS) for freshwater protection and biodiversity conservation are gaining popularity. ROPFs can play an important role in protecting natural watersheds from diffuse pollution, catalysing social benefits and integrating landscapes, including in urban areas The climate crisis can largely be described as a water crisis, so good water management is becoming increasingly urgent. Good water governance implies a participatory, transparent approach, especially when it comes to finding mutually acceptable solutions between different sectors or - even more relevantly - between countries. In the case of transboundary waters in the pan-European region, all shared water bodies are regulated by existing arrangements in only 20 countries, of which only 19 are States Parties to the Water Convention. It is noteworthy that most countries claim that such arrangements include groundwaters, but the extent to which joint management of transboundary aquifers is effective is not evident.

Spatial, sectoral and temporal information is crucial for generating knowledge, developing strategies and monitoring water actions. Water resources management therefore implies data and up-to-date information, transparency and dialogue between government and stakeholders. There is a positive trend in the pan-European region towards information and communication technologies linking science and policy. Many geographic information systems are well established at the level of individual river basins, although much remains to be done, in particular at the transboundary level. At the country level, detailed information exists at different levels in the pan-European region; heterogeneous territorial realities in a number of countries may conceal deficiencies in water management at local and regional levels, necessitating water statistics. Other difficulties stem from conceptual reasons: ecological assessment of water quality and determination of hydromorphological loads require knowledge that is not yet available in some regions.

Water-related services, including water and sanitation (selected Sustainable Development Goal indicators) Indicators 6.1.1 of the Sustainable Development Goal indicators 6.1.1 (proportion of the population using safe drinking water services) and 6.2.1 (proportion of the population using safe sanitation...) belong to a group of indicators that have been identified to ensure availability and sustainable use of water and sanitation for all (Goal 6). In particular, indicator 6.1.1 aims to contribute to achieving universal and equitable access to safe and affordable drinking water for all by 2030 (target 6.1), while indicator 6.2.1 is used to contribute to universal and equitable access to adequate sanitation for all by 2030 and to end open defecation, with particular attention to the needs of women and girls and people in vulnerable situations (target 6.2). Based on information available in the Global SDG Indicators Database128, which contains global, regional and country data and metadata on official indicators, average values for these indicators were calculated for each of the subregions within the pan-European space. It should be noted that, in order to ensure temporal consistency with the other indicators analysed in this assessment, it was decided to select 2017 for the analysis, as information is available for all indicators except for Sustainable Development Goal indicator 15.3.1 (ratio of degraded land area to total land area) for that year, and thus the assessment of the indicators has identical or similar time frames, thus ensuring temporal consistency in the analysis. At the same time, for some indicators, where available, as in the case of indicators 6.1.1 and 6.2.1, the latest values available in the SDG indicator database (i.e. for 2020) were calculated to identify any trend in values over this period, with an improving trend only for indicator 6.2.1 in all subregions except Central Asia where data are missing.

The countries with the highest proportion of the population connected to wastewater treatment plants (more than 90 per cent), most countries for which information is available, are above 70 per cent. The lowest values are found in Azerbaijan and

Albania (20 per cent and 17 per cent respectively in 2017). However, a number of countries did not provide information, and even the term "water treatment" is ambiguously understood due to differences in the degree of treatment or the lack of clear certainty about the presence of decentralised systems on the ground. Nevertheless, a global trend of improvement can be identified compared to the situation ten years ago, with a stabilising trend in recent years.

Freshwater quality and quantity (selected Sustainable Development Goal indicators) Indicator 6.3.2 (percentage of water bodies with good water quality) also belongs to the group of indicators that have been identified for Sustainable Development Goal 6. Specifically, this indicator aims to contribute to improving water quality by 2030 by reducing pollution, eliminating waste dumping and minimising the release of hazardous chemicals and materials, halving the proportion of untreated wastewater and significantly increasing the recycling and safe reuse of wastewater worldwide (target 6.3). This indicator tracks the percentage of water bodies (rivers, lakes and groundwater) in a country with good ambient water quality. For global reporting purposes, overall water quality is assessed on the basis of an index comprising data on five major groups of parameters (oxygen, salinity, nitrogen, phosphorus and acidification), from which it is possible to judge whether there is evidence of serious deterioration in water quality, including in the pan-European region, the methodology includes in situ measurements of these surface and groundwater quality parameters. Based on available information, it was found that data were not available for several countries in the pan-European region. It was therefore decided to present only the available values. There is a global trend towards stabilisation of the proportion of water bodies with good water quality in the environment. Despite this, some deterioration can be observed in a number of countries over this time period.Water management (selected Sustainable Development Goal indicators) Target 6.5 of the Sustainable Development Goals aims to achieve integrated water resources management at all levels by 2030, including through transboundary cooperation where appropriate. Indicator 6.5.2 measures the second part of target 6.5 by characterising the proportion of the transboundary water basin area covered by transboundary water cooperation agreements in force. Agreements are considered "operational" if there is a joint body, meetings between countries and information exchange at least once a year, and joint and coordinated management plans or objectives for the basin(s).

Nature-based solutions - from watershed protection to flood management: two diametrically opposed examples One type of investment that has received insufficient attention is focused on watershed protection, sustainable management and watershed restoration. These are natural infrastructures that can filter and recharge water to supply cities and other users, including farmers, industry and the environment itself. Land use within catchments is an important factor in determining whether catchments are healthy and can provide these environmental services. On average, catchments in Europe have been allocated to restoration and conservation

EUR 5.5 billion per year, and it is estimated that 99 per cent of the funding for these investments came from public sources. Some water service providers and cities are engaging with upstream parties in the catchments of their water sources, seeking to assist in changing agricultural and forestry practices or creating artificial wetlands. However, such investments remain limited due to regulatory barriers, perceptions of the high risk of such activities, or a general lack of understanding of what can be achieved from such investments. Nature-based solutions (NBS) may be a viable approach to support efforts to protect drinking water resources for many cities. According to a recent analysis, they have extensive potential, with 63 cities showing high feasibility potential for at least one type of ROPF and pollutant. Climate change, soil compaction and flood risks can be addressed with ROPFs and citizen engagement. The Glinsčica River basin in Slovenia lies within the boundaries of the city of Ljubljana. The expansion of Ljubljana has increased the area of impermeable surface in the valley of the Glinsčica River basin, which, combined with rising groundwater levels and increased heavy rainfall, has resulted in periodic flooding in parts of the city. A design process was initiated to develop ROPFs that would effectively reduce flood risk and address other societal issues

with users to collect information on the risk perception of the population and institutions in the area. For this purpose, workshops were held to capture the risk perceptions of the population. Stakeholders were then engaged to jointly develop and evaluate a dynamic model to measure the effectiveness of the ROPF in flood management in a business-as-usual scenario, allowing workshop participants to consider the potential effect of specific measures in terms of both flood risk reduction and co-benefits.

D. Coastal waters, marine ecosystems and seas

Marine pollution from both terrestrial (e.g. nutrients, plastics, chemicals) and marine (e.g. plastics, oil) sources remains a pressing problem in most marine regions. Beach and marine litter, of which plastic litter is a major contributor, is recognised as a serious global threat to coastal and marine ecosystems in most areas, including remote and sparsely populated areas such as the Barents Sea. Climate-induced changes in coastal and marine ecosystems include an increase in sea surface temperature of about 0.2 °C per decade in the North Atlantic and 0.5 °C per decade in the Black Sea (since 1981) and an observed decrease in surface water pH values (i.e. acidification) of about 0.02 pH units per decade in the marine regions surrounding the European Union (and in the oceans as a whole), except for variations in coastal zones, the nature of the impact of which has yet to be determined. However, marine protected area (MPA) coverage in 20 of the 37 coastal countries in the pan-European region is lagging behind target 11 of the Convention on Biological Diversity's Aichi Targets (at least 10% of coastal and marine areas covered by conservation measures), at 6.7% for the pan-European region as a whole. The proportion of sustainable fish stocks varies considerably geographically. Fish stocks in the Mediterranean and Black Seas continue to be significantly overfished, while the north-east Atlantic and the Baltic Sea show signs of recovery due to better management decisions. A holistic ecosystem approach to the management of coastal waters and marine ecosystems, which takes into account the combined effects of multiple pressures, gradually brings together social, economic and governance aspects. This approach is applicable both to the use of ROPF in building sustainable infrastructure to strengthen coastal resilience and climate resilient functions, and to the transition to blue sustainable tourism as one element of post COVID pandemic recovery.

Governments at all levels (local, national and regional) should take urgent action to reduce major pressures in order to halt the degradation of coastal waters, marine ecosystems and seas. Climate change, biodiversity loss and pollution threats are inextricably linked and constitute a "triple planetary crisis".

Additional efforts are needed to reach the benchmark level of 10 per cent of coastal and marine areas in the pan-European region, in particular in Eastern and South-Eastern Europe. Most countries in the European Union have already reached this level.

Coastal waters, marine ecosystems and seas, related indicators and data flows should be included as a separate theme in the ECE set of environmental indicators. Consideration should be given to using promising new developments in data (e.g.

Earth observations, artificial intelligence, citizen monitoring, models and new in-situ measurements) to improve spatial and temporal coverage, including the need for long time series data to understand the impacts of climate change. Policymakers should intensify efforts to complement inventories of several components of beach and marine litter with information on the composition and sources of litter to enable the development of more effective measures. In particular, joint efforts should be made in areas where the need for action at the subregional level has been recognised, such as the Caspian Sea, for which there is no reliable information on the presence or quantity of litter discharged into the coastal or marine environment.
Oceans play a critical role as climate regulators and buffers against the effects of climate change, to the detriment of their productivity and the health of marine ecosystems. The widespread degradation of coastal waters, marine ecosystems and oceans is a clear manifestation of the triple planetary crisis and the closely linked threats of climate change, biodiversity loss and pollution. At the global level, two-thirds of the oceans are significantly impacted by anthropogenic activities that create multiple pressures, ranging from excessive inputs of nutrients and hazardous substances (including plastics, microplastics and nanoplastics), unsustainable fishing (including illegal, unreported and unregulated (IUU) fishing) and habitat destruction through coastal development (including for tourism) to natural resource extraction. Other detrimental environmental changes resulting from climate change include ocean warming, ocean acidification and deoxygenation, which adversely affect species diversity and abundance of marine species.

"Blue economy", which is steadily growing and posing challenges for environmental sustainability, includes ocean-based income-generating activities such as fishing for food species, shipping, seabed mining, offshore hydrocarbon exploration and exploitation, tourism and recreation. Interest in seabed mining is growing and is fuelled in part by the increasing demand for minerals and rare earth elements, in particular cobalt needed for electric vehicle batteries, which is one of the measures to mitigate climate change. The systemic nature of these challenges creates an urgent need for integrated and ecosystem-based management approaches supported by spatially focused assessments and analyses of multiple drivers and cumulative impacts.

Despite the specific environmental and socio-economic characteristics and governance structures of the pan-European marine regions, a number of similarities can be identified among the main trends and challenges they face. The assessment uses a combined approach, combining existing knowledge at the marine region level with national data reported under Sustainable Development Goal 14 "Conserve and manage oceans, seas and marine resources for sustainable development".

The pan-European area comprises 37 coastal ECE member States and the following marine regions: the Baltic Sea, the Black Sea, the Caspian Sea, the Mediterranean Sea and the north-eastern Atlantic Ocean. With the exception of the Caspian Sea, a

wealth of knowledge and information has been accumulated for these marine regions through publications and indicator work undertaken by EEA and the governing or executive bodies of the regional maritime conventions.
Other marine (sub)regions included in the assessment, such as the Aral Sea, the Barents Sea, the East Siberian Sea, the North Sea and the Norwegian Sea, are not systematically discussed. Information on the Caspian Sea is mainly contained in the Tehran Convention's State of the Caspian Sea Environment Report. Of the 37 coastal countries in the pan-European region, 22 are member States of the European Union. A new indicator is playing an important role as a tool for measuring ecosystem health and halting biodiversity loss in all ecosystems, including marine ecosystems.
European Union Biodiversity Strategy 2030. In parallel, the Marine Strategy Framework Directive was adopted; Commission Decision aimed at achieving or maintaining an adequate state of the environment in the four regional seas of the European Union by protecting and restoring the marine environment and phasing out pollution. The Marine Spatial Planning Directive makes a key contribution to the implementation of of the Marine Strategy Framework Directive on aspects related to the use and management of ocean space. There is a direct link between the theme of coastal waters, marine ecosystems and seas and the two themes of the Conference. For example, the use of ROPF in building sustainable infrastructure improves the overall coastal resilience and climate resilience of the coastal zone. At the same time, this approach addresses multiple challenges, such as sea-level rise, flood defence and coastal erosion leading to loss of land, assets and livelihoods, and harmonises coastal development with habitat and environmental protection.
With more than half of the European Union's tourist hotels located in coastal areas, marine and coastal tourism is the backbone of the blue economy, particularly in the Mediterranean region, which accounts for about one third of world tourism. The COVID-19 pandemic severely affected the prospects for marine and coastal tourism, as well as many other closely related sectors, that the recovery from the COVID-19 pandemic will fuelling ambitions and trends towards more sustainable tourism.
Pollution of the seas from land-based sources includes discharges of domestic waste, mainly in the form of plastic litter, sewage and waste from industrial activities. Huge investments in large-scale projects and the construction of new or modernised wastewater treatment plants have led to an overall reduction in discharges of untreated wastewater into the seas, particularly in parts of the Black, Caspian and Mediterranean Seas. The semi-enclosed Baltic and Black Seas have historically been known for their high susceptibility to eutrophication, the enrichment of water with biogenic nitrogen and phosphorus due to limited exchange of water with external seas.
Contaminating marine litter includes beach and floating litter, seabed litter, litter in biota and micro litter, represented by pieces of plastic less than 5 mm in diameter,

known as microplastics. Microplastics are becoming a growing concern as they accumulate in the food chain and thus pose a risk to marine biota and human health. The presence of marine litter is observed throughout the pan-European area, including the sparsely populated Barents Sea region. With the exception of the north-east Atlantic, where marine litter is of equal importance, most litter comes from land-based sources. There is no reliable information on the amount of litter discharged into the coastal or marine environment of the Caspian Sea, despite the severity of the problem.

One of the major pressures affecting the sustainability, health, productivity and resilience of marine ecosystems is fisheries. Overexploitation of commercial fish and shellfish stocks continues in all marine regions of the pan-European area. The state of fisheries in the north-eastern Atlantic Ocean and the Baltic Sea has improved considerably, with clear signs of recovery of commercial fish and shellfish stocks. In the Mediterranean and Black Sea, however, the situation remains critical and shows no signs of improvement. This is due to increased fishing pressure, significant gaps in knowledge on the status of fish and shellfish stocks, and difficulties in the Mediterranean Sea in implementing management measures for the common stock. In the Caspian Sea, fish stocks are also declining as a result of overfishing and unregulated fishing. IUU fishing is one of the factors negatively affecting local economies and coastal livelihoods and threatening marine ecosystems.

Marine biodiversity is in sharp decline, with the rate of decline exceeding that of terrestrial species. Red List assessments for the European Union's marine regions show that of 1,196 marine species, 9 per cent are threatened with extinction and 3 per cent are near threatened. Birds, mammals and turtles are particularly endangered, with more than 20 per cent of species at risk of extinction. 18 red-listed sturgeon species throughout Europe and Asia have been recognised as endangered. Beluga in the Caspian Sea is on the Critically Endangered species list along with all other commercially important Caspian fish species, which are major producers of wild caviar. The resilience of marine ecosystems is further reduced due to changes in temperature and decreases in ocean oxygen content, as well as ocean acidification as a result of anthropogenic climate change. These changes in environmental conditions indicate that significant systemic changes are occurring in European Union marine regions 150. Rising sea surface temperatures are altering species151 ranges, abundance and seasonality, affecting marine food chains. Awareness of the role of the oceans in meeting climate goals is growing at the policy level, and more governments are committing to larger-scale ocean programmes. The European Union Biodiversity Strategy 2030 emphasises the need to increase the conservation coverage of European Union marine areas to 30 per cent, creating ecological corridors to help reverse biodiversity loss and contribute to climate change mitigation and resilience. In addition, the European Union's Nature Recovery Plan includes a proposal for legally binding restoration treaties.

At the global level, 51 countries, including 17 ECE member States, have committed to protecting at least 30 per cent of marine areas by 2030 through the "30 per cent by 2030" initiative Global Ocean Protection Alliance.

Following a participatory process (3rd International Forum on Ocean Governance, April 2021), the European Union has launched a revision of its International Ocean Governance Agenda, which is an integral part of the European Green Deal and the European Union's measure to achieve Sustainable Development Goal 14 (on marine ecosystems). Other initiatives at the regional or global level are aimed at raising awareness of marine debris pollution, the sustainable blue economy and environmental efforts. Understanding of marine issues continues to improve through the deployment of innovative sensors and autonomous observation platforms that enhance observation programmes through improved coordination and integration.

4. Indicators Development Goal 14 calls for the establishment of an appropriate system of indicators for a pan-European assessment of coastal waters, marine ecosystems and seas.

Marine pollution: beach litter density This indicator reflects the number of litter units per 100 metre stretch of beach in the maritime regions of the European Union. Data for the Caspian Sea are not available. Data are obtained from the EEA's Marine Litter Watch database, which operates on citizen science principles. Values are consistent with beach litter densities reported in regional assessments, particularly for the Baltic and Black Seas. Plastic is the most common type of litter and accounts for about 70-83 % of marine litter, and in some areas more than 90 %.Most assessments do not allow conclusions to be drawn about trends over time in the dynamics of marine litter pollution. This is due to survey limitations and methodological problems in interpreting marine litter data. The abundance of beach litter is highly dependent on water currents, prevailing winds and beach exposure.

United Nations (FAO) indicator 14.4.1 of the Sustainable Development Goals (proportion of fish stocks within biologically sustainable limits), which measures the sustainability of marine fisheries by the abundance of fish stocks within biologically sustainable limits, supplemented by data for four European Union marine regions on the proportion of assessed stocks meeting the basic criteria of good ecological status (GES) set out in the Marine Strategy Framework Directive . A fish stock whose abundance is at or above the maximum sustainable yield is classified as biologically sustainable. Conversely, when the abundance of a stock does not reach the level of maximum sustainable yield, the stock is considered biologically unsustainable.

Fish stocks in the Mediterranean and the Black Sea continue to be significantly overfished, while the north-east Atlantic and the Baltic Sea show signs of recovery due to better management decisions. Climate change impacts: mean acidity (pH) of seawater measured at an agreed group of representative sampling stations This indicator combines data reported by ECE coastal countries under indicator 14.3.1

of the Sustainable Development Goals (mean acidity (pH) of seawater measured at an agreed group of representative sampling stations) and compared with the global annual mean surface ocean pH. This indicator is used to monitor the carbon system by measuring four parameters: pH, total dissolved carbon, partial pressure of carbon dioxide, and total alkalinity. It is up to each country's government to decide which measurement sites to select, provided that measurements are made regularly at the same sites to record changes in parameter values. Aggregated values at the regional level can be obtained once values have been reported from at least half of the coastal countries.

Observations of ocean acidification over the past 35 years indicate an increase in ocean acidity of 0.052 pH units. At the national scale, the trend is more complex and shows large variations in the coastal zone. Long-term observations are needed to detect signs of ocean acidification, especially in coastal zones. Global mean annual surface ocean pH values from the Copernicus Marine Monitoring Service, based on a reconstruction method using in situ and remotely sensed data and empirical relationships, Climate change impacts: mean sea surface temperature anomaly, which reflects the mean annual sea surface temperature (in °C) correlated with the mean temperature of the global ocean and the four European seas. Warming has become noticeable, but it has occurred particularly rapidly since the era of satellite observations, which have provided more complete data. The trend in sea surface temperature is about 0.2 °C per decade in the North Atlantic and 0.5 °C per decade in the Black Sea. According to the Intergovernmental Panel on Climate Change158 , the average sea surface temperature has increased by 0.6 °C. Depending on the emissions scenario, sea surface temperatures are projected to continue to rise, albeit at a slower rate than land-based air temperatures.

"The Black Sea is recovering, but pollution by chemicals and marine litter is still a major problem", this case study refers to the period up to and including 2030. For decades, the Black Sea has been the most polluted marine region in the European Union. The Black Sea has undergone unprecedented degradation, with widespread nutrient loading causing an extensive dead zone. The main sources of nutrients are effluents from the agricultural sector (fertilisers and animal waste) and domestic and industrial waste. Three rivers, namely the Dniester, Dnieper and Danube, are the main source of nutrient, chemical and litter pollution in the Black Sea.

The EMBLAS project series contaminant monitoring programme has identified extremely high concentrations of chemicals in marine waters, biota, fish and shellfish. Traces of caffeine, pharmaceuticals and illicit drugs have been found in water samples, with pharmaceuticals, especially antibiotics, posing the greatest threat. The rate of floating litter (90.5 units/km2) was the highest among European Union seas and almost double that of the Mediterranean Sea. Microplastics have been detected in samples taken from seabed sediments. Over the past 20 years, the Danube has undergone extensive European Union-funded clean-up work. The construction of downstream treatment plants has prevented the discharge of

untreated sewage into the river, and as a result, its water quality has improved over the past 15 years. Other improvements include a reduction in industrial and agricultural discharges. The ecosystem of the north-western Black Sea shelf is recovering, as evidenced by the return of the once abundant red alga Phyllaphora. All of this is a prime example of a source-to-sea approach to coastal and marine management. "Green and Blue Recovery of Coastal and Marine Tourism in the MediterraneanThe Mediterranean basin has welcomed more than 400 million international tourists, with the tourism sector contributing up to 15% of regional GDP. Tourists are attracted by the landscapes and rich biodiversity, cultural heritage and traditional lifestyles, combined with favourable environmental conditions such as mild climate, beaches and clean seawater. . As one of the global hot 154
164 biodiversity points, the region is at the same time subject to critical levels of habitat loss due to unsustainable resource exploitation, pollution, climate change and invasive marine species. Negative impacts of tourism on the coastal and marine environment are mainly the result of the construction and operation of built infrastructure (resorts, residential developments, ports and marinas, facilities, etc.) and marine or coastal recreational activities (marine tourism, golf courses, water sports, etc.). The large spatial and temporal variations in tourism activity, which is concentrated mainly along the coastal strip and peaks in the summer season, dramatically increase the amount of potentially unmanaged waste as well as the discharge of under-treated urban wastewater. More than 75 per cent of the annual waste volume is generated during the summer period.

A key challenge is to promote blue sustainable tourism practices in coastal and marine areas that promote positive externalities for the environment, sector workers and local communities. The Mediterranean tourism sector has been hit hard by the travel restrictions caused by the COVID-19 pandemic. The sector is now at a crossroads: will it return to previous trends of unsustainable growth and mass tourism patterns or make a dramatic transition to more sustainable tourism patterns? The massive investments envisaged in ambitious green inclusive recovery plans offer a unique opportunity to rebuild for the better and transform the tourism sector, and contribute to the prosperity of the region. These interventions must be multilateral, involve diverse actors and deliver environmental and socio-economic benefits.

E. Biodiversity and ecosystems

Over the last 30 years, the total forest area in the pan-European region has increased by 33.5 million ha. With the exception of the Russian Federation, the relative share of particularly biodiversity-rich native primary forests has remained stable at around 3% of the total forest area between 2000 and 2020. Forest fragmentation remains an important pressure factor. Beyond forests, ecosystem health remains a concern, with no clear positive trend. Only a small proportion of habitats assessed at European Union level have a good conservation status, and the

general picture is likely to be similar outside the European Union. Over the last 30 years, the area of Protected Areas (PAs) in the pan-European region has almost tripled, hence the main PA-related policy objectives in the region have been met.
In the pan-European region, land acquisition for urban and infrastructure development continues. Although land acquisition has decreased in most EEA member countries, and in Eastern Europe even 155
reverse process, land acquisition practices and soil compaction remain a concern in many countries.
Governments should ensure that positive trends in forest areas are maintained. They should take additional measures to conserve remaining indigenous forests and their ecological functions, for example, by promoting management standards aimed at conserving high conservation value forests and by increasing forest connectivity. Efforts should be made to consolidate and improve the expanded network of protected areas in the ECE region through investments in management effectiveness, ecological representativeness and connectivity. The full range of management types should be utilised, as well as other effective conservation measures in these areas, to further strengthen territorial conservation networks.
Governments should take measures to further and progressively reduce land acquisition, and measures should also be taken to address the conversion of natural ecosystems to agriculture and habitat degradation resulting from agricultural practices unfavourable to biodiversity conservation, including, for example, better targeting such measures with subsidies and other incentives, integrate biodiversity conservation into all sectors and policies, refrain from the use of subsidies and other incentives, integrate biodiversity conservation into all sectors and policies, and reduce the use of subsidies and other incentives.
Biodiversity, which encompasses diversity within species, between species and between ecosystems, plays an essential role in sustaining the Earth's life support systems, enabling conservation measures to address social problems and maintain quality of life.
Ecosystem services are recognised as the basis for sustainable socio-economic development.
The Pan-European region is characterised by significant overlap with the Palearctic region and its extensive biomes of boreal coniferous and temperate deciduous forests, temperate grasslands and deserts, Mediterranean forests and Arctic tundra, as well as important marine ecosystems. It includes the largest continuous forest, grassland and peatland ecosystems on the planet. They act as critical carbon sinks, provide ecosystem services and underpin the economies of the region.
Policy goals and targets as well as the global policy framework for biodiversity in the broader context of sustainable development are defined by the relevant Sustainable Development Goals, in particular Goals 15 and 14. Countries in the pan-European region co-operate under various multilateral environmental agreements (MEAs). The main MEA on biodiversity is the Convention on

Biological[156] diversity in 1992. Its most recent Strategic Plan for Biodiversity, which has been implemented, was developed on the basis of the Aichi Biodiversity Targets. Other relevant MEAs include the Convention on the Conservation of Migratory Species of Wild Animals, the Convention on International Trade in Endangered Species of Wild Fauna and Flora, the Convention on Wetlands of International Importance especially as Waterfowl Habitat, and the Convention on the Conservation of Wild Fauna and Flora and Natural Habitats in Europe.

A major policy challenge related to biodiversity is to ensure its effective conservation and sustainable use. This implies addressing the drivers and root causes of pressures on species and terrestrial, marine and other aquatic ecosystems, including oceans, and increasingly requires restoration efforts. Strategies include adopting a mix of ambitious policies (regulatory approaches, economic instruments and voluntary approaches), mainstreaming biodiversity into economic and sectoral policies, eliminating illegal exploitation and trade in biodiversity elements, and eliminating illegal, unreported and unregulated (IUU) fishing. In this regard, it is crucial to enforce existing laws and regulations in order to put an end to illegal activities. Biodiversity conservation and restoration also require reforming and eliminating environmentally harmful subsidies and strengthening the role of biodiversity-related taxes, fees and charges. The strategic plan of the Convention on Biological Diversity has been only partially implemented and biodiversity loss continues According to the Global Biodiversity Outlook 5 report, only 6 of the 20 Aichi Biodiversity Targets, which are the core document specifying Sustainable Development Goals 14 and 15, have been partially implemented at the global level, none of which have been fully implemented.

For the pan-European region, the ECE environmental indicator D-3 on forests and other forested land shows that efforts to combat deforestation and forest degradation have been successful. This has been accompanied by a relative increase in the area under afforestation. large undisturbed ecosystems, both forest and other types of ecosystems, including wetlands, continue to degrade globally. Trends in ecosystems and habitats in the pan-European region may be similar: in the European Union, only 15% of habitat assessments indicate a satisfactory conservation status and 81% indicate an inadequate or unsatisfactory conservation status.

One of the drivers of ecosystem loss and degradation is the conversion of land from natural to artificial land cover. Over the past 20 years, the intensity of such land conversion has declined in most (but not all) countries in the pan-European region, as also evidenced by ECE indicator E-1 on land conversion.

The risk of extinction is still increasing, although conservation efforts have probably prevented it from rising even more dramatically. Going forward, 24% of species in well-studied taxonomic groups will remain at risk of extinction unless the drivers of this process are drastically reduced. Climate change is putting additional pressure on biodiversity by interacting with existing pressures. Species richness in agricultural landscapes and productive forests continues to decline; agricultural practices are among the main drivers of biodiversity loss at global and pan-European levels. Although European productive forests have become more diverse in terms of tree species composition, recent studies show that overall tree species richness in Europe is increasingly at risk, primarily from invasive species. Similar trends can probably be seen in the case of the pan-European region; the State of Nature in the EU report notes a deterioration in the average conservation status of bird populations. Species associated with agricultural land show a particularly negative trend.The area of protected areas has increased, but there is a need to further improve the effectiveness of their contribution to conservation objectives

Protected areas continue to be a key tool for reducing biodiversity loss. The area of protected areas on land and in the sea has increased significantly in recent years, including in the pan-European region. Marine Protected Area (MPA) data is also supported by the ECE D-1 indicator for terrestrial protected areas, so there remains considerable scope to improve the representativeness, connectivity and management effectiveness of PRs, and to strengthen compliance with existing PR legislation. There is a need for a broader policy response to biodiversity loss that reflects its implications for human well-being and sustainable development Over the past 10 years, efforts to mainstream biodiversity into policy, poverty reduction and development planning in most countries have been largely piecemeal rather than systematic. One positive example is the increasing use of environmental-economic accounting methodologies in some countries. Overall, little progress has been made over the past decade in eliminating, phasing out or reforming subsidies and other potentially biodiversity-damaging incentives, or in developing positive incentives for biodiversity conservation and sustainable use. This is also true for the pan-European region.

Resource mobilisation for biodiversity has improved in only a few countries. Mobilised resources are still insufficient to meet financial needs and continue to be outweighed by financial support for activities harmful to biodiversity. This is also true in the context of forestry, including reforestation. In contrast, in at least some countries there is an improved understanding of financing needs and gaps. The status and trends of biodiversity and ecosystem services are fundamental to human health and well-being and sustainable development. Human encroachment into natural systems and trade in wildlife disrupt the ability of these ecosystems to regulate themselves, increase the frequency of human contact with wildlife and can lead to the spread of infectious diseases.

WHO has organised a global study to elucidate the origin of the SARS-CoV-2172 virus. The theme of the Ninth "Environment for Europe" Ministerial Conference, "Greening the Economy in the Pan-European Region: Working towards Sustainable Infrastructure", responds to the need to mainstream the environment, including biodiversity and ecosystems, in all sectors. This conference theme is directly related to the E-1 indicator (land acquisition), as improving the environmental sustainability of infrastructure development depends in part on reducing its spatial footprint. Tourism activities depend on the state of biodiversity in the areas where they take place, on the one hand, and impact it on the other. By "applying the principles of circular economy to sustainable tourism", the ecological footprint of tourism activities in biodiversity-rich tourism areas is reduced, including pressures from waste generation, eutrophication and over-exploitation of resources. In turn, this enables the provision of cultural ecosystem services and thereby enhances human well-being and development opportunities in these areas. Expanding responsible travel to natural areas in line with ecotourism principles brings together conservation, community and sustainable tourism. Terrestrial protected areas (ECE indicator): overall status from satisfactory to good

The status of data availability for this indicator is very good in the case of EEA member and cooperating countries and satisfactory to good in the case of most other countries, the area of protected areas in the pan-European region has increased significantly over the last 30 years, with a 60 % increase in the last 10 years. The proportion of PRs in the European Union and Western Europe is now well above the Aichi Target 11 target of 17 % coverage, but is lower in other sub-regions. The High Ambition Coalition for Nature and People now sets a larger target of protecting at least 30% of the Earth's land and sea surface by 2030. The extent or effectiveness of biodiversity protection within protected areas, or their overall contribution to reducing global biodiversity loss, depends on the effectiveness of protected area management.

Forests and other wooded land (ECE indicator): overall status from satisfactory to good This indicator measures the total area of forests and other wooded land, its ratio to the total area of countries, the proportion of natural forest area and plantations, the contribution of forests dedicated to production, soil or water conservation and the protection of ecosystem services and biodiversity.

The share of indigenous forests, which tend to be particularly rich in biodiversity, remained stable at a low level of 3 per cent of the total forest area between 2000 and 2020.

At the same time, planted forests have become more important in absolute and relative terms, with their relative share increasing from 5.7 per cent in 1990 to 7.6 per cent in 2020. However, this does not mean that the expansion of planted forests is usually at the expense of indigenous forests; as indicated in the previous paragraph, the total forest area has increased.

Over the past 30 years, forest targeting has been characterised by a diversification from a narrow focus on production in 1990 to a broader range of desired outcomes, including soil, water and biodiversity protection. This diversification of forest designation can be interpreted as a management response to improve the quality of existing forests, including in terms of biodiversity conservation. The area of forests designated for water and soil protection more than doubled from 9.3 per cent to 18.8 per cent, while the area of forests designated for biodiversity conservation doubled from 1.9 per cent to 4.1 per cent.

Land acquisition: overall status from satisfactory to good, this assessment uses a modified version of ECE indicator E-1, based on the European Environment Agency's indicator "Land acquisition in Europe" (i.e. complete conversion of land from natural to non-natural land use categories). This indicator captures only a fraction of all the links that exist between land use change and biodiversity. Although agriculture is considered a natural land use, pressures on biodiversity from habitat loss or degradation are often associated with land conversion to agricultural land use or changes in agricultural practices.

The performance on this indicator is very convincing for EEA member and cooperating countries, while there are some gaps with regard to the completeness and consistency of land acquisition data in other ECE member States.

Net land acquisition has persisted in all subregions, although its rate has been declining. Land acquisition data for European Union accession countries since 2004 show a peak in the period 2006-2012 (0.11 per cent) and a subsequent decline (0.09 per cent in the period 20122023), possibly a consequence of the adoption of European Union policies and standards. The magnitude of land acquisition in other ECE countries decreased significantly between 2012 and 2018. However, this trend indicates considerable variation among EEA countries; there are also countries where the rate of land acquisition continued to increase throughout the period 2000-2018.

The data on land acquisition and conversion to other land use categories that were received from EEA member and co-operating countries are difficult to compare with data from other countries. This is due to differences in methodology between EEA members and co-operating countries on the one hand, and between EEA members and other ECE member States on the other. This incomplete comparability of data from other ECE member States is due, inter alia, to the limited availability of reliable remotely sensed data and consistent criteria for their analysis, the degree of consistency of national monitoring efforts, as well as apparently to changes in land classification in the early 2000s in some member States. This creates the need for further allocation of funds to establish uniform land cover classifications - ideally in line with the Corine land cover system - and to strengthen monitoring capacity, commitments to submit consistent national information to the Common Environmental Information System (CEIS), and a thorough updating of actual land cover categories with historical data in order to obtain reliable information on the trend of land cover in the region. Examples include cultural heritage areas, military training areas and sustainably managed productive forests that provide biodiversity benefits. These areas, which in many countries occupy a large proportion of the land area, have in the past largely remained in the background and attracted only limited resources and efforts to enhance the benefits of their biodiversity. This has begun to change with the adoption of the Strategic Plan for Biodiversity 2010-2030 of the Convention on Biological Diversity and the inclusion of other effective area-based conservation measures in Target 11 of the Aichi Targets; these changes are likely to be further developed in the post-2020 system of global biodiversity actions.

Other effective area-based conservation measures represent a significant but largely untapped opportunity to expand and consolidate area-based conservation networks in the pan-European region. They could make a significant contribution to enhancing overall ecological representativeness, linking existing protected areas and attracting additional actors to help improve biodiversity status.

For the European Union and countries that have signed association or partnership agreements with the European Union and are transposing European Union water legislation into their national legislation, the Water Framework Directive and the Floods Directive could, in principle, lead to the introduction of land and water management practices that fulfil the criteria of other effective conservation measures on a district-by-district basis. National forest categories in many countries in Eurasia, the Caucasus and Central Asia, such as "protective forests" (i.e. forests designed to protect groundwater reserves or to protect against landslides on slopes), also provide significant biodiversity benefits and could be recognised as other effective area-based conservation measures.

States should systematically explore and utilise the process of applying other effective conservation measures on a district-by-district basis to further strengthen their territorial conservation networks.International cooperation to prevent the impact of linear infrastructure on migratory mammals in Central Asia Many of the iconic migratory mammals of the Central Asian steppes, such as saigas, gazelles and kulans, are globally threatened with extinction, partly due to the significant increase in the number of migratory mammals in the Central Asian steppes. This relates directly to the first theme of the Conference, "Greening the economy in the pan-European region: working towards sustainable infrastructure". To reduce and mitigate these pressures, UNECE member States in Central Asia are cooperating through various initiatives under the Convention on the Conservation of Migratory Species of Wild Animals, including the Memorandum of Understanding on the Conservation, Restoration and Sustainable Use of Saiga and the Central Asian Mammal Initiative. These initiatives aim to remove barriers to migration, develop and support regional ecological networks and, 162

ultimately to maintain animal migrations in the region as one of the last global "migration hotspots". ECE Member States in the Central Asian region should continue to cooperate in the management of linear infrastructure facilities, minimising their impact on migratory mammals. F. Land and soil

Land use and land-use change in the pan-European region is still largely driven by agriculture, but the situation varies from country to country. In Eastern Europe and Central Asia, agricultural production is growing and rapidly approaching Soviet levels, while domestic demand has fallen as livestock numbers have declined. Analysis of current land use dynamics shows only a moderate increase in cultivated areas in zones with fertile soil (steppe and forest-steppe) and no signs of agricultural recovery in marginal (forest) zones. At the same time, the utilised area of agricultural land in the European Union is expected to continue to decline smoothly until 2030, albeit at a slower rate than in the previous decade. Land acquisition in the European Union has slowed down but remains a challenge. Between 2000 and 2023, 78 % of land acquisition in the European Union affected agricultural areas, i.e. arable land and pasture, as well as heterogeneous agricultural land. The main drivers of land acquisition and soil compaction in the European Union during this period were industrial and commercial land use, as well as the expansion of residential areas and construction.

Soil organic carbon (SOC) content, the carbon stored in soil organic matter, is the most important characteristic of soil and soil health because of its role in improving soil aeration and water-holding capacity, providing nutrients, maintaining its biodiversity and mitigating climate change. Soils with high carbon content tend to be more productive and better able to filter and purify water. GHGs play a major role in climate change, representing both a threat and an opportunity to help achieve the goals of the Paris Agreement. In Eastern Europe, for example, large-scale land conversion has transformed agricultural land from a source of small amounts of atmospheric CO2 emissions to a major sink of atmospheric CO2. Conservation agriculture practices in the pan-European region can play an important role in sequestering carbon, maintaining or enhancing soil productivity and preserving important soil functions (such as water regulation and biodiversity).

Soil erosion is a consequence of land use dynamics and has different characteristics in different parts of the region. Field

measurements in the European Union countries show that the average soil erosion rate is 0.2-3.2 tonnes ha-1 year-1 per country. In Eastern Europe, the average soil erosion rate has decreased over the last 30 years due to the mass retirement of arable land and climate change. In the Russian Federation, the total volume of washed away soil and erosion rates have decreased by 56.1 % and 15 %, respectively, over the last 30 years due to widespread retirement of arable land and reduced spring runoff. In Central Asia, wind erosion is the predominant type of land degradation, with limited involvement of irrigated and rainfed arable land due to its relatively small area and relatively low erosion rate. In most of the affected areas, further erosion reduction can be achieved through the introduction of conservation agriculture.The European Union, following changes in production, public awareness and consumer behaviour, is paying increasing attention to food safety through the development of local, organic, GMO-free and other certified products, leading to more sustainable agricultural practices. Countries in Eastern Europe and Central Asia see a need to prioritise self-sufficiency in staple foods, which may lead to less sustainable agricultural practices.

Governments in the pan-European region should intensify efforts to provide better guidance to farmers on the use of soil conservation practices in areas with degraded (eroded) soils. Simple models (based on the universal soil loss equation) already exist to allow farmers to explore different options for reducing erosion rates on their plots at an economically acceptable cost; however, these methods cannot be applied on a wider scale or to all soil types and further research and development is required. Policymakers should endeavour to maintain a reasonable balance between the accumulation of ERP to increase crop yields and its retention in the soil to mitigate climate change, as this is crucial for the implementation of global sustainable initiatives such as the 4 per 1000. Pan-European land policies should ensure that land degradation is reduced, while measures to combat soil compaction should be developed and implemented. In addition, governments should focus on ensuring consumers' rights to healthy (i.e. free of pesticides and residues of antibiotics, hormones or steroids) food and a healthy environment (including animal welfare), stable food prices and low household food expenditure. This can be achieved by promoting environmentally sound agricultural practices and a reliable food supply (domestically produced and imported) and, where appropriate, by redirecting investments in storage and transport.

In the face of intense rural exodus, more active measures should be taken to reverse the depopulation trend through income diversification, such as through rural tourism development and attracting new settlers. Recognizing the biodiversity value of low-intensity farmland, the European Union provided agri-environmental subsidies to support farming in marginal areas, but the economic impact of existing European Union programmes to support rural tourism was modest and their results depended on the specific characteristics of the areas. Countries in Europe and Central Asia that are Parties to the United Nations Convention to Combat Desertification (UNCCD) share the ambition to achieve a neutral land degradation balance (NLDB) by 2030. Compensation schemes are a new component of the NBDR approach, meaning that land degradation should be compensated by restoring or rehabilitating degraded land elsewhere. However, the methodology associated with the NBSAP targets is incompletely developed.

Most terrestrial carbon (1,500 Gt) is contained in soils, where it is more than twice the amount contained in vegetation or the atmosphere. The soils of the EEA member countries contain about 5 per cent of the world's soil organic C stocks, while soils in the Russian Federation alone contain about 21 per cent. Increasing the LEU content of soils in the pan-European region could make a positive contribution to mitigating GHG emissions globally, but almost 75 per cent of the Russian Federation is located in the permafrost zone, where LEU stocks could be released with climate warming, thus contributing to increased GHG emissions.

EEA member countries recognise agriculture as a critical factor in maintaining the biodiversity of extensive farmland habitats and early successional habitats such as heathland and grassland. The biodiversity of low intensity farmland may be higher than that of restored, semi-improved and woodland areas, and farmers in these areas are producers of both food and ecosystem services. The abandonment of such areas is therefore perceived in the European Union as a serious threat to biodiversity. Not only the decommissioning of arable land, but also the depopulation (or "devastation") of rural settlements needs to be reversed.

Although the role of soil is multifaceted, including water cycling, nutrient and pollution regulation, and as a habitat, the primary human use of land and soil resources is food production. Soil produces 90% of all food, feed and fibre. There is a shift in production and consumer behaviour in the European Union and Western Europe towards a preference for local, organic, GMO-free and other certified products. The resulting changes in agriculture should be extended to the rest of the pan-European region and to subregions whose food security strategies do not sufficiently emphasise the consumer's right to healthy food. Land and soil degradation is a challenge, including in the pan-European region, and the demand for land is increasing. Land degradation is often caused by a combination of poor land management, unsustainable agricultural practices, pollution and deforestation.

The Soil Strategy 2030, adopted by the European Union, defines an overall framework and concrete measures to protect and restore soils and ensure their sustainable use. It sets out a strategic vision and targets for achieving healthy soils by 2050 and concrete measures for the period up to 2030. The strategy, inter alia, specifies measures relating to soil and the circular economy and proposes the option of safe and sustainable utilisation of dredged soil based on the principles of the closed cycle and limiting land acquisition and soil compaction in circular land use. The restoration and/or remediation of land, including industrial sites and contaminated sites, provides an opportunity for sustainable urban development and reduces pressure on undisturbed land resources.

Healthy soils are essential for food production. In most EEA Member States, information on SSS was derived from field soil surveys conducted by different national or regional agencies, making data comparisons difficult. Estimates of the most complete POC observation network indicate loss of POC in all ecosystem types and land-use classes. The cause of such losses is likely to be accelerated decomposition of organic matter as a result of temperature increases caused by climate change. Support through the European Union's Common Agricultural Policy could slow the process of arable land retirement and rural depopulation in this grouping, but is unlikely to reverse it. In Eastern Europe and Central Asia, some 58 million hectares of arable land have been drastically converted and are unlikely to be fully recovered because of the rapid depopulation of marginal rural areas and the lack of supportive policies like the Common Agricultural Policy in those countries. Numerous field studies show a significant reduction in soil erosion on no-till land; more carbon is also sequestered after no-tillage than after conventional ploughing. However, there is no clear national or regional policy on conservation agriculture. Conservation agriculture in the pan-European region has shown very limited growth compared to other regions of the world (e.g. 2.5 million ha of agricultural land in the European Union is no-tillage). After switching to no-tillage, farmers face a certain shift in the balance: on the one hand, yields are often lower; on the other hand, input costs are also lower due to the limited use of machinery and fertilisers and reduced labour per unit area. Farmers following no-tillage methods often resort to regular applications of high doses of herbicides, although longer-term benefits are possible with certified organic products. Rural tourism can play an important role in revitalising abandoned rural settlements. There is a need to shift the focus of policy makers from arable land abandonment to the 'emptying' of thousands of villages across the pan-European region, as low yields are unlikely to cause people to move out of villages, while intensive rural exodus can certainly lead to land abandonment. With the development of new communication technologies, isolation and lack of employment opportunities are no longer reasons for out-migration from small villages and mountain villages, as the response to the COVID-19 pandemic with the temporary relocation of urban residents to rural areas clearly demonstrated. Analyses of the many existing projects to rehabilitate abandoned villages show that, among the various approaches, rural tourism has the greatest potential for success.

The proportion of degraded land and soil erosion has been identified by the European Parliament as "probably the most serious environmental problem in Europe". Most land degradation studies assess areas in terms of potential erosion risk, as field measurements of actual erosion rates, especially at large scales, are difficult to carry out. At the global level, the UNCCD assessment methodology covers all three supporting indicators: land cover change, land productivity change and carbon stock. UNCCD Parties provide information on the total area of degraded land and the confidence level of the assessment, while the International Fund for Conservation of Nature provides full coverage using remotely sensed data.

Organic carbon content in topsoil, the Soil Protection Framework Directive provided for the identification of areas in Europe threatened by a decline in soil organic matter below a certain critical level and the development of appropriate measures to prevent such a decline. "Critical" POC concentration of 2 per cent (or 3.4 per cent of soil organic matter according to the standard conversion factor) is the most frequently mentioned threshold in policy documents. The European Commission's Roadmap for Resource Efficiency in Europe has proposed a target of preventing the decline of POC levels in general and increasing them by 2030 for those soils that currently contain less than 2 % POC 190. Recent scientific publications have emphasised the importance of the clay fraction of soil organic matter rather than the strict requirement of 2% POC concentrations.

Arable land area, the exact threshold level of change in agricultural land area has not been defined, although any reduction in area is by default seen as a negative factor in terms of food security. Over the past decade, the long-term trend of decreasing arable land area in the European Union has continued, albeit at a slower rate. A positive trend has emerged in recent years. However, a reversal of this positive trend is possible in the coming decade. It is interesting to note that in Eastern Europe and Central Asia, current land use dynamics also showed some increase in cropped area, especially in the fertile areas of Kazakhstan, the Russian Federation and Ukraine. Portuguese "montado" and Spanish "dehesa": the survival of agriculture on marginal lands The Common Agricultural Policy supports agriculture on marginal lands through agri-environmental subsidies under the second pillar of work on rural development. About 4% of European Union subsidies are directed to "less favourable for farming" areas that are assumed to have high levels of biodiversity 195. Some experts challenge this policy, expressing the wish that subsidies for the development of marginal land should not be linked to agricultural activities. Nevertheless, there are several positive examples where farming on marginal lands has both environmental and economic benefits. Two of the best examples are the Portuguese "montado" and the Spanish "dehesa" farms

These agroforestry systems are dominated by cork oak and sharp-leaved oak, which produce cork as a forestry product and acorns for livestock, respectively. Between the trees, farmers establish pastures and sow cereal crops. The biodiversity of these
168
systems are very high, and they have retained many of the main characteristics of the original vegetation. In addition, because of this multifunctionality and large spatial scale of operations, many of these farms are economically viable.

G. Chemicals and waste

Chemicals and waste management is at the heart of addressing many of the current challenges faced in the transition to a carbon-free and sustainable economy. Often there is either a lack of capacity in the pan-European region to make informed decisions on chemicals and waste issues, or insufficient integration of expertise into decision-making processes.

Government policymakers, industry and the public do not have easy access to information and knowledge that can help make results-oriented choices.

Chemicals play a vital role in today's economy and are essential to paving the way towards a green economy. Yet it remains difficult to fully identify the range of human exposure to hazardous chemicals. No set of exposure-focused indicators are regularly monitored in the region. In addition, there is a lack of information on the impact of chemicals on the effectiveness and economic viability of circular economy models such as recycling.Despite waste management hierarchy placing the greatest emphasis on waste prevention, the amount of waste generated continues to grow across the region. Waste generation is increasing even where there is strong political commitment to the principles of the circular economy, such as in the European Union and other Western European countries.

A particular problem is waste electrical and electronic equipment (or e-waste), which contains both hazardous and valuable components. The average e-waste generation rate is stabilising in the region as a whole, but continues to increase rapidly in economically less developed subregions. Collection and recycling rates of e-waste are extremely low in all subregions; recovery rates are also low. This misses an important opportunity to realise economic benefits for the region and reduce its dependence on the supply of vital raw materials, which is a bottleneck in the transition to a sustainable future economy.

Recycling rates vary significantly between countries in the region and are particularly low in Eastern Europe and Central Asia. Only a few countries in the European Union and Switzerland have recycling rates above 45 per cent for municipal waste. The situation was improving in all subregions, but slowly, efforts should be intensified to staff public administrations with qualified personnel willing to interact with all sectors of society and to continue to improve access to reliable and detailed information to ensure sound chemicals and waste management. Chemicals and waste management must be better adapted to the challenges of today and the requirements of the coming transition period by optimising the balance of risks and opportunities.

Governments should endeavour to further promote the comprehensive and harmonised implementation of multilateral environmental agreements (MEAs), including the Protocol on Pollutant Release and Transfer Registers to the Convention on Access to Information, Public Participation in Decision-making and Access to Justice in Environmental Matters (Aarhus Convention). In order to develop a more comprehensive picture of the adverse effects of chemicals on human health and the environment and to work towards addressing this issue, Governments should endeavour to establish a results-oriented and gender-sensitive region-wide monitoring scheme as a form of scientific and policy cooperation, should work towards the establishment of a mechanism involving all countries and sectors and aimed at identifying reference models and best practices, and should work towards the establishment of a regional monitoring scheme. Knowledge sharing will enable decision makers at all levels to realise the potential benefits of existing best practices, a resource-oriented pan-European e-waste partnership should be established with the objectives of efficient collection and management of recyclable materials to ensure recovery of valuable resources. The recovery of secondary resources from e-waste is an urgent priority, especially given the rapidly increasing amount of e-waste in Eastern Europe, South-Eastern Europe and Central Asia.

In order to reduce waste, Governments should support efforts to prevent waste generation and to manage minor and major repairs and remediation, including through the use of financial incentives such as tax breaks. These waste prevention efforts will improve resource efficiency. In addition, Governments in the pan-European region should adopt an approach leading to a "recycling" - or resource-efficient - economy and strengthen the management of raw materials, including, for example, through the application of the Resource Classification Framework and the United Nations Resource Management System.

Chemical use and waste generation are closely linked to living standards and economic prosperity. It is estimated that between 40,000 and 60,000 industrial chemicals are traded globally and are used, inter alia, in agriculture, health care and the production of goods such as electronics, textiles, furniture and toys. Chemicals also have an important role to play in the transition to a green economy, as they are components of resource-efficient technologies and products. However, some chemicals are hazardous to the environment and human health. Chemicals in air, water and soil can affect individual species, alter biodiversity and undermine the resilience of ecosystems. Harmful exposure to chemicals can adversely affect human health through a wide range of effects, including disruption of the immune, endocrine and reproductive systems, genetic effects and the development of chronic diseases such as cancer, cardiovascular disease and asthma.

The accumulation of large volumes of waste is associated with the inefficient use of resources in unsustainable consumption and production practices in modern society. Some wastes have hazardous properties and their proper management is an essential element in reducing chemical pollution. Other waste streams waste materials and energy and add to environmental pressures, such as microplastics entering the food chain, with detrimental effects on biodiversity and human health. At the same time, sound and value-based solid waste management can make a significant contribution to climate change mitigation, potentially eliminating 15 to 20 per cent of GHG emissions globally.

The challenge facing the pan-European region is twofold: to protect the ecosystem services available to current and future human society, and to address the link between environmental degradation and economic prosperity. Meeting these challenges requires the adoption of more sustainable consumption and production patterns, as well as the sound management of chemicals and waste as an integral component of the transition to a green economy. Risks and opportunities need to be well understood and responded to with effective measures.

The production capacity of the global chemical industry was 2.3 billion tonnes, making the chemical industry the second most economically important manufacturing industry in the world. Trade in chemicals is expected to increase significantly in the future; the number of new chemicals is also increasing. Of the 345 million tonnes of chemicals consumed in the European Union in 2016, 62% were in categories classified as 171
hazardous to human health and 35 per cent as hazardous to the environment. In the latest European Environment Report: State of the Environment and Future Outlook, the potential combined effects of different chemicals were identified as a particular concern. A complete picture of the exposure and impact of hazardous chemicals on the environment and human health is difficult to obtain because of the complexity of the field, the large number and diversity of chemicals used, and the lack of a

common set of result-oriented indicators that are regularly monitored in the region. Methodologies for such risk assessment are still rather fragmented. The knowledge base for the European Union is extensive but still fragmented, while for other regions it is very limited.

The use and handling of chemicals is the subject of a whole body of legislation. The European Union has the most stringent regulations, with some 40 pieces of legislation in force. These include the European Union Regulation on Rules for the Registration, Evaluation, Authorisation and Restriction of Chemicals, which defines the main characteristics of listed chemicals. The European Union Sustainable Development Strategy for Chemicals was launched in October 2020 with the goal of a toxic-free environment; it aims to phase out the most harmful substances in consumer products and financially support the introduction of safe and sustainable chemicals. The Globally Harmonised System of Hazard Classification and Labelling of Chemicals sets standards for hazard classification, labelling and the development of Material Safety Data Sheets in all countries; its adoption has taken much longer than anticipated, but the region is now on track. In addition, the policy response to issues of particular concern, including lead in paint, has been facilitated by the Strategic Approach to International Chemicals Management developed by UNEP, which, together with the Responsible Care Programme of the chemical industry, has also contributed to capacity-building. The mandate of the Strategic Approach to International Chemicals Management having expired, planning for the post-2020 process provides an opportunity to further strengthen multilateral cooperation and disseminate systems to ensure that stakeholders have access to appropriate data and knowledge for decision-making, as well as adequate capacity at the implementation stage.

Several MEAs regulate the handling of substances of significant concern to human health and the environment. These instruments provide a solid framework, but the full range of benefits can only be realised if they are universally ratified across the region, which is not yet the case. Eight of the 54 countries in the pan-European region are not parties to the Rotterdam Convention on the Prior Informed Consent Procedure for Certain Hazardous Chemicals and Pesticides in International Trade. Only 37 countries in the region are parties to the Protocol on Pollutant Release and Transfer Registers.

With regard to waste management, significant differences remain between Western Europe and other subregions. A common problem is the continued increase in total waste generation in most countries, even though waste prevention is given the highest priority in the waste management hierarchy. The European Union and European Free Trade Agreement countries have national waste prevention programmes that often focus on promoting reuse and repair, but few programmes directly support market-based reuse options, such as recovery or production from recycled materials. The European Union Waste Management Regulations establish a fairly solid framework for the collection, valorisation or sound management of waste. Average recycling rates for municipal solid waste in the European Union have increased steadily over the last 10 years, and a new Closed Loop Economy Action Plan, part of the European Green Deal, has been in place since March 2020. Countries that have joined the European Union have shown remarkable progress in waste management, which demonstrates the effectiveness of its regulations. Countries in Eastern Europe, South-Eastern Europe and Central Asia have made some progress in municipal solid waste valorisation; however, overall recycling rates remain relatively low and change is slow. This suggests that circular economy models are not yet effectively operating in these subregions. However, some countries have initiated major waste management reforms, including the setting of recycling targets for municipal solid waste (e.g. Russian Federation, Uzbekistan).

The rapidly growing volumes of e-waste in Central Asia, Eastern Europe and South-Eastern Europe pose a particular challenge. In the European Union and Western Europe, the amount of e-waste is stabilising but at astonishingly high levels, with e-waste generation more than double the global average of 7.3 kg per capita. Of particular concern is the low collection rate of e-waste, even though collection is a prerequisite for valorisation. Even in the European Union, where advanced schemes are in place, less than 45% of the estimated e-waste generation was collected in 2023.

Closed-loop economy-oriented initiatives have also emerged in the region as a result of civil society or private sector efforts. Repair initiatives, sharing measures and recycling production schemes are just a few examples of new business models, sharing models and alternative production systems. They show that all sectors of society have begun to respond to the need for better resource management and waste prevention.

The introduction of circular economy models represents a valuable opportunity to ensure the future prosperity of the region. One promising element to support sustainable consumption is the introduction of a right to repair. In addition, urgent action is needed to end premature obsolescence schemes. Two models of the circular economy that have reached industrial scale are production from recycled raw materials and industrial symbiosis. Independent and transparent sustainability assessments are also important. International expert groups can help countries analyse their future needs for specific resources and how to meet them. "Green camouflage" that misleads consumers and exploits their environmental concerns can have serious detrimental effects and is unacceptable. Countries that wisely make the "green transition" today will enjoy a competitive advantage decades from now. Compliance with multilateral environmental agreements on hazardous wastes and other chemicals (Sustainable Development Goal indicator 12.4.1)

This indicator measures progress made in the sound management of chemicals and hazardous wastes in accordance with the provisions of the Rotterdam Convention on the Prior Informed Consent Procedure for Certain Hazardous Chemicals and Pesticides in International Trade, the Basel Convention on the Control of

Transboundary Movements of Hazardous Wastes and their Disposal, the Stockholm Convention on Persistent Organic Pollutants and the Montreal Protocol on Substances that Deplete the Ozone Layer. Compliance with reporting obligations under MEAs is monitored on five-year cycles (annual monitoring is not possible because MEAs provide for different reporting deadlines). While the region performs well with respect to the Montreal Protocol, the Stockholm Convention underperforms: all subregions, with the exception of South-Eastern Europe, perform worse than in the previous period, with an average compliance rate of less than 60 per cent. In the case of the Basel and Rotterdam Conventions, the average compliance rate in the region is 70-80 per cent; the European Union and South-Eastern Europe perform better than the other subregions. Other possible indicators include the implementation of pollutant release and transfer registers (or participation in the ECE Protocol on Pollutant Release and Transfer Registers) and adherence to the Globally Harmonised System of Classification and Labelling of Chemicals. Total waste generation per capita, this indicator characterises the total amount of waste (hazardous and non-hazardous) generated in a country per year in all sectors. Waste generation is an ECE environmental indicator; the final review report on the establishment of SENS showed good progress and is therefore a reliable indicator. The average waste generation per capita in the region increased by 31 per cent between 2012 and 2018 (see figure 35) and by 7 per cent if major inorganic waste is excluded. Most countries have seen an increase in waste generation. There are significant differences between countries; these can partly be explained by the fact that some countries are dominated by certain sectors of the economy. In Estonia, for example, a large proportion of waste is generated by the oil shale industry, which is a unique situation in the region. The large aggregate amount of waste in Eastern Europe and Central Asia is largely due to the amount of mining waste. Despite progress in reporting, it is not possible to calculate waste less major inorganic waste for all countries. Despite commitments by countries to promote waste prevention, total waste generation is increasing in the pan-European region and in all its subregions. Additional efforts are required. Benchmarks are needed to assess the amount of waste that can be prevented in different sectors. Economic instruments such as "landfill taxes" (on materials sent to landfill), collateral-refund systems, tax rebates or other fiscal incentives for innovative enterprises and extended producer responsibility should be urgently explored to incentivise waste prevention. E-waste generation per capita, e-waste contains both hazardous components and valuable resources such as vital raw materials. In the pan-European region, on average, around 15 kg of e-waste per capita per year population is consistently generated, with different trends across sub-regions.

This is mainly because volumes are stabilising or slightly decreasing in the European Union and Western Europe, while in Central Asia and Eastern and South-Eastern Europe they continue to grow rapidly. The level of e-waste generation in the region is significantly higher than the world average, with

Western European countries generating on average more than three times as much e-waste per capita as Central Asia. A precondition for the high-value valorisation of this material flow is separate collection. Nevertheless, even in European Union and Western European countries with collection and recycling infrastructure, significant amounts of e-waste are not included in formal collection and valorisation schemes. Recycling rates for municipal solid waste, there are significant differences in recycling rates for municipal solid waste between subregions, but some progress is being made across all subregions. In some countries of the European Union, recycling rates are the highest in the world. The average recycling rate for the European Union increased from 37.3 per cent in 2009 to 47.7 per cent in 2023. In five European Union countries, the recycling rate for municipal solid waste is still below 25 per cent. The most pronounced improvements are in Eastern Europe, South-Eastern Europe and Central Asia, where municipal solid waste recycling rates are below 25 per cent; actual rates are generally well below 25 per cent or even close to zero. A few positive examples stand out, notably Uzbekistan, where the municipal solid waste recycling rate is currently around 20 per cent (see case study below). Overall, the trend in the region is towards increased recycling and hence a circular economy, but progress is slow. Accelerating the transition requires strong commitment from policy makers, coupled with the allocation of adequate financial resources and a willingness to adopt successful schemes.

Reforming the waste management system Uzbekistan has initiated large-scale reforms of the environmental policy framework, including the introduction of new institutional structures for waste management and the introduction of a strategy for municipal solid waste management for 20192030. The coverage of the population with waste management services has increased from 22 per cent in 2016 to 53 per cent in 2023. The government has set a target of 100 per cent waste collection coverage by 2025; the strategy also aims to achieve recycling rates for municipal solid waste of 45 per cent by 2025 and 60 per cent by 2028. The country is on the right track; in 2019, the municipal solid waste recycling rate is close to 20 per cent compared to 9 per cent in 2017.

Recent studies have revealed the content of more than 6,000 different additives in plastic products. Only some of them polymerise in the plastic matrix, while many others can leach out and potentially impact the environment and humans. When plastics are processed, individual chemicals or mixtures of substances can inadvertently enter new products as contaminants, creating new risks in value chains. Such cross-contamination has been identified, for example, in children's toys and food contact products.

H. Environmental financing and public spending on environmental protectionDespite the negative environmental impacts of fossil fuels, all countries continue to subsidise fossil fuel extraction to varying degrees. International Monetary Fund (IMF) projections suggest that these subsidies will continue until at least 2025, with indirect subsidies increasing until then, and environmental tax revenues increasing in all countries in the pan-European region.

In 2023, European Union environmental tax revenues totalled €330.6 billion, up 52 per cent in nominal terms from 2002. In all countries in the pan-European region for which data are available, public expenditure on the environment has increased since 2000, closely following the growth in gross domestic product (GDP).

The last five years have seen an increase in the use of green bonds as a tool for financing environmentally friendly projects. These bonds are used by both the private sector and national governments. In the pan-European region, the European Union countries are the leaders in the use of green bonds, while countries in other regions have also started to use such instruments. There is a severe lack of quantitative data for Central Asia and South-Eastern Europe. This complicates attempts to assess progress in environmental protection and environmental financing. The lack of reliable data also means that it is impossible to reliably calculate the investment and operating costs of achieving environmental goals and to use these data in policy development.National environmental policies in the pan-European region should aim to eliminate harmful subsidies and rapidly shift to more environmentally friendly energy sources.

Environmental taxes are one of the most effective instruments for incentivising economic actors to reduce various types of pollution and protect the environment. Compared to green subsidies, which provide the same incentives, they have the added advantage of allowing governments to generate revenues that can be used to reduce the

market-distorting taxes within the economy and/or financing of public environmental expenditures. Countries are encouraged to increase the use of these or equivalent instruments, such as quota trading mechanisms. Future public environmental expenditure should be seen in the broader context of environmental and public finance. Subsidies always distort markets and increase public sector spending. The need for subsidised environmental finance should therefore be periodically reviewed in the light of the polluter pays principle.

In addition, it is important to conduct regular impact assessment analyses to better target subsidies so that they deliver real benefits where and when they are needed.Governments in the pan-European region should promote green finance, in particular the green bond market, through a range of policy measures, including demonstration bond issuance, dissemination of clear green bond guidelines, and favourable regulatory policies In Central Asia and South-Eastern Europe, there is an urgent need to improve data collection systems in line with internationally recognised standards, such as those of OECD and Eurostat. For example, data collection on environmental expenditures should follow internationally recognised methodologies and classifications. In particular, it is important to specify and report data on which organisations spend money on environmental protection, how much, for what purposes and who finances these expenditures. To achieve the goals of the

Paris Agreement and protect the environment while ensuring an adequate quality of life for their citizens, countries need a major environmental and energy transition. At the global level, the OECD estimates that between 2016 and 2030, $95 trillion in public and private energy investments will be needed to support growth and sustainable development. At the global level, the OECD estimates that between 2016 and 2030, $95 trillion of public and private investment in energy, transport, water and telecommunications infrastructure will be needed to support growth and sustainable development, or about $6.3 trillion per year. This would be about $6.3 trillion per year. According to the same source, making these investments climate compatible would require an additional US$ 0.6 trillion per year - and this is a small additional US$ 0.6 trillion per year. This is a small incremental cost compared to the expected benefits. The European Union's Green Deal plans to invest a total of €1 trillion until 2030, or about €125 billion per year.

Governments must provide leadership for these necessary transformations by pursuing policies that reconcile private interests with the common good. Public spending alone will not be sufficient. Sound environmental, fiscal and investment policies are therefore essential to maximise the impact of public spending and attract private investment. The pan-European region comprises countries with widely differing political, economic and social conditions. However, all countries should share the goals of environmental protection and climate change mitigation. In particular, it is important to establish the right fundamental environmental policies to align incentives across the region. There is also an urgent need to accelerate the review of inefficient fossil fuel subsidies and broaden the basis for carbon tariffs, with a focus on tracking the impact of implemented policies and sharing policy experiences.

At the global level, the achievement of environmental protection and climate change mitigation goals is still a long way off; the recently released UNEP report "Measuring Progress: Environment and the SDGs" indicates that negative trends persist on a number of indicators. The pan-European region is no exception. For example, despite the European Union being a leading region in the environmental field, key targets of its Seventh Environmental Action Programme are currently unachievable. At the national level, environmental targets are often not met: for example, even in environmentally advanced Sweden, 15 of the 16 national environmental quality targets set by Parliament to be achieved by 2030 have not yet been met.

These observations emphasise the need for countries in the pan-European region to further strengthen their environmental policies and increase investments in environmental protection and climate change mitigation. Environmental financing instruments should be fully utilised.

In line with these objectives, public spending on the environment and revenues from environmental levies have increased in the region since the early 2000s. Similarly, green finance and green bonds have become increasingly common, with the European Union leading the way. However, fossil fuel subsidies are still in place and are projected to continue until at least 2025. Environmental tax revenues, the environmental tax revenues used in this assessment (from the IMF's climate change indicators and the Eurostat database) should be considered as the lower boundary of the assessment, as they do not include environmental fees and charges; however, they do include taxes on energy, transport and pollution.

In the European Union, on average, revenues from environmental taxes have remained at around 2.2-2.5 per cent of GDP since 2000. Nevertheless, there are clear contrasts between individual countries within the association. For example, since 2015, Croatia's environmental tax revenue has exceeded 3.4 % of GDP, while in Germany, Ireland and Luxembourg such revenue is less than 2 % of GDP. In Western Europe234 , environmental tax revenues averaged 2.5-3 % of GDP between 2000 and 2007, subsequently stabilising at around 2 % of GDP. Analysing the total revenues received shows that in Iceland, Norway and the United Kingdom, revenues fell sharply between 2007 and 2008, undoubtedly due to the financial crisis. Data for Switzerland are only available from 2008 and show that since that year, revenues from the environmental tax have been around 1.4 per cent of the country's GDP.

Data on environmental tax revenues for most of the period 20002019 are available for two other countries, Serbia and Turkey. In Turkey, revenues from the environmental tax increased sharply between 2000 and 2003, rising from 2.4 per cent to about 4 per cent of GDP. They stabilised at around 3.5 % of GDP in the subsequent period, before falling to around 2.3 % of GDP in 2018 and 2.2 % of GDP in 2019 (thus amounting to around €15.5 million in both years).

On the other hand, the amount of environmental taxes collected in Serbia has been steadily increasing. Between 2005 and 2018, these revenues increased from €631 million to €1,791 million, i.e. by 184 per cent . In these two countries, the share of environmental tax revenues in GDP is higher than in both the European Union and Western Europe. As noted above in the main findings, there is a lack of data for most countries outside Western Europe.

Public expenditure on the environment includes public expenditure on biodiversity and landscape protection, environmental research and development, pollution control, and waste and wastewater management. This figure represents the minimum amount spent annually in the countries of the pan-European region, as only public expenditure is taken into account. Total environmental expenditure is therefore likely to be higher, as the private sector also contributes to environmental protection. In the European Union, for example, in 2020, governments spent €70 billion on environmental protection, corporations spent almost €157 billion (i.e. more than twice as much as governments) and households spent about €60 billion236. However, for most non-European Union and Western European countries, data on total (i.e. public and private) environmental expenditure are unfortunately not available. European Union countries spend on average the equivalent of 0.8 per cent of GDP on environmental protection. This is the highest share in the pan-European region, followed by Western Europe. In all other countries, the share of public environmental expenditure in GDP is smaller Eastern European countries subsidise fossil fuels at higher rates than countries in other regions. This result is mainly due to the significant amount of subsidies provided by the Russian Federation, which totalled more than €520 billion in 2019, i.e. around 35% of the country's GDP.

The high level of fossil fuel subsidies can be explained mainly by two factors:

First, countries whose economies are partly dependent on fossil fuel production have economic incentives to subsidise them. For example, the three countries with the highest share of fossil fuel rents in 2023 according to the World Bank - namely Azerbaijan (25 per cent of GDP), Kazakhstan (29 per cent of GDP) and the Russian Federation (35 per cent of GDP) - are also among the countries that heavily subsidise fossil fuels in relation to their GDP - 33.4 per cent, 29.4 per cent and 35.2 per cent, respectively.

Second, direct fossil fuel subsidies are typically implemented as a poverty alleviation measure to reduce the burden of transport and energy costs on poor households, and are therefore more common in poor countries. Capital mobilisation through green bondsGreen bonds were created to finance projects with environmental and/or climate benefits and can be issued by sovereign governments, regional and local governments, and private sector entities. Proceeds from the issuance of these bonds are used for green projects, but are secured by all assets of the issuer. The green bond market has seen exponential growth since its inception around 2007, with aggregate issuance reaching a symbolic threshold of $1 trillion in December 2023. US$1 TRILLION. Certified green bonds have been shown to be effective in reducing GHG emissions in the private sector. While how such bonds can be utilised by governments requires further study, it is important to monitor the dynamics of green finance in general, and in particular the dynamics of green bonds. In addition, the availability of green and climate finance may influence the optimal level of more traditional policy instruments, such as carbon taxes. The European Union countries are leaders in the green bond market.

Croatia's environmental policy is largely driven by its accession to the European Union. While some indicators suggest that the country is making considerable efforts to ensure environmental protection and green growth, there is still room for improvement. In particular, Croatia can reduce the existing diesel cost differential (e.g., by raising taxes on diesel to the level of taxes on other fuels) and increase absorptive capacity. One institution that plays a key role in environmental financing is the Environmental Protection and Energy Efficiency Fund. It acts as a hub for collecting environmental fees and charges and managing programmes and projects that promote environmental protection, energy efficiency and renewable energy. Funds for such projects come from foreign foundations, international organisations, financial institutions and bodies and national and foreign entities. In particular, within the framework of the European Union, a total of €10.7 billion has been allocated to Croatia from European structural and investment funds. In addition, within the framework of the social cohesion policy, the country has received funding in the amount of EUR 8.6 billion for the entire period 2014-2020. Some of these funds are earmarked for environmental protection and energy efficiency.

However, when it comes to the use of European Union funds, the authors of a recent report by the S-GI Network point to difficulties in absorbing the funds. According to the National Strategic Framework Programme, which governs the use of European Structural Funds and the Cohesion Fund, Croatia must spend almost €10 billion by 2023 on waste management, water management and air protection - the three most important environmental issues in the European Union accession negotiations. Nevertheless, SG&A Network notes difficulties during policy implementation, mainly due to the inconsistent Public Procurement Act. The uncertainty caused by the interpretation of the law is presented as the main problem affecting the absorption of European Structural and Investment Funds in Croatia. According to the European Commission, Croatia is still among the five countries with the lowest disbursement rates.

Croatia has one of the highest environmental tax revenues as a percentage of GDP in the European Union. In 2019, environmental taxes amounted to about 3.5 per cent of GDP, compared to the European Union average of about 2.35 per cent. According to the latest assessment by the European Commission, Croatia provides a number of examples of sound fiscal measures to protect the environment. For example, the country levies a "forest public function levy", which is paid annually by companies and other commercial and industrial organisations. In addition to funding reforestation work in karst areas, part of the levy is spent on demining (10 per cent), firefighting (5 per cent) and scientific work (5 per cent). However, as in all other countries in the pan-European region, fossil fuels are still subsidised. such subsidies amounted to USD 1.3 billion. THESE SUBSIDIES AMOUNTED TO US$ 1.3 BILLION. In addition, the country has not yet fully eliminated the "diesel differential" - the difference between diesel and petrol prices - which represents an indirect subsidy for diesel.

Turkey's ecological environment is under pressure due to population growth, industrialisation and rapid urbanisation. These pressures have resulted in a range of environmental problems such as desertification, deforestation, water scarcity, degradation of nature and marine pollution. To address these problems, the country has adopted new laws and institutional practices as part of its efforts to comply with European Union environmental standards.

Turkey has a relatively high share of environmental taxes as a percentage of GDP (3.4 per cent on average over the period 2002-2017, a figure that has fallen slightly since then), mainly due to high taxes on petrol and diesel. However, transport taxes, while creating some green incentives, tend to push less affluent consumers towards older, more polluting cars245. A review of transport tax schemes would therefore be advisable. Although the country is still heavily dependent on fossil fuels, the share of renewable energy in the country's energy mix is increasing, mainly due to the government's green tariffs. Eurostat data allow for a more detailed analysis of environmental expenditures, showing a very high level of private sector activity, spending 50-100% more than the government on environmental protection.Make greater use of instruments to encourage private sector investment in environmental projects, including public-private partnerships, green banks and green bonds.With regard to fossil fuel subsidies, the bulk of harmful subsidies are tax breaks on petroleum products and heating subsidies These should be phased out and replaced with support measures to move towards greener alternatives.

Case study: carbon pricing post-pandemic affected all countries and caused economic crisis in many of them. However, despite the undoubtedly negative effects of the pandemic, this presents an interesting opportunity to use policy instruments to support economic recovery consistent with environmental objectives. As governments focus on stimulating and stabilising economies, the design of such recovery packages will play a crucial role in the planet's climate and economic future. Along with other measures, a carbon price can play a role in supporting sustainable economic recovery primarily through three mechanisms, namely supporting green industries, encouraging investment and raising incomes.

First, carbon pricing helps to support sustainable industries and the competitiveness of low-carbon products, which can provide opportunities for additional green jobs in line with many of the targets in the Sustainable Development Goals. Second, a carbon price can incentivise investment in and revenue mobilisation for low-carbon, carbon-neutral and carbon-negative technologies.

Third, carbon pricing could provide much-needed revenue for governments to support additional stimulus programmes and investments. So far, however, a significant proportion of stimulus spending has not been channelled into green recovery. Low-carbon or green projects receive only a small proportion of the allocation for economic recovery. For example, the Green Stimulus Index shows that only 12 per cent of the nearly $15 trillion in stimulus spending by the G20 countries is going to low-carbon or green projects. However, the time has come to rethink post COVID recovery policies to maximise their environmental benefits.

Measures that should enable this to happen include:

- bailout programmes for shabby corporations to include green terms;
- loans and subsidies for green investments;
- subsidies for green research and development.

## CHAPTER 5

**5 Green Infrastructure Systems, Sustainability health saving life cycle.**

Sustainable infrastructure systems (sometimes referred to as green infrastructure) are systems that are planned, designed, constructed, managed and decommissioned in a way that ensures economic and financial, social, environmental (including climate change resilience) and institutional sustainability throughout the life cycle of the infrastructure. Sustainable infrastructure can include built infrastructure, natural infrastructure, or hybrid infrastructure containing elements of both. This will not only help to improve service quality, but also to create modern information systems across the pan-European region.Resilience to climate change, preservation of ecosystem services, environmental restoration and biodiversity protection are key factors in planning future infrastructure projects. Achieving these goals while providing urgently needed infrastructure services will require the implementation of nature-based solutions. Material efficiency and the circular economy are at the heart of a sound sustainable consumption and production strategy. New technological advances in resource efficiency, recycling and reuse (including through increased modularity of infrastructure project components) should be considered as key elements in the planning, design, construction and operation of infrastructure projects. A. Greening the economy in the pan-European region: working towards sustainable infrastructure

Sustainability should be mainstreamed as early as possible in the strategic planning phase. While sustainability should be addressed throughout the life cycle of a project, the earlier it is taken into account, the more benefits it can bring. If policy makers start to consider sustainability as early as possible, they can create the right policy, regulatory and institutional environment to better integrate sustainability in later phases. As project timelines approach, the opportunity to make effective political, technical or economic changes diminishes. However, decision-making processes remain fragmented, reducing opportunities to identify synergies at the national and sectoral levels and linkages between infrastructure sectors. To achieve more sustainable infrastructure outcomes, this fragmented approach needs to be abandoned.

Investments in sustainable infrastructure are recognised as one of the strategies with the greatest impact on a better recovery from the COVID-19 pandemic; this is due to their critical role in creating jobs and short-term economic growth and long-term development in line with global commitments to sustainable development, such as the Sustainable Development Goals and the Paris Agreement. The lack of structures to prepare economically sound sustainable infrastructure investment projects, as well as technical and institutional capacity to plan and prepare sustainable infrastructure projects, and the urgent need to stimulate economic development and job creation around the world, is pushing decision-makers towards "business as usual" projects. Infrastructure needs are now variable and changing faster than ever before. Thus, sustainable infrastructure must be flexible, interconnected, and rely on real-time information to adapt to changing conditions. To have real-time data, citizens in general, and especially users of infrastructure systems, must play an active role in the process of data collection (using various technologies and mobile apps in particular) and periodic reporting of satisfaction Sustainable infrastructure systems (which are sometimes referred to as "green infrastructure") are systems that are planned, designed, built, managed and decommissioned in a way that provides economic and financial, socially Sustainable infrastructure can include built infrastructure, natural infrastructure or hybrid infrastructure containing elements of both. This will not only help to improve service quality, but also to create modern information systems across the pan-European region.Resilience to climate change, preservation of ecosystem services, environmental restoration and biodiversity protection are key factors in planning future infrastructure projects. Achieving these goals while providing urgently needed infrastructure services will require the implementation of nature-based solutions.Material efficiency and the circular economy are at the heart of a sound sustainable consumption and production strategy. New technological advances in resource efficiency, recycling and reuse (including through increased modularity of infrastructure project components) should be considered as key elements in the planning, design, construction and operation of infrastructure projects. Sustainable infrastructure must be environmentally responsible, socially inclusive and economically viable. It is important to ensure that the needs of all stakeholders have been identified and addressed. The multifaceted nature of sustainable infrastructure is addressed in the UN Environment Assembly resolution on green and sustainable infrastructure, which also mentions some of the previously noted elements (including the importance of the circular economy, infrastructure sustainability, environmental protection and nature-based solutions). A common definition of sustainable infrastructure should be developed in the pan-European region, this will enable reporting and quantification of progress across countries and sub-regions. Significant data gaps have been identified both in the proposed social, environmental, institutional, economic and financial indicators and in quantifying the contribution (positive or negative) of infrastructure development and the achievement of the indicators proposed in this assessment, existing tools to promote sustainable infrastructure development, including the ECE Protocol on Strategic Environmental Assessment, should be utilised and an integrated and full life-cycle approach should be ensured, with a A life-cycle approach should help align short-term and long-term goals; for example, investments in traditional carbon-intensive energy sources may meet short-term needs but lock in unsustainable development patterns and prevent countries from achieving the goals of the Paris Agreement and the Sustainable Development Goals, closing an already small window of opportunity to achieve a sustainable future.

Significant capacity gaps remain, preventing the large-scale deployment of sustainable infrastructure. Additional resources should be directed towards providing the institutional and technical capacity needed to plan, design, execute, operate and decommission sustainable infrastructure projects. Developing a common understanding of what "sustainable infrastructure" means and defining a common strategy for quantifying progress across countries can help fill these capacity gaps. ROPFs can be used to complement, replace or maintain traditional grey infrastructure, thereby contributing to closing the gap in infrastructure access, quality and sustainability in climate resilience. ROPFs can thus play an important role in enhancing climate resilience and ensuring the provision of sustainable infrastructure services. There is a wealth of research and other material on the potential and opportunities for ROPFs to improve community resilience; however, in some cases, lack of demand and incentives have hindered their realisation. In the short to medium term, governments in the region should utilise economic and financial incentives to support the implementation of ROPFs. Special incentives and capacity development will be required to catalyse and implement circular economy strategies at the regional and national levels. These incentives should be consistent with the work already done in relation to the European Union Taxonomy and the Pan-European Green Economy Strategic Framework on sustainable consumption and production patterns, as well as the coherent definition of nature-based solutions. To ensure that the needs of all stakeholders are identified and met, it is essential that environmental and social impact assessments are carried out. These assessments should include, among other things, a gender analysis that recognises the specific needs of women. This will facilitate the integration of gender perspectives into the planning, design, construction and operation of infrastructure. For decades, infrastructure development has been considered the foundation of economic growth and development. However, in recent years, the world has realised that the potential benefits of infrastructure development do not always materialise. Environmental degradation, loss of biodiversity, social displacement and increased GHG emissions are some of the unintended consequences of unsustainable infrastructure. In order to meet climate and development goals while "leaving no one behind", it will be vital to bridge the infrastructure gap, which will require investments of US$6.9 trillion per year until 2030. Countries in the pan-European region face similar challenges as energy demand continues to rise, climate-related hazards become more frequent and intense, and there is a growing need to improve social welfare and equity. These and many other factors will drive the need to develop more resilient infrastructure Climate change and resilience, GHG emissions in the pan-European region continue to rise. With infrastructure construction and operation accounting for 70% of all GHG emissions, infrastructure development must be at the centre of any sensible climate strategy. Infrastructure development will play a dual role in achieving a more climate resilient future, firstly as a climate change mitigation strategy and secondly as an adaptation strategy. Given the significant share of infrastructure across sectors in total GHG emissions, it is crucial to transform existing production models with less carbon-intensive options. In addition, large areas in the pan-European region already regularly suffer from the effects of climate change, including, for example, heat waves, prolonged droughts, sea level rise or floods. Infrastructure solutions are thus widely recognised as a key climate change adaptation strategy. For many decades, an additional beneficial effect of infrastructure was considered to be its ability to provide strong, reliable barriers to protect populations from unwanted perturbations such as flooding. However, this approach has changed dramatically and has been supplemented by ROPFs, sometimes referred to as "green infrastructure "It has now become clear that traditional "grey" infrastructure is often unable to cope with the increasing impacts of climate change. Thus, the combination of ROPF and a comprehensive understanding of the ecosystem services that nature provides, together with the predictability of traditional grey infrastructure options, offers a broader ('green-grey') range of synergies that will better match the multiple solutions needed depending on the context. Coping with the crisis and creating jobs The COVID-19 pandemic caused an unprecedented global economic downturn. This crisis exposed gender inequality, global gaps in the availability of basic services, and the lack of flexibility and resilience of infrastructure systems. According to the International Labour Organization (ILO), the crisis-induced job shortage will reach 75 million in 2021, falling to 23 million in 2022.

Moreover, lost employment growth will only be restored by 2023. However, the pandemic also creates a rare opportunity to build a "better-than-ever" recovery, laying the foundation for a sustainable and green future through investment in sustainable infrastructure. Investment in infrastructure is likely to be a key element of recovery efforts in many countries, in part because of the potential for job creation. In addition, ensuring that infrastructure investments are climate resilient and do not increase potential risks and vulnerabilities will reduce the direct economic losses from climate-related disasters, while minimising the indirect costs caused by the cascading effects of disruption to critical services and economic activity.

New technologies and innovations, the pandemic showed the interconnectedness of the world and that, in real life, existing infrastructure systems are in many cases fragile, not fit for purpose and even obsolete. Thus, the health crisis combined with the crisis of inequality and the lack of flexibility of infrastructure systems caused a domino effect, amplifying the devastating effects of the pandemic. Even now, as digital communication technologies update their operating systems every couple of months, the planning, design, construction and operation of multi-million dollar infrastructure projects that are rigid, inflexible and expected to operate without any change for decades continues. It is therefore not surprising that countries are looking to meet the changing needs for temporary healthcare facilities, telecommuting and the next generation of transport systems such as electric or driverless cars. To better meet future infrastructure needs, there is a need to ensure that the infrastructure sector focuses on delivering infrastructure services rather than being locked into projects. A problem-orientated approach fosters innovation, creates opportunities to explore new technologies, and encourages better solutions. For example, it is important to frame the problem as "the need to improve the supply of safe drinking water" rather than "building more water treatment plants". The second, more traditional option limits the ability to integrate non-traditional and more sustainable alternatives, such as ROPF, to solve the problem at hand. Data-driven decision-making, geospatial design and modelling will be critical to improve understanding of the complexity of a future world where human needs, environmental and social impacts, and planetary boundaries must be part of developing the best possible solution.

Migration is a massive phenomenon driven by the search for better opportunities around the world. Shifts in urbanisation patterns have intensified in recent years as a result of climate change, violence and conflict. The International Organisation for Migration estimates that there are 272 million international migrants worldwide, i.e. 3.5% of the world's population, exceeding projections for 2050. Europe has traditionally been a major destination for international migrants, receiving some 82 million international migrants, and Asia some 84 million; together they accounted for 61 per cent of the world's international migrants in the year in question. Given the difficulty of predicting mitigation patterns due to the close link to economic crises, political instability and conflict, the lack of predictability puts significant pressure on existing infrastructure such as hospitals or drinking water systems, making it impossible to provide the necessary services for the increased number of users. In view of this, it is crucial to ensure that the infrastructure planning process takes a long-term perspective at the outset, including demographic changes such as population ageing and potential migration processes that may lead to changes in urbanisation patterns and hence increased demand for infrastructure. Improving social wellbeing and equality. Creating and maintaining a healthy and safe environment is a key objective of sustainable infrastructure. In view of this, the direct and indirect safety and health impacts of "non-green solutions" must also be considered. Exposure to air, water or soil pollution and other toxic hazards can have long-term effects on human health and well-being. To guarantee well-being and equity for all potential infrastructure users, the special needs of certain groups, such as women, must also be considered. Stakeholder engagement processes, public consultation and gender mainstreaming strategies should underpin every infrastructure project, helping to identify and minimise the risk of social exclusion. Climate change, population growth, rising inequalities and the protection of biodiversity are just some of the challenges that humanity will face in the coming years. In response to these challenges, global initiatives have emerged in recent decades to support more inclusive, responsible and sustainable development models. Examples include the 2030 Agenda for Sustainable Development and its

Sustainable Development Goals. All these initiatives, while addressing different themes, have one thing in common: a paradigm shift towards a more sustainable model of development is needed to meet the critical challenges of the twenty-first century. This new paradigm can only be achieved through coordinated action involving governments, public and private institutions, academia and civil society. The ongoing pandemic has highlighted the tremendous opportunities that resilient infrastructure offers for "better-than-new" recovery in the era of post-pandemic recovery.

In this regard, the role of sustainable infrastructure is now widely recognised as a driver of both inclusive growth and productivity and accelerating the transition to a low-carbon and climate resilient economy. However, global efforts to stimulate a green economy and develop more sustainable and resilient infrastructure were discussed before the pandemic, so the question arises as to how states can ensure that this critical period of awakening does not pass without meaningful results and action? An important first step in this regard is the Pan-European Strategic Framework for a Green Economy, developed in 2016 by the ECE Committee on Environmental Policy with the support and cooperation of the ECE secretariat, UNEP and many other key players.

The main objective of the Pan-European Strategic Framework is to guide the pan-European region in the transition to an inclusive green economy by 2030, in line with the Rio+20 outcomes and the 2030 Agenda. Under the framework, the pan-European region will develop along the following lines

a model that ensures economic progress, social equity and sustainable use of ecosystems and natural resources, which ensures that the needs of present generations are met without compromising the needs of future generations. The implementation of the framework is supported by the Batumi Initiative for a Green Economy (BIG-E), which covers the period 2016-2030 and includes voluntary commitments by countries and public and private organisations to a green economy. To date, over 30 countries and organisations have submitted more than 100 commitments under the BIZ-E platform264.

Achieving all of these ambitious goals requires cooperation among countries, as well as normative and policy instruments that support and encourage the transition to a more sustainable development path. Equally important, all these efforts must be undertaken at an early stage of the development process. A good example illustrating the importance of these elements is the Convention on Environmental Impact Assessment in a Transboundary Context (Espoo Convention, adopted in 1991), which requires parties to assess the environmental impact of certain activities at an early stage of planning. The Espoo Convention is based on the idea that adverse environmental impacts and threats do not recognise national boundaries. Accordingly, it imposes an obligation to consult between parties on all major projects that may have adverse environmental impacts on a transboundary scale, which helps to reduce environmental threats and potential damage. The

Espoo Convention laid the foundation for the international introduction of strategic environmental assessment, a systematic decision-support process aimed at ensuring that environmental and other aspects of sustainability are effectively integrated into policies, plans and programmes. The COVID- 19 crisis has not only exacerbated countries' budgetary constraints, but also reinforced the need to invest in sustainable and more resilient projects. Mobilising finance for sustainable investments can have a major impact on the implementation of sustainable development projects. Instruments such as thematic bonds - mainly green, social and sustainable bonds - can make a major contribution to supporting the Sustainable Development Goals and sustainable recovery from the effects of the pandemic. However, sustainable finance had been part of the international discourse for years before the pandemic. The Paris Agreement (Art. 2, para. 1(c)) included a commitment to "align financial flows with a trajectory towards low-GHG-emitting development and resilience to climate change". In addition to existing commitments, initiatives such as the European Union Taxonomy have been introduced over the last couple of years. The taxonomy is a classification system that establishes a list of ecologically
sustainable economic activities. In addition to its importance for sustainable post-pandemic recovery, the taxonomy also plays a role in meeting the European Union's climate, energy and European Green Deal commitments. The mobilisation of financial resources and the strengthening of policy frameworks must be accompanied by capacity development initiatives. This will ensure that countries have the technical and institutional capacity to integrate these changes into their infrastructure policies. Most recently, in a resolution on green and sustainable infrastructure, the United Nations Environment Assembly called on Member States to integrate the UNEP International Best Practice Principles for Sustainable Infrastructure into national policies, to implement existing tools and frameworks, to cooperate internationally to strengthen different approaches (including financing) and to take into account the role of digital infrastructure.

The progress of sustainable infrastructure initiatives, given the wide range of actors involved in the lifecycle of infrastructure projects, has led to the development of numerous initiatives to identify indicators to quantify progress towards sustainable infrastructure. The various approaches identified range in scope and purpose, from general aspirational principles, safeguards and best practices, infrastructure sustainability rating systems and schemes, to reporting guidelines. General principles are intended to outline promising directions for action on a global scale in most cases they are published by international groups. Examples of such principles are the G20 Principles for Investing in Quality Infrastructure, the UNEP International Best Practice Principles for Sustainable Infrastructure, the OECD Policy Compendium of Best Practices for Investing in Quality Infrastructure, and the OECD Guidelines for Investing in Quality Infrastructure: Supporting Sustainable Recovery from the Crisis COVID-19.

These environmental and social considerations provide the basis for a better understanding of possible unintended consequences and other risks associated with infrastructure development. Examples of well-known and widely used safeguards and risk management frameworks are the International Finance Corporation Performance Standards and the Equator Principles. Most MDBs have their own safeguards policies as a basis for due diligence processes. Infrastructure resilience rating systems and schemes, numerous infrastructure resilience rating frameworks have been developed in different geographical regions. The purpose of these frameworks is to provide comprehensive guidelines and criteria for assessing projects against more than 50 indicators.

The application of these tools is in many cases linked to the attainment of a sustainability certificate or award. A significant number of frameworks and criteria for quantifying sustainable infrastructure have been developed, but various stakeholders recognise the need to consolidate and harmonise approaches and the recently established Financing for Accelerating Sustainable Transition - Infrastructure framework.

In order to monitor and communicate the sustainability performance of a project - not necessarily an infrastructure project - several reporting guidelines have been developed over the past few years, including the Global Reporting Initiative and the Dow Jones World Sustainability Index .Due to the complexity of infrastructure development, the diversity of its sectors and the different stages of its life cycle and stakeholders involved, a significant number of tools and frameworks for quantitative assessment have emerged This has led to a need for access to information and a better understanding of the use of currently available tools in order to find the one that best suits the user's needs. In this regard, Deutsche Gesellschaft für Internationale Zusammenarbeit has created the "Sustainable Infrastructure Tool Navigator " platform to help users identify the most appropriate tools for their needs and goals. This new initiative provides access to a comprehensive database of sustainable infrastructure tools, which users can browse by keywords or by applying, inter alia, filters by tool type, sector and infrastructure lifecycle stages. The initiative has recently been supported by UNEP on a partnership basis.

The comparative analysis covers six profile frameworks: (a) Pan-European Strategic Framework for Greening the Economy;

(b) A common set of agreed indicators for sustainable MDB infrastructure;

(c) UNEP Best Practice Principles for Sustainable Infrastructure; (d) G-20 Principles for Investing in Quality Infrastructure;

(e) Financing for Accelerating Sustainable Transition - Infrastructure (FAST-Infra);

(f ) The European Union taxonomy of sustainable activities.

These systems are compared in the following main categories: environmental sustainability and resilience; social sustainability; institutional sustainability; and economic and financial sustainability.

The comparative analysis highlighted several key issues:

a) In the category "Environmental Sustainability and Resilience", almost all of the tools selected mention greenhouse gas emission reduction, climate change mitigation and adaptation, environmental conservation and circular economy, or resource efficiency.

This category shows the greatest consistency between systems;

b) in the Social Sustainability category, all but one framework mentions equality, inclusion and/or gender considerations. At the same time, however, considerations of human and labour rights, health and well-being, and resettlement are not always included;

c) in the institutional sustainability category, transparent and anti-corruption practices are mentioned in two thirds of the instruments analysed. In addition, some frameworks also cover accountability procedures such as sustainability certification, sustainability disclosure or sustainability and compliance policies;

d) less homogeneity was found in the category "Economic and financial stability". Some frameworks refer to the need to guarantee positive economic returns and job creation. In contrast, others consider the importance of mobilising innovative sources of finance and taking externalities into account. The comparative analysis has led to the suggestion of indicators, sub-indicators and units of measurement.

Quantification of indicators in the pan-European region: trends identified

An infrastructure project is sustainable if various environmental, social, institutional and economic considerations are fulfilled throughout the life cycle of the project. However, due to the multi-dimensional nature of sustainability and the lack of an agreed baseline at the pan-European regional or sub-regional level, information on infrastructure sustainability indicators is limited or non-existent. Therefore, after identifying the most commonly used sustainability indicators and the information available at country and regional level, each indicator has been analysed.

Indicator 1, Climate Change Adaptation and Mitigation, aims to reduce GHG emissions while ensuring the resilience of infrastructure projects and integrating strategies 195

climate change adaptation and mitigation throughout the cycle. Due to the broad scope of this indicator, it is divided into two sub-indicators:

1.1 "Reducing GHG emissions "

1.2 "Disaster Risk and Strategies for Disaster Risk Reduction".

According to the United Nations SDG Indicators Database for quantifying progress on Sustainable Development Goal indicator 13.2.2 "Total greenhouse gas emissions per year", net GHG emissions in the pan-European region increased if 2014 is taken as the base year. Between 2014 and 2023, two subregions of the pan-European region (the European Union and Western Europe) showed positive progress in reducing GHG emissions. However, the subregions of Central Asia, Eastern Europe and South-Eastern Europe experienced an overall increase in GHG emissions, leading to an increase in emissions for the region as a whole. Looking at the progress made under sub-indicator 1.2 "Disaster risk and disaster risk reduction strategies" and based on the United Nations Statistics Division (UNSD) data on the Sendai Framework monitoring system, all subregions, and thus the pan-European region as a whole, have increased the adoption and implementation of disaster risk reduction strategies. Thus, indicator 1 as a whole shows mixed results and more efforts should be directed towards adaptation to and mitigation of climate change. B on climate change. Additional efforts should be directed towards gathering information on adaptation strategies to be used in countries and regions. Adaptation strategies include using nature-based solutions, working to reduce flooding, restoring hydrological connectivity, designing or planning infrastructure for the potential impacts of climate change, building capacity to adapt to new risks, and diversifying energy supplies. Due to the complexity of some of these topics, the proposed indicators are only first steps towards measuring a more comprehensive resilient climate infrastructure strategy. Further data collection on regional adaptation strategies should be undertaken to include additional indicators.

Indicator 2, Environmental Conservation and Biodiversity Protection, aims to prevent negative impacts and/or restore biodiversity and the environment while preserving ecosystems and ecosystem services throughout the life cycle of an infrastructure project. This indicator is quantified through two sub-indicators:

2.1 "Protecting biodiversity" and 2.2 "Protecting ecosystem services".

Biodiversity protection is quantified in accordance with Sustainable Development Goal 15 and its indicator 15.9.1. (a) "Number of countries, 196

that have set national targets in their national biodiversity strategy and action plan in line with Aichi Biodiversity Target 2 on biodiversity in the

within the framework of the Strategic Plan for Biodiversity 2011-2030 or similar and monitor progress towards such targets". According to information published by UNSD, each country in the pan-European region has developed its own strategic biodiversity plans and action plans. The achievement of this target does not necessarily mean that biodiversity targets have been met, but it does indicate that national strategies are in place. It should be noted that very little information is currently available at national, sub-regional or regional level on the impact of infrastructure development on biodiversity disturbance. Sub-indicator 2.2 "Protection of ecosystem services" was quantified according to Sustainable Development Goal indicator 15.3.1 "Proportion of degraded land to total land area". According to the ECE SDG Dashboard, there are significant differences in land degradation between countries: from 97 per cent in Tajikistan - due to erosion caused by overgrazing, poor irrigation maintenance and salinisation - to only 1 per cent degraded land in Belarus and Finland. Similar to the biodiversity situation, there is little or no information on the percentage of land degraded due to infrastructure development or other relevant information to quantify the services provided by natural ecosystems in different countries.

Indicator 3 "Closed-loop economics" addresses the importance of proper resource utilisation throughout the lifecycle of an infrastructure project. Based on the available information and its linkage to infrastructure development, the most appropriate unit of measurement has been identified as the "Construction and demolition waste recycling rate". Only limited information was found at the level of the pan-European region. However, this indicator is part of the European Commission's set of indicators for the circular economy. Detailed information is therefore available at the European Union level. According to the latest information published by Eurostat, the average recycling rate of construction and demolition waste remains almost constant at 87 % in 2014 and 2016 and 88 % in 2023. The data collection process applied in the European Union can be extrapolated to the level of the pan-European region to quantify this indicator.

Indicator 4, Gender Equality and Empowerment, aims to promote social inclusion, gender equality and the protection of human rights by promoting economic empowerment and ensuring social mobility and equal opportunities for all. Based on the availability of data, the following unit of measurement is proposed - "Gender employment gap in the pan-European region". According to the latest information published by the International Labour Organization (ILO) in the ILOSTAT database 2021, there are significant differences between sub-regions. For example, the gender employment gap in the South-Eastern Europe subregion is currently 21.2 per cent compared to the Western Europe subregion (6.4 per cent) and the European Union subregion (9.9 per cent). The gender gap in employment shows a positive trend, having narrowed in most subregions. This is the case for the European Union, where the gender gap in employment fell sharply from 20.8 per cent in 1990 (first available data) to 9.9 per cent in 2023, or the Western Europe subregion, where the gap narrowed from 18.2 per cent in 1990 to 6.4 per cent in 2019. The dynamics in the Central Asia and Eastern Europe subregions go against this trend, as the gender gap in employment in these subregions increased by 1.5 and 0.9 per cent, respectively, between 1990 and 2023. The gender employment gap in the pan-European region narrowed from 19.2 per cent in 1990 to 14.4 per cent in 2023; there is still considerable room for improvement.

Indicator 5, Life Cycle Cost Accounting, is a key element of the sustainability framework. This indicator considers the net economic and social returns of infrastructure over the life cycle of a project (including positive and negative externalities). Externalities are specifically mentioned in the Pan-European Strategic Framework for a Green Economy. One of their nine focal areas (FA.2) aims to promote the internalisation of negative externalities and the sustainable use of natural capital. However, there is only limited evidence on quantifying the impact of externalities in the region. The first step in this direction is cost-benefit analysis. Hence, the criterion for quantifying this is the number of countries that conduct cost-benefit analyses for the infrastructure sector. According to the OECD questionnaire on the challenges and application of cost-benefit analysis for pre-feasibility studies of capital investment, cost-benefit analyses in major infrastructure projects that have participated in the preparation of this feasibility study. However, only one third of these countries did so because of statutory requirements. Furthermore, traditional cost-benefit analyses do not include sustainability considerations (such as climate risk) and externalities (such as the cost of pollution, ecosystem services or biodiversity protection). Thus, having a cost-benefit analysis should not be an end goal, but rather a useful step towards a more comprehensive analysis of infrastructure development throughout its life cycle. Indicator 6, Access to Basic Services, aims to improve physical and economic access to basic services, ensuring healthier living conditions and well-being. Given the scope of this work and data availability, services such as access to drinking water, sanitation, electricity and 2G, 3G or 4G mobile networks are considered to quantify this indicator.

Access to drinking water is quantified in accordance with Sustainable Development Goal indicator 1.4.1 "Proportion of population living in households with access to basic services". According to data published in 2023 by the WHO/UNICEF Joint Monitoring Programme for Water Supply, Sanitation and Hygiene, access to basic drinking water services is roughly similar across the pan-European subregions and in all cases exceeds 90%. In this respect, the Western Europe subregion is the only subregion with full access to such services, followed by the European Union (98.6 per cent). In almost all countries, access in rural areas is more than 75 %.

When considering the proportion of the population using basic sanitation services, the information collected shows a greater heterogeneity of results compared to the previous sub-indicator. The results range from 82.3 per cent access in rural areas of Eastern Europe to 99.5 per cent in urban areas of South-Eastern Europe and Western Europe. Together, the percentage of the population using basic sanitation services in the pan-European region is 96.3 %. At country level, the lowest percentage of access to sanitation (72 %) is found in rural areas in two countries. Access to electricity is also relevant when considering basic services. This sub-indicator is quantified in accordance with indicator 7.1.1 of the Sustainable Development Goals and refers to the proportion of the population with access to electricity. According to UNSD, the pan-European region has full access to electricity, with the exception of Central Asia (99.9 per cent).

The last sub-indicator considered under access to basic services is the "proportion of the population covered by a mobile network".

The provision of mobile networks is covered by indicator 9.C.1 of the Sustainable Development Goals and refers to the percentage of residents living within range of a mobile cellular signal. While 2G offers limited voice services, 3G and 4G provide high-speed, reliable and high-quality access. The ECE statistical database shows that 2G mobile networks cover almost the entire population of various pan-European subregions in 2023. 3G coverage in 2023 varied by region between 83.8 and 99.3 per cent. In comparison, in the case of 4G, there was greater variation, ranging from 63.1 to 98.3 %. Compared to previous years, the proportion of the population covered in the pan-European region by 2G networks does not change. At the same time, there is a significant increase in 3G and 4G coverage between 2012, the earliest year for which data are available, and 2023, the latest year for which data are available. In 2012, the percentage of the population covered by 3G networks was 77.7 per cent, 17.6 per cent lower than in 2023. In the case of 4G networks, the difference is even greater: while in 2012 the percentage of the population with access to 4G was 22.6 per cent, in 2023 this figure has risen to 83.6 per cent, an increase of 61 per cent

Indicator 7, Transparency and Anti-Corruption, aims to ensure that the planning, design, construction and operation of projects are transparent so that relevant information is available to all stakeholders. The quantification of this indicator corresponds to Transparency International's Corruption Perception Index, where 0 represents the highest level of corruption and 100 the lowest. According to Eurostat, this indicator is part of the Sustainable Development Goal indicator set of the European Union and is used to monitor progress towards indicator 16.5.2 of the Sustainable Development Goals.

According to the results published in the Corruption Perceptions Index 2020, Western Europe is the sub-region with the lowest level of corruption (76.2), followed by the European Union (63.7).

However, in each of the other subregions, the score is below 40, meaning that the public sector is perceived as more corrupt than in the Western subregions. In this respect, the subregion with the highest perception of corruption (27.8) is Central Asia, followed by South-Eastern Europe (38.2) and Eastern Europe (39.9). Ratings for previous years are only available for the European Union. Comparing the 2019 and 2020 scores shows that in most European Union countries the level of corruption perception has slightly decreased or remained the same. However, if we take a much broader time frame, the situation is quite different: 17 out of 27 countries have seen an increase in the perception of corruption.

Indicator 8, Fiscal Sustainability and Innovative Financing, aims to ensure the financial sustainability of assets throughout their life cycle. This includes mobilising innovative sources of capital on a large scale. Significant work has been done in various sub-regions to mobilise finance for more sustainable and resilient projects. An example is the European Green Deal investment plan, which will mobilise European Union funding and create a favourable framework to stimulate public and private investment, for the transition to a climate-neutral, green, competitive and inclusive economy. The unit of measure proposed for this indicator corresponds to indicator 13.a.1 of the Sustainable Development Goals, and its objective is to mobilise finance to meet the international commitment to allocate $100 billion to climate-related costs. The proposed indicator is in line with indicator 13.a.1 of the Sustainable Development Goals and aims to mobilise finance to meet the international commitment to provide $100 billion for climate-related costs. According to the European Environmental Information and Observation Network (Eionet) and the European Commission's Directorate-General for Climate Action, the European Union's contribution in 2023 is €16.206 billion, a 37% increase compared to the base year of 2014. Only limited information is available for some other pan-European sub-regions. This indicator does not cover the full amount of funding for sustainable development. However, it is a first step towards financing other key aspects of sustainability, such as biodiversity protection and social inclusion.

Overall, these indicators reflect the current situation of sustainable infrastructure in the pan-European region, based on information currently available . Further work will be needed in the future to refine these indicators (e.g. quantifying progress in implementing adaptation strategies in different countries) and to focus the indicators more specifically on infrastructure. The work done should be considered a first step towards a sound sustainable infrastructure agenda.

Naples - Bari (Italy) railway line: the first project in Europe be certified by the Envision sustainability rating system Railway systems are a key element of the long-term transport strategy defined by many countries around the world. However, these linear projects can often have potential harmful environmental and social impacts and, among other risks, are exposed to climate change. Thus, applying the concept of sustainable infrastructure can help to identify opportunities for improvement and existing shortcomings affecting the sustainability performance of infrastructure projects. This case study presents an overview of the application of the Envision rating system, one of the most widely used methodologies for quantifying infrastructure sustainability, and its application to the Naples-Bari railway line (Italy), the first Envision-certified project in Europe. The Naples-Bari section is part of the Scandinavia-Mediterranean railway corridor of the Trans-European Transport Network. This project aims to improve services by increasing speed, accessibility, capacity and interconnectivity with other modes of transport, including ports and airports. This €6.2bn project will comprise a multi-use corridor where synergies with other infrastructure sectors such as energy and telecoms are also being considered. Envision's application and validation of the project covers a shorter section of 21 kilometres (Frasso - Telesino - Telese - San Lorenzo).

The holistic approach to sustainability enabled by the application of Envision early in the project has resulted in the highest sustainability performance, a Platinum Award. Some of the benefits of integrating sustainability indicators into this project included selecting the route in a way that minimised environmental impact. Applying environmental indicators early on in the project identified areas of high environmental value, floodplains and agricultural land used for wine production, allowing them to be bypassed in the route design. Specific climate change and resilience considerations, as well as local authority involvement were also identified as part of the project appraisal with Envision. According to the project team, the application of sustainability tools and its indicators allows for "an innovative approach to design to be favoured. Designers working in accordance with the environmental sustainability criteria of the [Envision] protocol also tend to look for According to the Sustainable Infrastructure Institute (SII) definition. The tool is divided into 64 sustainability and resilience criteria in five main categories: quality of life; governance; resource allocation; natural world; and climate and resilience. new and creative solutions to achieve high quality goals with less waste, better utilisation of natural resources and use of innovative materials. "3 The Lower Danube Green Corridor: floodplain restoration for flood protection More than two decades ago, the governments of Bulgaria, the Republic of Moldova, Romania and Ukraine joined forces to develop the Lower Danube Corridor project. This 1,000 kilometre corridor project is intended to have positive effects in terms of flood protection, water purification and climate change mitigation, while at the same time restoring areas of high ecological value. As defined in the Declaration of Co-operation for the Lower Danube Green Corridor, signed in Bucharest by the Environment Ministers of the four countries, the project envisages "a minimum allocation of 773,166 ha of existing protected areas, 160,626 ha of proposed new protected areas and 223,608 ha of areas where restoration of the natural floodplain is proposed". Currently, 70% of the floodplain in this section of the river has been lost or damaged. In principle, 25 % of the total floodplain area could be restored as a result of this project. The restoration of former wetlands could allow the storage of up to 1.6 billion m3 of water, significantly minimising flood risk in the area. In terms of economic feasibility, floodplain restoration along the Lower Danube Green Corridor is estimated at €183 million, with annual revenues associated with ecosystem services estimated at €111.8 million per year.In addition to the previously mentioned project benefits (flood risk prevention, natural connectivity, etc.), the restoration of ecosystem services and the use of ROPF provide significant positive impacts of additional externalities. These include the key role of wetlands as carbon sinks, the restoration of biodiversity in the zone of influence, the development and protection of economic zones and the reduction of water pollution in floodplains and wetlands.This project illustrates the importance of environmental restoration and the positive externalities associated with protecting natural assets. Solutions in green infrastructure help mitigate the inevitable impacts of climate change, environmental degradation and biodiversity loss

B. Applying circular economy principles to sustainable tourism

A pan-European tourism economy based on circular economy principles would be more resilient to and better prepared to respond to crises - economic, health, epidemiological or environmental challenges faced by the region. The circular economy is important for sustainable tourism development and can contribute to the achievement of the Sustainable Development Goals; in particular, it will accelerate the transition to a green travel and tourism economy. Despite the increasing efficiency of tourism, its rapid growth is having increasingly tangible impacts that are increasingly leading to environmental and social problems. The closed-loop principle should be the basis of a strategy to transform and rebuild the tourism sector after the COVID-19 pandemic. Policymakers must therefore ensure transformation on this basis by providing the necessary tools and moving away from business as usual.

The circular economy, despite its dependence on social aspects such as green jobs and welfare, mainly covers the physical environmental issues of energy and resource utilisation and the closing of resource cycles. Sustainable tourism development is orientated towards a broader perspective of economic development within social and environmental constraints. Therefore, the circular economy is a necessary but not sufficient element of sustainable tourism development.

A circular economy is an economic system in which the (linear) concept of "end-of-life" is replaced by the reduction, reuse, recycling and recovery of materials in the production, distribution and consumption processes. Apart from individual cases, due to the complexity of the tourism value chain, which includes many sub-sectors, the application of the principles of such an economy in tourism is still its infancy. Owing to the cross-sectoral nature of tourism, the concept of tourism based on the principles of the circular economy, while complex, has the potential to become a driving force in other sectors. The extended and end-to-end tourism value chain offers numerous opportunities for longer, higher quality and reusability of materials and products used for the provision of tourism services, value creation, partnerships, as well as the reduction of waste to as close to zero as possible .

Key areas of tourism that are closely linked to both the Sustainable Development Goals and the circular economy are energy consumption and emissions in transport, hotel and catering operations, waste management at tourism facilities, including in hotel and catering operations (e.g. food and plastic waste), water use and wastewater management in general, and resource use in construction, interior decoration and domestic facilities. Opportunities may be most obvious in the construction and operation of hotels and restaurants, including the utilisation of (food) waste. Clean aviation fuel (electrofuels) opportunities are utilised on a very small scale. Many sharing economy initiatives currently have too many consequences that are contrary to the principles of the circular economy, such as additional construction or large kilometres travelled.

Whereas the impacts of tourism have been measured in economic terms for decades, the development of indicators for sustainable tourism, let alone monitoring circularity, is still under development, but the process is hampered by a number of challenges. Currently, there are no indicators in the pan-European region that provide clear information on the extent to which closed-loop principles are being utilised in tourism and on trends in this area. There is therefore an urgent need to redefine how success will be measured in the future. On several common aspects of circularity, classification definitions vary from State to State. Finally, even basic tourism statistics tend to be incomplete and, due to differing definitions, there are problems in their utilisation, with detailed statistics needed for accurate

closed-loop monitoring being lacking. Digitalisation offers opportunities for better and more uniform measurement and monitoring, but depends on the availability of uniform and up-to-date data on the circular economy in the tourism sector.
Governments should intensify efforts to help reduce energy consumption and GHG emissions, in particular in the context of tourism, as this can be achieved by
204
They should also invest in low-emission transport infrastructure. They should also invest in low-emission transport infrastructure. A broad-based commitment to the Glasgow Declaration: Commitment to a Decade to Combat Climate Change in Tourism can contribute to these efforts and enable the harmonisation of climate action by all stakeholders in the tourism sector, including Governments, civil society and other actors. This requires, inter alia, the expansion of international rail transport infrastructure and long-distance transport itself, the development of electric vehicle charging infrastructure at tourist destinations, the introduction of closed-loop concepts related to the use of water, waste and materials, and the greater integration of closed-loop principles into policies and financing. In addition to reducing energy consumption and emissions in transport, such reductions in tourism can also be achieved by promoting the use of renewable energy in tourist accommodation, restaurants and attractions. In general, it is recommended that best practices in the circular economy be shared and initiatives such as the Global Initiative to Combat Plastic Use in the Tourism Sector, led by UNEP and UNWTO, be promoted in the tourism sector. Governments in the pan-European region should take advantage of these opportunities to prioritise domestic tourism when developing recovery plans in the aftermath of the COVID-19 pandemic, as it is more resilient to crises and has a lower impact on the climate, and tourism destinations are closer and easier to incorporate into a closed-loop model than international medium- and long-distance tourism products. Policymakers and entrepreneurs in the region should apply the principles of the circular economy throughout the tourism value chain. Treating tourism as a value chain can accelerate the transformation of tourism into a circular economy industry and enhance its long-term viability and sustainability.
Tourism, due to its interlinkages with other economic activities and direct interaction between producers and consumers, has the potential for long-term positive impacts beyond the sector itself. Financial support can help tourism regions to establish adequate (recycling and other) infrastructure to cope with large seasonal fluctuations in material flows.
Member States and ECE governing bodies should select a limited number of specific tourism indicators with key impacts relevant to the measurement of the circular economy in tourism for inclusion in the ECE statistical databases. Indicators demonstrating the extent to which the tourism economy is consistent with the circular economy model should be harmonised and used to monitor sustainability in tourism, ensuring their compatibility with the Sustainable

Development Goals. The development of circular economy indicators could follow the approach taken by UNWTO in the framework of the Sustainable Tourism Statistical Measurement Programme (ST-MPI) initiative. This programme is being developed jointly with the United Nations Statistics Division (UNSD) and is intended to become the next United Nations standard for measurement in the tourism sector and to be used by countries as an aid to provide reliable, comparable and integrated data to better guide sustainable tourism decisions and policies (including the Sustainable Development Goals).

Other areas of focus may include:

a) Further integration of existing measurement systems (Tourism Satellite Accounts, the System of Environmental-Economic Accounting, the European System of Tourism Indicators and the SP-ITI) to create a platform to measure the extent to which the tourism economy is sustainable and/or follows a closed-loop model;

b) Continued work on the selection and measurement of indicators for the Sustainable Development Goals, including the development of an additional set of indicators to judge the extent to which the tourism economy is in line with the circular economy model;

c) Advancing the development of subnational tourism statistics, recognising the importance of localised information for tourism decision-making.

There is a growing consensus that the recovery of the tourism sector after the COVID-19 pandemic should be based on the principles of sustainability (people, planet and prosperity) as the key to resilience, and that the circular economy as a strategy to achieve a green transformation of the sector plays a critical role in doing so.

Over the past half-century, mining has tripled, and it is the extraction and processing of natural resources that is responsible for more than 90 per cent of biodiversity loss and water scarcity, and about 50 per cent of climate change impacts.288 Critical resources are already becoming scarce, ecosystem services are increasingly degraded, and it is increasingly difficult to offset anthropogenic pollution and waste. Critical resources are already becoming scarce, ecosystem services are increasingly degraded, and anthropogenic pollution and waste are increasingly difficult to offset. In recent decades, tourism, having become a major economic sector, has come to play a significant role in this development, with the number of tourists visiting other countries reaching 1.5 billion in 2023.

UNWTO estimates that tourism accounted for 4 per cent of global GDP. Tourism includes various resource-intensive components, including flights, accommodation, restaurants and attractions, but also facilitates social exchange and intercultural dialogue. Prior to the pandemic, tourism activities were based on the traditional paradigm of a linear economy with climate and environmental impacts. There is a high risk that this linear paradigm will continue after the pandemic and that the opportunity for a green transformation in the tourism sector will be missed.

Environmental issues in which tourism plays a significant role are energy use and emissions, biodiversity loss, water use, over-consumption (of food as well as other environmental and social aspects) and waste generation. The share of tourism in global $CO_2$ emissions is estimated at 5 %, of which 75 % is attributable to tourism transport (air transport 40 %, road transport 32 % and other transport 3 %), 21 % to accommodation and 4 % to tourism activities. Due to its high altitude impact, air transport also has a significant non-$CO_2$ impact on climate change. According to a study conducted later on a larger scale, tourism accounted for about 8 % of global emissions in 2013. In 2016, transport-related emissions from tourism alone were estimated to account for 5 % of global emissions, and are projected to increase by 25 % by 2030 under the current ambitious scenario. Under another (developed before the COVID pandemic) scenario of maintaining the current state of affairs, global tourism would exceed the full carbon budget of all sectors and households needed to stay within the maximum temperature rise agreed in the Paris Agreement by 2060-2070. This is due to the high energy consumption of the tourism sector, in particular for transport and hotel stays, which increases with increasing class of service.

Route length and mode choice are key drivers of tourism transport emissions. UNWTO and the International Transport Forum (ITF) forecast that by 2030, the number of domestic and international trips will reach 15.6 billion and 1.8 billion, respectively. The number of trips made by land-based modes will increase by 70% (almost 5 billion trips) and emissions from these trips will increase by 12% (from 691 million to 775 million tonnes of $CO_2e$), accounting for 44% of total emissions (up from 50% in 2016). In contrast, the number of tourists travelling by air (both international and domestic) is expected to account for 33% of the total in 2030, but air transport will account for 56% of all emissions. The nature and extent of growth will depend on tourism development in the post-Pandemic COVID-19 period.The use of water for tourism in a number of destinations poses challenges, as travelling to warm countries 207

during the dry season, with high water consumption for swimming pools, accommodation facilities and attractions, as well as, for example, in the production of artificial snow for winter tourism. This adversely affects water availability and groundwater levels and puts additional strain on often inadequate infrastructure.

Food consumption in the tourism industry - an estimated 75 billion meals per year - generates a range of environmental problems. For example, the average level of food waste in the hospitality industry is estimated at 40 per cent and in restaurants at 60 per cent. UNEP estimates that international tourism will account for about 200 Mt of waste in 2050, which seems a conservative estimate as international tourists in Europe already generate 1 kg of solid waste per day. Waste generated by the tourism sector, including plastic waste, can overload local waste treatment and disposal infrastructure, especially during the high season and in locations where infrastructure is not yet well developed. There are various global initiatives to address waste, including in the tourism sector, such as the Global Initiative to Combat Plastic Use in the Tourism Sector. Tourism is a factor in the decline of biodiversity through land conversion, overexploitation of natural resources for food, materials, fresh water and recreation, spread of invasive species, interference with wildlife, pollution from sewage, sewage, solid waste, use of fertilisers and pesticides and indirectly through its share of GHG emissions. At the global level, the share of land use for tourism is still small. But at the local level, tourism can have serious impacts and generate many problems with land rights and land allocation, including competition with nature and agriculture and problems with landscape quality. However, tourism can also contribute to the protection of biodiversity through nature conservation.To these environmental concerns has been added relatively recently the problem of overtourism, which describes situations "in which the impacts of tourism at certain times and places exceed the limits of physical, environmental, social, economic, psychological and/or political capacity". The main drivers of over-tourism are often related to factors that cause some of the above-mentioned environmental problems, such as tourism density, air travel intensity and the proportion of beds on online rental platforms.

As COVID-19 pre-pandemic models show, energy consumption and associated emissions, as well as water use, land use and food consumption, will double in 25-45 years. This will increase the already significant anthropogenic pressures on a number of the planet's carrying capacities and

is contrary to policy objectives, such as those set out in the Paris Agreement and the Sustainable Development Goals. In many ways, tourism itself will be affected by these pressures: for example, climate change can alter the comparative attractiveness of destinations, causing changes in tourist flows, worsening water and snow shortages can affect the supply of tourism products, and extreme weather can damage tourism infrastructure, which ultimately also translates into lower revenues and reduced contributions to national and local economies.

While attempts to move towards a more sustainable tourism development have been made at all levels for at least two decades, they have not yet been successful on a large scale and cannot keep up with the effects of overall volume growth. UNWTO recognises that approaches "such as the circular economy, which encourage business models based on renewable resources, longer and more diverse product life cycles, collaborative consumption and interconnected value chains, can play an important role in developing and improving resource management systems not only in the tourism sector, but also in the sustainable development of destinations". In essence, the concept of the circular economy is seen as a business model alternative to the traditional linear model of economic development, with the environment playing a key role. According to the dominant definition, the circular economy is "an economic system in which the concept of 'end-of-life' is replaced by reduced use, alternative reuse, recycling and recovery of materials in the processes of production, distribution and consumption. It functions ... to achieve sustainable development, thereby simultaneously ensuring environmental quality, economic prosperity and social justice for the benefit of present and future generations", and is thus a strategy to accelerate green transformation and sustainable tourism development. Its classic "3 R's" principles (Reduce, Reuse, Recycle) are often expanded to a "ladder" or R-structure of up to 10 principles or strategies (Refuse-Rethink-Reduce-Reuse-Repair-Refurbish-Remanufacture-Repurpose-Recycle-Recover).

The main advantages of the circular economy lie in its potential to promote sustainable development and reduce environmental stress while creating economic benefits and jobs. Technological and, to an even greater extent, cultural barriers have been found to be the most significant factor slowing the transition to circularity. The United Nations Development Programme (UNDP) and UNEP identify tourism as one of the few sectors that is key to the economic development of all countries, while providing opportunities for climate change mitigation through resource efficiency and furthering the transition to a circular economy. They recommend that tourism be viewed through the lens of circular economy or value chain concepts to identify and assess its interdependence with other sectors, such as those selected for the climate agenda. Within a circular economy approach, measures can be developed that incentivise (climate) efforts in all those sectors on which tourism depends. For example, tourism is closely linked to food production, distribution and utilisation. UNDP sees particular potential for applying circular economy principles to the tourism sector in countries where it is a strong component of the economy. The circular economy is considered a very promising area for contributing to a number of Sustainable Development Goals, in particular Goal 7 on energy, Goal 8 on economic growth, Goal 11 on sustainable cities, Goal 12 on responsible consumption and production, Goal 13 on combating climate change, Goal 14 on marine ecosystems and Goal 15 on terrestrial ecosystems. The main challenge for policies related to the circular economy is to ensure the effective definition and implementation of its principles in the tourism sector, in particular since the entire tourism chain is a fusion of segments of several other sectors, from construction to transport, and is predominantly a service sector. Policy awareness is also a challenge, as the published survey of 73 national tourism strategies

UNWTO and UNEP found only one reference to circular economy principles. However, several countries, such as Spain and Slovenia, mention tourism in their circular economy strategies or roadmaps.

3. Status, Key Trends and Recent Developments, estimated that the global circularity gap (Circularity Gap Report 2020) is 8.6 per cent, down from 9.1 per cent in 2018, while 17 per cent is required to close the global emissions gap316. Progress in the development of the circular economy in the pan-European region is not uniform. ECE reports an increase in resource efficiency in the region, while domestic material consumption per unit of GDP has decreased by about 10 per

cent, total output has increased by 40 per cent. There are also significant differences among ECE member States in this respect: the average decrease in domestic material consumption of 3.1 per cent in the European OECD countries contrasts with an increase in the Eastern ECE countries. During the same period, the overall material intensity in the ECE region continued to rise, increasing by 18 per cent, partly due to increased imports of raw materials to substitute for domestic production. ECE also points to the important role of ECE member States in the global demand for materials and the consequent responsibility of these countries - as part of the transition to more sustainable consumption and production - outside the ECE region317. This issue is also extremely relevant for international tourism, where resources are mainly consumed abroad and many of the products consumed are imported. The consumption of material resources in the ECE region largely reflects the economic level of States: less developed countries experience high levels of growth with high levels of resource consumption, while more developed countries, whose economies are dominated by the services sector, are characterised by lower material intensity. The use of material resources and the complex interactions and feedback loops between human and natural systems in the ECE region are described in the publication "Interconnected natural resource areas in the ECE region".

In the European Union, the recycling rate (recycled materials as a percentage of total materials used) has increased from 8.2 % in 2004 to 11.2 % in 2017, although the rate has remained virtually unchanged since 2012. One of the world leaders in recycling is considered to be the Netherlands (24.5 %), while, for example, Norway (2.4 %) lags far behind the global average. In March 2020, as part of the European Green Deal programme and in order to align it with new strategies, the European Commission presented a new action plan for a circular economy, developed after the previous version. In its action plan on the circular economy, the European Commission states that "scaling up the circular economy to include the rest of the economic players in addition to pioneers will make a decisive contribution to achieving climate neutrality by 2050 and removing the resource dependency of economic growth, while ensuring the long-term competitiveness of the [European Union] and leaving no one behind".

Achieving this transition requires accelerating the shift to a regenerative growth model that returns more to the planet than it takes from it, moving towards consumption retention

resources within the planet's capacity and therefore aim to reduce its consumer footprint and double its recycling rate in the coming decade." The action plan includes proposals for product design, closed-loop production processes, waste reduction and consumer empowerment. The European Parliament also had its say, adopting a resolution on the action plan, which calls for additional measures and aims to achieve a fully circular economy by 2050. The resolution emphasises the important contribution that the circular economy can make to achieving the goals of the Paris Agreement and the Convention on Biological Diversity, as well as the Sustainable Development Goals. The principles of the circular economy have yet to take their place in the European Union's tourism-specific policies, as the current framework within which the Commission operates dates back to 2010. The Council of the European Union encourages European Union member States to take into account a number of challenges and opportunities when developing tourism strategies and policies, which include, inter alia, "sustainability, including resource efficiency, the circular economy, seasonality, and the management and distribution of growing tourism flows". Policies should contribute to the European Union's climate goals, the Paris Agreement and the Sustainable Development Goals. It is likely that aspects of the circular economy will be taken into account in the "Tourism Transition Process" as the basis for a new European Agenda for Tourism for the period 2030-2050. There are still very few examples of the application of circular economy principles in tourism both worldwide and in ECE member States. Tourism products are highly diversified, often cross-sectoral and usually include a number of components such as accommodation, transport, programme of activities, food and beverages. The tourism value chain is complex. A vast number of businesses and organisations are responsible for all these components of tourism, and the tourist often combines them into the final product. Thus, the large-scale application of the principles of the circular economy to tourism final products may not be easy. The individual component option is more realistic, but in the long run a whole value chain approach will have a greater impact. In tourism, there have long been businesses that are familiar with the principles of the closed-loop economy and, by replacing property rights with access, offer shared-use structures and product-service systems. Airbnb and Uber, for example, are well known. Such initiatives are currently associated with a range of negative impacts, including additional building construction and additional vehicle mileage, as well as various other environmental, social and tourism revenue leakage issues. Examples of sharing without such externalities are found in the transport sector (bicycle and, to a lesser extent, scooter hire schemes). Examples are also found in the case of traditional accommodation facilities (hotels corresponding to the concept of the circular economy). The UNEP and UNWTO Global Initiative to Combat Plastic Use in the Tourism Sector includes commitments such as engaging the tourism chain in the transition to making all plastic packaging reusable or recyclable or compostable, making investments to increase recycling rates and reporting on targets. Sometimes these can be simple and effective measures, such as ensuring the availability of potable tap water in public places, reducing tourists' reliance on bottled water and preventing packaging waste.

The COVID-19 pandemic has hit tourism hard, especially international tourism. According to UNWTO, international tourist arrivals fell by 74% globally in 2020 due to travel restrictions and various socio-economic challenges. During the first three quarters of 2021, international tourist arrivals were still 76% below 2019 levels. It is estimated that the collapse of the international tourism market alone in 2020 would mean a loss of US$1.3 trillion in export earnings and a loss of US$1.5 trillion in export revenues. It is estimated that a collapse of the international tourism market alone would mean a loss of US$1.3 trillion in export earnings and the threat of losing around 120 million jobs. There is a growing consensus in academia and policy circles that rebuilding the sector must be done in a sustainable manner to mitigate impacts and ensure resilience. UNWTO recognises that the COVID-19 crisis "has brought into focus the importance of local supply chains and the need to rethink how goods and services are produced and consumed, two key elements of the circular economy. By adopting circular economy principles and further improving resource efficiency in the tourism value chain, the tourism sector has the opportunity to embark on a path of stable and sustainable growth". Thus, in order to move towards a circular economy in tourism, UNWTO recommends investing in the transformation of tourism value chains, integrating circular economy processes, prioritising circularity for sustainable food and moving towards plastic recycling in tourism.

UNWTO concludes that a consensus is emerging in tourism circles that post-pandemic recovery must also include addressing the underlying causes of the phenomenon and the challenges to achieving sustainability. However, there is little time left for a real transition, as many countries and tourism-dependent businesses are desperate to resume operations after various knockdowns, and consumers are eager to spend holidays away from home. There is a danger of a return to the traditional model with consequences for (additional) investments in building a sustainable closed-loop tourism economy. In terms of energy consumption (and emissions), the faster recovery of domestic tourism that has been observed in some countries is positive from the point of view of the circular economy.

The first European Union action plan for the circular economy proposed a simple and effective monitoring system. The European Commission introduced a new set of indicators, including the Closed-Cycle Economy Monitoring Indicator Framework, which has been adopted by Eurostat. The Framework, which includes 10 indicators, some of which are broken down into sub-indicators, is designed to measure progress in building the circular economy in a way that covers its various aspects at all stages of the life cycle of resources, goods and services. The indicators cover four thematic areas: production and consumption; waste management; secondary raw materials; and competitiveness and innovation. The list is purposely structured to be concise and specific. While emphasising existing data, the list leaves room for areas where new indicators are being developed, such as green public procurement and food waste. The European Commission's indicators are largely limited to recycling of materials with a focus on waste, partly due to the availability of reliable data, but also due to the lack of other options. In a resolution adopted in 2021, the European Parliament calls on the Commission to propose binding European Union targets for 2030, which will be monitored through new indicators to be adopted by the end of 2021 as part of an updated Framework List of Indicators for monitoring the circular economy. The European Commission links these new indicators to the pillars of its action plan, while wishing to ensure a link between the circular economy, climate neutrality and the pursuit of zero pollution. In previous decades, the impact of tourism was measured in economic terms, but now there is a need to rethink the way in which success is measured, which means strengthening the measurement of social and environmental aspects, with circular economy indicators playing an important role for the latter. UNWTO, with the support of the United Nations Statistics Division (UNSD), has initiated the creation of the Statistical Programme for Measuring Sustainable Tourism Indicators (SP-STI). The objective of the SP-STI is "to develop an international statistical for measuring key aspects of the role of tourism in sustainable development, including economic, environmental and social aspects".339 The last stage of the SP-STI development is the development of a statistical programme for measuring sustainable tourism indicators. In the last phase of the development of the SP-STI reported on, four main accounts were identified: water, energy, GHG emissions and solid waste flows. As the literature on the application of circular economy principles in tourism is still in its infancy, there are very few direct references to indicators for measuring the circular economy in tourism, apart from the UNWTO and UNEP recommendation, which states that "the implementation of circular economy principles implies the reliable measurement and monitoring of the impact of economic activities on sustainable development". Effective indicators should be relevant to the main issues covered and (statistical) data for evaluation should be available and comparable over time and across geographical, economic and political regions. Other sources recommend avoiding overly broad indicators (sets of indicators). While this may be politically and scientifically attractive, it is not always feasible. It is also recommended not to make the choice too difficult by suggesting to focus on a small set of meaningful key indicators, prioritising them through a participatory process to make them actionable and allow for follow-up. Indicators for monitoring tourism development on closed-loop principles could be developed in the policy process associated with the establishment of a pan-European Common Environmental Information System (CEIS). Digital platforms are widely seen as an opportunity to harmonise indicators, allowing a comprehensive picture that takes into account economic, socio-cultural and environmental aspects. In proposing appropriate indicators to measure and monitor the process of building a circular economy in tourism in ECE member States, one should start by identifying the key challenges in the tourism chain that are relevant in terms of their environmental impact, contribution to the Sustainable Development Goals and potential for applying circular economy principles. This is quite close to the definition of "hotspots" in the hotspot analysis framework promoted by the UNEP Life Cycle Initiative344. UNEP considers an environmental impact a hotspot if it accounts for more than 50 per cent of the total life-cycle impact across all stages of the life cycle of a good or service in any particular impact category (e.g. GHG emissions, energy or water consumption, waste), ensuring that the majority of the impact is accounted for.

In the remainder of this section, a simplified approach is used to develop provisional indicators at the national level, in which the main tourism elements are mapped to key categories of environmental impacts. Accordingly, indicators can be derived from these "hotspots", i.e. when the contribution of a particular

215

The contribution of the tourism element to the impact category is much more significant or more relevant than that of other tourism elements. In "warm spots", this contribution is significant but less relevant than in hot spots, and in "cold spots" it is almost or not relevant. In the course of this analysis, based on the specific literature on environmental impacts, which is briefly summarised in the general context sub-section above, several hotspots have been identified in relation to hotel operations, origin-destination transport, and events and activities. Service providers, while not having a direct impact, can serve as a driver. Several hot and warm spots can be identified as priority areas in the tourism chain with the potential to integrate closed-loop principles. These are the operation and construction of accommodation facilities and restaurant and bar activities, where such potential can be found in all impact categories except biodiversity. These range from the use of renewable energy to water conservation, building with closed-loop principles, utilising closed-loop food chains, increasing reuse and recycling and, as a result of some of these steps, reducing emissions. Similar potential can be identified for different activities. In transport, the greatest potential lies in saving energy by reducing distances and improving energy efficiency, as well as switching to renewable energy sources, resulting in lower emissions.

The final step is to identify preliminary indicators and measure their evolution in order to determine whether the tourism economy is now in line with closed-loop principles. Where applicable, such indicators may overlap with indicators of sustainable tourism development. In discussing indicators, the following subsections present preliminary indicators for monitoring the circular economy in tourism, indicating the origin of each indicator or the corresponding database. Each indicator is discussed from the perspective of the status and trends in ECE member States, data comparability and availability. Due to data limitations, sometimes only selected ECE member States from each subregion (European Union, Western Europe, Eastern Europe, South-Eastern Europe and Central Asia) are compared to show how the circular economy has evolved over the last decade. In most cases, although not always, bias towards the European Union due to lack of data has been avoided.

The development of indicators is hampered by a number of challenges. Currently, ECE member States do not have indicators that provide clear information on the application of closed-loop principles in the tourism sector, so a list of relevant indicators needs to be compiled and agreed upon. For several common aspects of the closed-loop, classification definitions vary from State to State. Despite recommended standards for the maintenance of tourism satellite accounts and, for example, the International Recommendations for Tourism Statistics, tourism data tend to be incomplete and difficult to compare. Data also vary in availability and quality across countries in the pan-European region. The most significant gaps are in data on modes of transport, transport lengths and almost all domestic tourism flows in terms of number of trips, arrivals, overnight stays, passenger-kilometres and modes of transport used. Finally, the detailed statistics needed for accurate closed-loop monitoring are generally not available. Digitalisation holds promise as an additional source of data and for better and more uniform measurement and monitoring, but this depends on the availability of uniform, high-quality and up-to-date data on the circular economy of tourism.

Waste reduction is one of the most important prerequisites for the transition to a circular economy, and tourism is a major source of waste generation at the local level. Tourist arrivals initially significantly increase municipal solid waste generation (per capita), up to a tipping point where an increase in tourist arrivals contributes to a decrease in municipal waste per capita, due to the counterbalancing technological effect associated with changes in the characteristics of tourism firms that arise when tourist arrivals increase. In order to achieve a circular tourism economy, special attention should be paid to countries with high tourism activity and high waste utilisation rates. Examples from the Netherlands, Norway and Turkey show that national municipal waste disposal rates (i.e. not used for composting, recycling or energy recovery) vary greatly between countries. In the Netherlands, 2.6 per cent of total municipal waste is disposed of, in Norway 9.7 per cent and in Turkey 88.4 per cent. And while in the Netherlands the share of waste disposal has halved since 2010, in Norway it has increased, mainly due to the growth of waste. In order to determine the real impact of tourism on waste generation dynamics in individual countries, information on more specific indicators should be collected in all countries. Multiplying the volume of waste by the share of tourism in national GDP348 gives a rough idea of the waste generated by tourism. This value can be considered a rough approximation of the ratio of the number of tourists to residents and tourist expenditure, which have been identified as drivers of municipal waste generation. For more detailed statistics, UNWTO proposes to apply its statistical programme for measuring sustainable tourism indicators (SP-STI) and tourism information may require direct input from the tourism industry, for example with an estimate of the amount of solid waste generated per tourist arrival. The European Tourism Indicators System (ETIS) proposes to measure the percentage of recycled waste per tourist against the total recycled waste generated per permanent resident per year. In future policies, tourism revenues could be used to invest in recycling facilities (including composting, and such pilot projects already exist) or to limit the maximum tourism capacity, if necessary to manage the amount of waste, tourism enterprises could be encouraged to actively reduce waste generation by prohibiting the use of disposable and non-recyclable goods and packaging and encouraging restaurants and hotels to give away free of charge unclaimed hh

There is strong evidence that tourists on holiday consume significantly more water than at home and compared to locals. Water consumption in the tourism sector is closely linked to energy production and food preparation, and is best restricted at tourist accommodation where most of the consumption occurs. In order to close the water cycle, it is necessary to endeavour to meet all demand from renewable water sources, including closed-loop water use. Therefore, fossil water sources (groundwater and glacial water) should not be utilised. As the main tourist flows occur during the warm and dry season, many (summer) tourist destinations suffer from water scarcity. In destinations where there are concerns about the availability of water to support tourism activities, it is not sufficient to record water consumption in the tourism sector alone. It is also necessary to keep records of water supplies and to record their change. The provisional indicator proposed to assess the degree of tourism water supply lock-in is based on the work of Gössling et al. and consists of two (national) sub-indicators: the share of water consumed in the tourism sector; and the share of renewable sources in total water supply (stocks). These indicators vary across the pan-European region;

the share of water consumed in the tourism sector is often high in Mediterranean countries, while the share of renewable sources in water supply varies. The share of water from renewable sources depends on the degree of water scarcity and therefore varies greatly between countries. The use of national indicators may mask water scarcity at regional and local scales. Based on current trends,

218

demand for freshwater in tourist destinations is increasing, putting pressure on renewable resources, and water scarcity is becoming an increasing problem due to climate change. In order to bridge the gap between the existing views of academia and industry practice, it is recommended that more comprehensive water management indicators that take into account the water situation in a particular area, the infrastructure planning process and its operation are used. These could be linked to the principles of the circular economy, such as indicators such as renewable water consumption per guest night (peak season), solar thermal and photovoltaic panels installed per bed, energy consumption per guest night. Future policy measures could focus on the mandatory application of water-saving technologies and the formulation of a water utilisation plan for arid regions, taking into account the need for water allocation for tourism, agriculture and the local population. Furthermore, studies have shown that informing tourists about the consequences of excessive water consumption and water scarcity issues can have a positive impact on reducing water consumption. Examples already exist, for example the municipality of Valencia in Spain measures the water footprint of tourism. In addition, advanced methods of obtaining water may become indispensable for tourism in the coming decades.

Energy consumption in the hotel and catering sector The hotel and catering sector accounts for 21 % of tourism-related emissions and is the main consumer of energy at tourist destinations, excluding transport.

The energy consumption of tourists and locals can vary greatly, in particular depending on the class of accommodation and the facilities of the accommodation. On the other hand, the emissions associated with energy consumption can be reduced through the use of renewable energy and energy-saving technologies.

Therefore, the share of energy from renewable sources in the total final energy consumption at tourist destinations can serve as an indicator of the closed loop of non-transport energy consumption in the tourism sector. The ECE SDG dashboard includes data on renewable energy sources for each ECE member State360. To better define the energy consumption of the tourism sector, the ETIS system proposes to measure annual renewable energy consumption compared to the total energy consumption of a tourism destination per year.

One limitation when comparing areas or countries is that the share of renewable energy in the energy mix varies greatly from country to country. For example, in Iceland 81.1 per cent

of energy production is from renewable sources, while Turkmenistan uses 99.9 per cent non-renewable sources. The average share of renewable energy sources in the energy mix of ECE member states is 21.5 per cent. The history of energy supply development defines the status quo; depending on the countries, there have been both positive and negative trends in the use of renewable energy sources. Future policies should aim at stimulating the switch to renewable energy sources, including in remote tourist destinations, and include appropriate requirements or incentives for the introduction of energy saving technologies in new facilities or modernisation.

Energy consumption in tourist transport and their role in climate change

Tourist transport is almost entirely dependent on fossil fuels and is the main source of CO2 emissions from tourism, with aircraft also having a significant non-CO2 impact on climate change and a 'radiative forcing' or heating effect caused by GHGs in the atmosphere. The shoulder between the permanent tourist residence and the tourist holiday destination accounts for the bulk of the tourist itinerary and hence energy consumption and emissions. In order to identify closed-loop measures in this hotspot, it is important to know what mode of transport tourists arrive and return by: aeroplane, car, cruise ship or a more environmentally friendly mode of transport such as bicycle, bus or train. The more tourists use these greener modes of transport and travel shorter distances, the more energy can be saved and emissions prevented. Compared to air transport, the opportunities to decarbonise transport through the use of renewable energy are also much greater for other modes of transport. The choice of travel mode is related to the availability of transport modes and the psychological preferences of a country's citizens.

Since the required energy consumption indicators for tourism transport are not routinely produced, it is suggested to analyse the share of domestic travel and the share of international travel by air. An increasing number of countries are voluntarily participating in the Carbon Offsetting and Reduction Scheme for International Aviation (CORSIA).With some caveats, in the case of large countries, domestic tourist travel tends to have lower emissions than foreign travel due to shorter distances and less use of air transport. In 2019, 73.3 % of trips made in ECE Member States were domestic, with the share strongly dependent on the size of the country, the number of domestic trips made within the European Union was 0.4 % higher than trips made outside the European Union.

48.6 % of inbound tourism in ECE member States was by air, with 49.3 % of tourism trips outside the European Union travelling by air, compared to 46.1 % . Between 2012 and 2019, outbound tourism using air transport increased by 34.8 % in these countries, with air travel accounting for 61.5 % of the total increase in outbound tourism.

Future policy measures should in most cases encourage investment in infrastructure for low-emission transport modes, such as rail, instead of air transport, and in the expansion of domestic tourism. In addition, the concept of climate-smart tourism should be promoted, as it aims to reorient international promotional investments in favour of less carbon-intensive options, such as longer stays. The construction and maintenance of tourism facilities (e.g. accommodation) is resource-intensive, a challenge that may well be addressed based on the principles of a circular economy. As these aspects have not yet been measured. In order to make the construction and maintenance of tourism facilities more circular, it is suggested to partly use recycled building materials and reclaimed furniture, to rent expensive machinery on long-term leases and to use easily repairable materials and interior finishes; however, these are difficult to use as indicators, in some cases the circular processes in construction are used for marketing purposes Future policies should support the use of recycled materials and furniture.

Sustainable tourism plans are extremely important and allow for the alignment of destination strategies with national sustainable development goals and for moving the level of application of closed-loop principles in tourism beyond mere impact reduction. In addition, some international processes - such as those defined in the ECE Protocol on Strategic Environmental Assessment - will help to reduce impacts and thus reduce the challenge of ensuring the implementation of closed-loop principles. The integration of sustainable development and circular economy policies into national tourism policy plans can be assessed to measure the sustainability of tourism and the degree of circularity in the sector. UNWTO and UNEP sustainable consumption and production models for tourism and characterised the scope of reporting on sustainable consumption and production.

According to the report, biodiversity and sustainable land use issues are present in

sustainable tourism development reports from around the world.
However, water efficiency policies are not covered and closed-loop principles are mentioned only once. Other gaps identified in the study relate to the integration of energy efficiency, emissions and waste management. The picture is similar with regard to sustainability. Specific guidance on how sustainability issues should be addressed in practice is found in country policies in only 55 per cent of cases. In order to implement closed-loop processes in tourism destinations, future policies should encourage the funding of marketing organisations that draw not only on the principles of sustainable development, but also on closed-loop systems and opportunities in their tourism development plans, learning from experiences with closed-loop tourism. Furthermore, policymakers should identify barriers to the development of a circular tourism economy and propose policy frameworks to overcome them, as well as inter-agency cooperation, in particular between tourism and environmental authorities, but also with other entities, including transport and energy authorities. International aviation has been identified as one of the sectors that is difficult to align with climate goals, despite the fact that European Union aviation is part of the European Union Emissions Trading Scheme. The production of electrofuels is based on a well-known energy-to-liquids process: jet fuel production (Jet A) using CO2, water and a significant amount of renewable energy. The source of CO2 can come from large industry, but eventually it can be captured directly from the air. In the latter case, it becomes possible to completely close the carbon cycle (hence the sometimes used term "closed cycle paraffin"). Compared to other environmentally friendly aviation fuels, the production of electrofuels requires 80 per cent less land, very little water and does not damage raw materials, nature or agriculture. The production of electrofuels for the (international) aviation industry is an ideal transnational example of applying the principles of the circular economy to tourism, which also contributes directly to international climate change mitigation goals in line with Sustainable Development Goal 13 (Combating Climate Change).
Various projects are currently under development. In the Netherlands, Shinkero, in co-operation with the Port of Amsterdam, Schiphol Airport, KLM and Skyenergy, is planning a commercial plant using waste CO2 and clean hydrogen at the Port of Amsterdam. Together with KLM, Schiphol Airport and SCV Energy, Skyenergy is also building an electrofuel plant in Delfzijl, the Netherlands. Zenid's initiative with Uniper, Rotterdam-Hague Airport, Clymeworks, Skyenergy and the Rotterdam-Hague Airport Innovation Programme involves the construction of a demonstration plant in Rotterdam to produce clean paraffin using CO2 captured from the air as feedstock. Norwegian consortium Norsk e-fuel plans to build a commercial facility to produce hydrogen-based renewable aviation fuel. KLM announced that a passenger flight had been flown using partially clean synthetic paraffin produced from CO2, water and renewable energy from the sun and wind.
However, the production process requires a very large amount of energy, which

may further widen the gap between the demand for renewable electricity and its supply, attempts to increase which have so far been unsuccessful, and the resulting fuel will be two to six times more expensive than Jet. Electric fuels cannot enter the market without a very substantial tax on paraffin produced from fossil fuels and/or subsidies, or without a mandatory requirement to use fuel blends with a gradual increase in the share of electric fuels, up to 100 per cent in 2050. Such a requirement would be the most direct and reliable way to reduce aviation emissions to zero by 2050, with the associated costs borne by airlines and hence passengers (polluter pays principle). Requirements to use fuel blends are already included in national air transport policies in Germany, the Netherlands, Norway and Sweden. The European Union has proposed a new "Fit for 55" regulatory package that includes a requirement to switch to fuel blends containing sustainable aviation fuels. In 2018, The Circular Hotels Leaders Group emerged in the Netherlands. The group, which currently comprises 12 hotels located mainly in Amsterdam, has already taken many steps towards environmental sustainability or is on the cusp of doing so. The group is exploring closed-loop business operations and shows that co-operation, in addition to knowledge, can open up new opportunities in this area. These include, but are not limited to, joint procurement and the pooling of waste streams for beneficial uses. One of the best-known examples is the Jakarta Hotel .

In Haarlem and Rotterdam in the Netherlands, similar groups have been established in the restaurant business (Circular Restaurants Leaders Group) to build on the experience of this hotel group. Each group in Haarlem and Rotterdam consists of about 20 restaurants that are also working on closed-loop solutions. Preventing food waste is an important challenge, but it is not the only focus. An important focus of this project is on closed-loop procurement (from sustainable local ingredients to zero-waste clothing and alternatives to plastic straws), packaging, menus, kitchen organisation, waste management and contact with guests.

In Spain, the Impulsa Baleares Foundation, in line with the recommendations of the One Planet Framework for Responsible Tourism Recovery, has created its own strategic framework of closed-loop principles for the hotel sector. It is designed to enable the adoption and monitoring of best practices in the sector, to stimulate the creation of closed-loop linkages throughout its production chain and thus contribute to closing gaps in the implementation of global principles related to environmental sustainability and tourism at the local level. The framework also proposes a set of criteria to enable hotel companies to track their progress in implementing closed-loop principles, using 81 key performance indicators that are directly linked to 125 business lines to incentivise the adoption of closed-loop best practices.

Selected indicators of environmental sustainability and circular economy, Jakarta Hotel, Amsterdam

1. Construction

- The Building Research Establishment's Environmental Assessment Method (BREEAM) - rated 'excellent' BREEAM is a method of certifying a sustainable built environment.

2. Energy consumption

• There are 1700 m2 of solar panels installed on the roof and on the solar side of the building.

• The winter garden cools the entire space inside the complex by 5 °C, so air conditioning is rarely required.

• Water from the Ei waterway surrounding the hotel was used to cool the building on all of its floors.

• A geothermal heat pump uses natural heat to heat the hotel's water.

3. Utilisation of water resources

• Irrigation system using rainwater and domestic water for watering the garden and plants.

• Water saving shower heads and taps to reduce water consumption by guests.

• All plastic water bottles (except those in the mini-bars) have been replaced by water filtration machines that purify tap water.

4. Food supply and disposal channels

- The hotel's restaurant and bakery mainly use local ingredients. Food waste is pressed into dense blocks which are used as compost.

5. Disposable plastic products

• Tough stance on single use plastic items, no plastic bottles sold.

• Re-fill toiletries bottles instead of using travel versions.

The Danish island of Bornholm is committed to environmental sustainability and carbon neutrality. Based on the Sustainable Development Goals, the municipality has defined eight development goals. This strategy for the development of this tourist destination, which makes no specific reference to the objectives of a circular economy, is close to being an example of a possible development of a tourist destination based on circular principles in its broad scope, systematic approach and goal of achieving carbon neutrality. The strategy was developed by the municipality, a tourism marketing organisation and a number of local actors, which allowed for

to achieve a successful transition over the past 13 years. This example shows how long-term strategies, jointly developed by key stakeholders, can have a major impact and support the transition to a circular economy.

The Bornholm goals for sustainable and carbon neutral development:

1. Business: making environmental sustainability good business.
2. Evidence-based environmental sustainability: document and track the green transition.
3. Carbon Neutral (in 2025 in energy production, in 2032 all waste becomes a resource, in 2035 a zero-emission society).
4. Mobility: make land transport environmentally friendly.
5. Housing: make sustainable housing part of our cultural identity.
6. Food: to take an avant-garde position in Danish organic food products.

7. Nature: Ensure that the protection of natural resources is of vital importance to all.
8. Social inclusion: ensure that everyone in Bornholm becomes part of the "bright green island".

Environmental governance relates to environmental and natural resource decision-making and the forms of interaction that take place between different actors, whether State, private sector or civil society, at different levels, which for the purposes of this assessment are limited to the regional, subregional and national levels. The fundamental principles of environmental governance include participation, rule of law, transparency, responsiveness, consensus, equity and inclusiveness, efficiency, effectiveness and accountability. Of primary interest here are decisions, often taken by consensus, that promote environmentally sustainable development. As the Ninth Ministerial Conference "Environment for Europe" is being held at the same time as a meeting of environment and education ministers, and because of the importance of education for shared and informed decision-making, this chapter also looks at education for sustainable development (ESD).Furthermore, given the importance of respecting human rights for good governance, Rights can be seen in terms of substantive rights, including the right to a clean, healthy and sustainable environmentZBB, and procedural rights, including the right to a clean, healthy and sustainable environmentZBB, and procedural rightsZBB.

The 2030 Agenda for Sustainable Development can also be seen as a framework for good governance, as such governance is key to the realisation of the 17 Sustainable Development Goals. However, it is more difficult and incomplete to identify good environmental governance indicators based on the 2030 Agenda. Not only do the indicators address environmental governance to a limited extent, but there is also a severe lack of data on relevant indicators.

Commitments to promote gender equality and women's empowerment are a key part of the 2030 Agenda and the Sustainable Development Goals, whose universal adoption demonstrates global recognition of the importance of gender equality and women's empowerment in achieving sustainable development. Effective environmental governance must therefore also consider and analyse the gender implications of environmental policies and programmes.

B. Intergovernmental bodies

1. Regional and subregional levels The highest-level regional environmental meeting is the Ministerial Conference "Environment for Europe", prepared by the ECE Committee on Environmental Policy; the outcomes of the Conference become the region's substantive input to the work of the United Nations Environment Assembly.Supporting environmental governance at the subregional level are many other international bodies, including:

a) The Green Economy and Environment Action Programme Task Force, established under the Environment for Europe ministerial process and serviced by the OECD, which focuses on supporting countries in Eastern Europe, the Caucasus and Central Asia in aligning their environmental and economic objectives;

b) The Executive Committee of the International Fund for Saving the Aral Sea, which promotes co-operation between Central Asian governments on water resources and environmental management. One of its subsidiary bodies is the Interstate Commission on Sustainable Development;

c) European Union bodies, including the European Environment Agency (EEA), whose task is to provide reliable independent information on the environment through its European Environmental Information and Observation Network (Eionet) linking member countries (European Union members as well as Iceland, Liechtenstein, Norway, Switzerland and Turkey) and cooperating countries (Western Balkans). With the dissolution of the Regional Environmental Centre for Central and Eastern Europe, only two (sub)regional centres remain: for the Caucasus and for Central Asia.

2. Treaty bodies

The region's multilateral environmental agreements (MEAs) also provide a forum for environmental governance through their treaty bodies, including governing bodies, working groups and bodies responsible for implementing or complying with such agreements. These agreements include the ECE environmental treaties, as well as, for example, the Barcelona Convention, the Agreement on the Conservation of Small Cetaceans of the Baltic and North Seas, the Framework Convention for the Protection and Sustainable Development of the Carpathians and the Alpine Convention aimed at the protection and sustainable development of the Alps. Although the number of participants exceeds the 50 per cent level noted in the GEO-6 regional report, being a contracting party to these agreements and participating in the meetings of their governing bodies is not sufficient to ensure better environmental governance.

Nevertheless, the effectiveness of such agreements can be measured through implementation and compliance mechanisms, assessments of the achievement of their objectives and regular reporting under the agreements. For example, one of the obligations of parties to the Water Convention is to conclude transboundary water co-operation agreements. This commitment is in line with Sustainable Development Goal indicator 6.5.2 "Proportion of transboundary water basins covered by transboundary water co-operation agreements in force water-use"

In the case of the Espoo Convention and its Protocol on Strategic Environmental Assessment, the number of cases where their environmental assessment procedures have been applied to projects, plans and programmes is a good indicator of their effectiveness and improved management, but many parties to these agreements do not have centralized databases and there is no legal obligation to report on their practical application. Another indicator of the effectiveness of the Espoo Convention can be gauged from the work of the Committee for the Implementation of the Convention, clarifications were requested and found satisfactory in all cases, and two of the 33 parties to the Protocol were also approached by the Committee after finding that the legislation of one of the parties was not in conformity with the treaty. In the case of the Air Convention, one of the main obligations is the reporting of national emission inventories. Emission inventories submitted by parties to the Convention show reductions in emissions of air pollutants in the region in more than 90 per cent of cases.

Regular reporting by countries of their emission inventories allows for the assessment of emission reduction trends and the impact of emission control strategies to support policy and decision-making. In this regard, the ECE scientific assessment report detailed reductions in airborne concentrations of dispersed particulate matter (PM) in measuring station areas in Europe and the United States by about one third and in Canada by 4 per cent between 2000 and 2023, resulting in the prevention of about 600,000 premature deaths annually. The Protocol on Pollutant Release and Transfer Registers requires parties to establish and maintain publicly accessible national PRTRs.

C. National institutions and legislation

At the national level, the weight of the national environmental policy body reflects the prioritisation of environmental protection in policy (in small Western European states, due to the small number of ministries, ministries often cover different areas, including environmental protection). One indicator of national legislation on environmental governance is the existence of national laws on environmental impact assessment (EIA) and strategic environmental assessment (SEA).

D. Civil society

The role of civil society in environmental governance is generally defined by three themes: public participation in decision-making, access to information and access to justice in environmental matters. These are the three key elements of the Aarhus Convention and the overall Sustainable Development Goal indicator on access to information (16.10.2, number of countries with constitutional, legislative and/or policy guarantees for citizens' access to information adopted and in place), which tracks fairly closely with the number of parties to the convention.

Indicator 16.7.2 of the Sustainable Development Goals (proportion of the population that considers decision-making inclusive and responsive, by sex, age, disability and population group) would provide a similar picture for the public participation component of decision-making, but data are currently sorely lacking. Access to justice is even more difficult to track. Countries should further develop specific mechanisms for collecting, coordinating, collating and processing information from various statistical sources, which is necessary for monitoring access to justice for members of the public in environmental matters. Countries should also include in their national monitoring systems indicators for target 16.3 of the Sustainable Development Goals ("promote the rule of law at the national and international levels and ensure equal access to justice for all") with disaggregated data related to environmental cases. Useful indicators of access to justice in

environmental matters might include the number of environmental courts or courts with environmental divisions or the number of environmental lawyers per capita.
The number of environmental defenders who have been killed or harassed and persecuted (in defence of human rights, their land and the environment) could be used to track progress on Sustainable Development Target 16.10 ("ensure public access to information and protect fundamental freedoms in accordance with national legislation and international agreements"), but in the pan-European region the number is fortunately small.
The Espoo Convention and its Protocol on Strategic Environmental Assessment promotes access to information through mandatory public notification of projects, plans and programmes that are likely to have a significant impact on the environment, and provides for public participation and due consideration of members of the public in decision-making and planning on such matters.
At the same time, challenges remain in the implementation of certain provisions relating to access to justice and public participation. Common obstacles to full and effective implementation of the Convention often include insufficient awareness among public authorities, financial constraints and a lack of human resources and technical tools, or the poor quality of those resources, combined with insufficient coordination among various environmental authorities, public authorities, NGOs and the . Some countries reported having made significant legislative changes to transpose the provisions of the Convention into national legislation.
However, the implementation process still varies from country to country, depending on, inter alia, legal traditions, governance structures and socio-economic conditions. With regard to access to information, only a few Parties to the Convention have updated and amended their national legislation, as most countries already adequately implement the provisions of the Convention in this area. However, some obstacles remain with regard to access to information, including difficulties in distinguishing between environmental and non-environmental information and in applying an appropriate procedure for dealing with requests from the public. Ensuring the rights of the public to environmental information, while taking into account rights related to trade and industrial secrets, statistical and personal data confidentiality, intellectual property and copyright, remains a challenge in many countries. Many parties to the Aarhus Convention have noted delays and non-compliance with deadlines in providing requested information, in relation to the COVID-19 pandemic. Some parties continue to note problems with procedures for dealing with "sham decisions" on access to information requests. Some parties reported obstacles leading to the provision of incomplete information, such as lack of database interoperability, incomplete and fragmented data. On the positive side, parties across the region reported significant progress in making environmental information available in electronic databases that are easily accessible to the public through open telecommunications networks.
This underlines the important contribution of CEIS to good environmental

governance. Numerous effective electronic tools, such as electronic databases, publicly accessible government e-services, websites and information portals, which are regularly updated and improved, are further developed in this area. Despite the progress made in this area, more efforts are needed in the countries of the subregions of Eastern Europe, Central Asia and South-Eastern Europe to establish and maintain more effective information and online environmental monitoring systems. This applies in particular to pollution registers and emissions.

Parties to the Protocol on Strategic Environmental Assessment and several non-parties reported that almost all had provided "timely public communication" of the draft plan or programme and environmental report and that this had been done through both official notices and electronic . In addition, in some cases it was indicated that other means were also used, such as publication in an electronic journal for official notices and in newspapers, as well as mailings. Most respondents defined the "public concerned" based on the geographic location of the proposed plan/programme and/or by providing information to the entire public, giving their representatives the opportunity to self-identify as the public concerned. Many also considered the nature of the environmental impacts of the plan or programme under consideration (significance, extent, accumulation). In order to effectively and efficiently communicate the regional/local plan or regional/local programme, information is disseminated at the regional and/or local level.

With regard to the implementation of the provisions of the Aarhus Convention on Public Participation in Eastern Europe, Central Asia and South-Eastern Europe, countries reported on recent legislative changes. In the case of some parties, these changes were aimed at establishing a legal framework for public participation in EIA and SEA processes and the issuance of environmental permits, while in others the focus was on improving existing relevant provisions. Similar trends in Eastern Europe, Central Asia390 and South-Eastern Europe were reported by parties to the Protocol on Strategic Environmental Assessment during the third review of the Protocol's implementation between 2016 and 2018.391 The Aarhus Convention and the Aarhus Convention on Biological Diversity, however, have not yet been implemented. Nevertheless, Aarhus Convention parties from these subregions noted many obstacles to the effective implementation of public participation. Parties from the European Union subregion, Iceland, Norway, Switzerland, the United Kingdom and the European Union continue to improve procedures for public participation in activity-specific decision-making processes and to expand the range of decisions and decision-making stages requiring public participation.

In terms of EIA procedures, parties to the Aarhus Convention are increasingly ensuring participation in the pre-assessment procedure, at the scoping stage and at the stage of the draft EIA decision prior to its adoption. Parties to the Protocol on Strategic Environmental Assessment reported that they had provided opportunities for the public to submit comments and opinions on draft plans and programmes in a number of economic areas that form the basis for obtaining consent for the development of projects requiring EIA, and that the public was increasingly involved in the pre-assessment, scoping and drafting stages of the environmental report. Interested citizens can do so primarily by submitting comments to the relevant authority or coordinator and by participating in public hearings.

Other types of decisions affecting the environment where the parties to the Aarhus Convention have made efforts to ensure public participation include construction and planning decisions, integrated environmental permits, decisions on environmental protection measures, decisions on whether to authorise projects that may have significant impacts on Natura 2000 sites, nature and landscape protection decisions, forest management decisions, environmental licensing, decisions on the extension of the operational life of the Natura 2000 network, and decisions on the use of the Natura 2000 network.

Under the Protocol on Strategic Environmental Assessment, all parties are required to ensure that comments received through public participation are given due consideration when adopting a plan or programme. The same applies to parties to the Espoo Convention for projects that may have significant adverse impacts. Other relevant instruments include the 2021 United Nations policy brief "Transforming Extractive Industries for Sustainable Development", which focuses on ensuring sustainable management of natural resources.Overall, the most challenging component for parties to the Aarhus Convention remains the implementation of its access to justice provisions.

The two issues most frequently cited by the parties were as follows:

-regulating the rights of environmental NGOs to seek judicial or administrative remedies in environmental cases (standing);

- financial obstacles.

Parties are aware of these difficulties and the information provided on the work undertaken shows their real interest in promoting the implementation of this component of the Convention. Some parties have amended their legislation as a result of developments in jurisprudence or on the basis of recommendations by the Aarhus Convention Compliance Committee.

Four positive trends have been identified during the current reporting cycle, namely:

a) Improving the admissibility of environmental litigation, representing public interest;

b) An increase in the number of cases in which courts and other supervisory bodies verify the substantive legality of contested decisions, actions or omissions;

c) Taking measures to remove or reduce financial barriers; (d) Promoting awareness and specialisation of the judiciary and other legal professionals in the field of environmental protection.

All reporting Parties indicated in their reports that their legislation provides for the principles of non-discrimination, equality before the law and protection from punishment, prosecution and harassment of persons exercising their rights under the Convention. At the same time, however, practice on the criminalisation, prosecution and harassment of environmental defenders varies considerably between Parties. Available research shows that women are often excluded from environmental decision-making This occurs at all levels:

- on a personal relationship level;
- at home;
- in private companies;
- at the local and national government level. E. Private sector

One indicator of private sector engagement is the number of companies publishing environmental sustainability reports (indicator 12.6.1 of the Sustainable Development Goals). A simple indicator is whether a company in a country publishes a minimum report, but the idea is rendered meaningless by the small number of such reports. As reporting improves, more meaningful data may become available. Another indicator related to private sector governance is the number of countries that have laws and regulations on mandatory corporate sustainability reporting

The rather limited amount of reporting on environmental, social and governance (ESG) aspects may to some extent be explained by the fact that in most countries in the pan-European region small and medium-sized enterprises (SMEs) are excluded from mandatory reporting tools, as SMEs constitute the majority of companies.

The European Union's Non-Financial Reporting Directive (NFRD) requires certain large and publicly traded companies to disclose material on environmental, social and human resources issues, such as anti-corruption, anti-bribery and human rights. The forthcoming Corporate Sustainability Reporting Directive , which will amend or replace the DNFO, should be a game changer for European Union member States, requiring all large and listed companies in the European Union to introduce mandatory environmental sustainability reporting standards, as part of the Protocol on Pollutant Release and Transfer Registers, which notes the lack of technical capacity of companies to monitor emissions and transfers of pollutants.

The report of the 2020 survey on lessons learned in the implementation of the Protocol on Pollutant Release and Transfer Registers395 indicates that PRTRs have evolved significantly since the adoption of the Protocol in 2003. PRTRs play an important role in ensuring transparency and public participation in environmental decision-making processes.

F. Gender issues

Gender mainstreaming is important for both men and women. The importance of gender mainstreaming in policies and programmes stems from the fact that the needs, responsibilities and roles of men and women are different. If policies and programmes are developed without analysing their impact on men and women, there may be negative consequences, especially for women. In addition, the male perspective is so entrenched in society that policies, programmes and infrastructure are often male-centred even when a gender-neutral approach is taken. As a result of

this so-called 'gender-blind' approach, policies and programmes are male-only.
In environmental governance, it is important to achieve gender responsiveness in order to address the needs and interests of both women and men equally and to mitigate the negative effects of discriminatory policies, strategies or programmes. In addition, such approaches ensure that environmental policies are equitable and benefits are distributed fairly.
As part of a just transition to a sustainable society, policies must be designed with women in mind, with the need for women to participate in decision-making. This is particularly relevant for functions that will be automated in the future and roles in the informal economy where women make up a significant proportion. Approaches to gender mainstreaming in environmental governance should also recognise differences in women's experiences. Discrimination on the basis of, for example, racism, social status, age or disability results in different life experiences for women. A one-size-fits-all approach to gender mainstreaming should therefore be avoided.
Although there is no common vision for gender mainstreaming in environmental governance in the pan-European region, some ECE subprogrammes have developed guidelines and have incorporated gender perspectives into their work. For example, the guidelines of the Committee on Housing and Land Management have been revised, recommending gender analysis in housing and urban development policies. The ECE Gender-Responsive Standards Initiative prepared a Declaration on Gender-Responsive Standards and Standards Development, which invites all standardisation bodies to mainstream gender into their procedures in order to ultimately promote gender equality. In addition, the nineteenth session of the Steering Committee of the Transport, Environment and Health Pan-European Programme on Transport, Environment and Health Steering Committee in October 2021 decided that further work on gender mainstreaming should be undertaken and integrated into the work plan The complexity of analysing environmental governance from a gender perspective is due in particular to the lack of baseline and disaggregated data demonstrating how environmental policies affect women. However, even non-disaggregated data is lacking for gender governance indicators. For example, data on Sustainable Development Goal indicator 5.C.1, which provides an indication of the proportion of countries with mechanisms to track and disclose public expenditure on gender equality and women's empowerment, is available in only 34 per cent of countries, while data on Sustainable Development Goal indicator 5.1.1, on the presence or absence of a legal framework to promote, monitor and enforce gender equality and non-discrimination, is available in fewer countries.
G. Analysing progress and identifying future steps The ECE and OECD peer reviews of environmental performance (EPRs) provide a mechanism for regular, impartial analyses of progress in environmental governance. The reviews also provide recommendations for improving environmental performance and

management, and describe the process for following up on recommendations made in the previous review.

EPRs conducted in the pan-European region since this work started more than 25 years ago. Over the past 25 years, the ECE and OECD methodologies have evolved. In the latest, fourth cycle of ECE reviews, interested countries will be offered the possibility of including a non-exus nexus option (e.g. water - food - energy - ecosystems, air - transport - health or water - soil - waste). The nexus approach would build on the principle of integrating governance and management across all components of the nexus to make recommendations aimed at enhancing policy coherence, synergies and mutual benefits, and at identifying concessions (or trade-offs) and reducing them over time. This approach is also expected to contribute to the transition to a green economy and improved resource efficiency. The implementation of the recommendations on non-vacuum interactions will require enhanced joint action and collective efforts by relevant institutions and stakeholders.

Recommendations from the environmental performance review and implemented by Member States reviewed by many countries reviewed three times 235

at intervals of 5-15 years. Each country review analyses the implementation of recommendations from the previous review. For example, in 2023, the overall estimated implementation rate for the two countries undergoing the third review, Kazakhstan and North Macedonia, was 70 per cent. In Kazakhstan, 28 (80 per cent) of the 35 recommendations from the previous review (in 2008) were implemented, partially implemented or in progress. In Northern Macedonia, 29 (63 per cent) of the 46 recommendations from the previous review (in 2011) were implemented, partially implemented or under implementation.

In both countries, full implementation of the recommendations from their second review was not yet achieved in 2023. Lack of capacity and resources, as well as gaps in legislation, institutional development and administrative organisation, and frequent changes in the institutional framework and/or public policy direction were identified as the main obstacles in the work of these countries in implementing the EPR recommendations. The ECE EPRs of the fourth cycle will cover topics similar to those of the third cycle reviews and will focus on environmental governance and finance, national-international cooperation, the state of environmental components and the state of the environment. The review of the results of the relevant targets of the Sustainable Development Goals and the green economy remains important. At the request of the country under review, the coverage of the green economy could be expanded to address the circular economy, the climate change pillar would be expanded and would continue to focus on, inter alia, climate change impacts on priority sectors, mainstreaming climate change adaptation in priority sectors, GHG abatement and low-carbon development. The fourth cycle EPRs will continue to address issues related to human rights and the environment, including mainstreaming the needs of vulnerable groups. The substantive content of the EPRs of the fourth cycle will continue to be decided on a flexible basis, taking into account the specific needs of each country under review. The evaluation of the implementation of the recommendations of previous EPRs will continue to feature prominently.

Education for Sustainable Development (ESD) equips people with the knowledge and skills to enable them to lead healthy and productive lives in harmony with nature and with concern for social values, gender equality and cultural diversity. Such education also empowers people to play an active role in environmental governance. The ECE Strategy on Education for Sustainable Development serves as a framework for ESD in the pan-European region. A questionnaire is sent periodically to ECE member States to collect information on the state of ESD in each region.

Country. Six issues are tracked against a set of 51 criteria. The General Assembly also adopted a resolution on ESD in the overall context of the 2030 Agenda for Sustainable Development. It called on the international community to provide inclusive and equitable quality education at all levels so that all people can have access to lifelong learning opportunities that help them acquire the necessary knowledge and skills to seize opportunities to participate fully in society and contribute to sustainable development. While existing policies and MEAs, institutions, the private sector and civil society are contributing to environmental protection and progress has been made in some areas across the region, the assessment of status and trends and the policy recommendations contained in the thematic chapters point to the need to further strengthen environmental governance and existing policies in the region and to make the necessary adjustments to address significant gaps and inequalities.

The environmental governance, environmental legislation and policy landscape in the pan-European region has evolved and become more integrated and coherent since the Eighth "Environment for Europe" Ministerial Conference (Batumi, Georgia), in particular as a result of developments under key mechanisms such as the 2030 Agenda for Sustainable Development, the Paris Agreement and other multilateral environmental agreements (MEAs). This landscape is based on a much-needed science-policy interface with key elements of monitoring, evaluation and knowledge building, and is enabled by partnerships and co-operation between stakeholders and countries in the pan-European region.

As emphasised in this assessment, while progress has been made in environmental protection in some areas, there are significant gaps that pose a threat to human health and the environment in the pan-European region, the environmental assessment has identified knowledge gaps in various areas including air quality, freshwater, marine ecosystems, land and soil. In addition, there are knowledge and data gaps in the area of chemicals and waste, including e-waste, and most countries lack common policy objectives on biodiversity, resource efficiency and waste prevention, and the development of sustainable infrastructure 237 and the circular economy. Monitoring and measurement of environmental indicators still lags behind most other sectors, and disaggregated information is scarce. The assessment also found that there is also room for improvement in integrated environmental planning and integrated policies, including with regard to environment and health, particularly in countries in the eastern part of the region.

In addition, the environmental governance system in the pan-European region remains partly fragmented in terms of policy application, institutional strengthening and legislative harmonisation, as evidenced by the incomplete participation of countries in existing MEAs, as well as in their implementation and reporting.

Tracking progress and evaluating the effectiveness of policies in the region also remains a challenge due to the lack of: a) data and information;

(b) Established standard procedures for assessing whether the policy is fit for purpose.

The indicators selected in the assessment provide only a limited indication of where progress has been made and what changes are expected in the coming years. Nevertheless, they provide insights into areas where urgent action is needed.The availability and accessibility of timely, relevant and reliable data are essential to ensure informed decision-making, transparency and public participation. . The lack of baseline data, especially for assessing the sustainability of infrastructure and the application of circular economy principles to sustainable tourism, illustrates the need to better integrate the environmental dimension of the Sustainable Development Goals and the socio-economic dimensions of sustainable development.

In addition to enhancing participation in existing MEAs and international policy mechanisms, including the Batumi Initiative for a Green Economy (BIG-E), there is a need to: (a) develop policies and set consistent quantitative targets to better address emerging issues, including the circular economy and sustainable infrastructure, to support the transition to sustainable development in the region, and (b) ensure better implementation of policies on the ground, for example by scaling up successful pilot schemes, mobilising and mobilising the private sector, and (c) ensure that policies are more fully implemented on the ground.

Strengthening the knowledge base in support of environmental policies is another critical condition for improving environmental management. Increased use of geospatial data and new technologies, including big data, artificial intelligence and, in particular, machine learning, as well as increased digitalisation, will enhance the efficiency and effectiveness of strategy integration, provided that they are well managed. Strong partnerships, both within and across borders, will be critical and will need to be further strengthened.Little time remains to ensure the successful implementation of the 2030 Agenda. As a recent assessment in the publication Sustainable Development Goals: How well the 2030 Agenda is being implemented shows, by 2030 the ECE region will have met only 23 of the 169 targets of the Sustainable Development Goals and only 7 targets related to the environment and climate change. For 57 targets, progress needs to be accelerated and for 9 targets, the current trend needs to be reversed. There is insufficient data to assess the fulfilment of 80 targets. It is therefore essential to maximise the use of existing instruments and initiatives in support of the Sustainable Development Goals in the coming years. If necessary, additional measures and more ambitious targets, e.g. on e-waste or resource efficiency, can accelerate the implementation of the political agenda.

The following courses of action have been identified as creating favourable conditions for a successful transition to a green and circular economy and for sustainable development in the region.

A. Improved strategies and implementation and scaling up of activities

1. Promoting participation in multilateral environmental agreements and harmonisation of policies and legislation Policy fragmentation across the region should be reduced in order to promote and participate in existing MEAs and support countries in ensuring coherence and harmonisation of legislation.

2. Accelerating the implementation of the Pan-European Strategic Framework for a Green Economy Greater participation in the Pan-European Strategic Framework for a Green Economy and the Batumi Initiative for a Green Economy is needed. Governments and public and private entities should intensify their activities through voluntary commitments in the form of green economy measures and include, inter alia, commitments to the circular economy and sustainable infrastructure development, including by promoting nature-based solutions. Successful pilot measures, including those illustrated in the case studies presented in the present assessment, can be scaled up or replicated.

3. Developing and adopting common harmonised policies in the pan-European region on emerging themes, including circular economy and sustainable infrastructure

To address emerging challenges related to increasing pressures on ecosystems and health, the development and adoption of systemic policy frameworks across the region in support of a green economy and the transition to sustainable development will be critical to keep pace with the pace of change in an increasingly complex world and to address emerging challenges. Possible areas of synergy include the adoption of common system policies with shared goals related to circular economy, sustainable infrastructure and resource efficiency. Policies should be gender-sensitive.

4. Strengthening mechanisms for monitoring the effectiveness of policies and legislation, including at the international level Tracking progress and evaluating the effectiveness of policies in the region remain challenging, and standardised procedures are often needed to assess whether policies are meeting their objectives and to address data and information gaps.

B. Investing in just transition and reorienting funding, in particular towards sustainable infrastructure, circular economy and nature-based solutionsThe pandemic has led to an unprecedented global economic downturn with high loss of life and employment in some sectors. It exposed gaps in knowledge, capacity, access to basic services and gender equality. However, the pandemic has also created an opportunity to redress resource exploitation, increased GHG emissions and other injustices that have negatively affected ecosystems and human well-being. Countries should seize this opportunity to invest in a just green transition.

1. Investing and redirecting finance to support a just transition Governments and private actors need to invest and redirect finance to support sustainable infrastructure, circular economy and especially nature-based solutions (NBS). While the transition will require large investments, the pan-European region will reap huge benefits in terms of both reduced pressures and impacts on ecosystems and nature, as well as the resulting health benefits and new economic opportunities. Where possible, investments in ROPFs should be prioritised in the interest of enhancing sustainability, with climate-friendly construction and operation.

2. Enhancing participation and access to information in environmental governance Effective environmental governance is based on broad participation, including public participation, and pluralistic governance, which are basic conditions for a just transition. In addition, participatory processes in planning, implementing and evaluating the effectiveness of actions to ensure a just transition, with a focus on the participation of vulnerable groups and access to justice as required, are necessary to ensure optimal solutions and support. Access to and availability of timely and reliable information is essential.

3. Investing in capacity development and education for sustainable developmentTransition to sustainable development requires developing and investing in the capacity and education of responsible authorities, the private sector and civil society.

C. Strengthening the science-policy interface and harnessing technology and innovation

The pan-European region is home to many outstanding scientific organisations, universities, research centres and individuals with the capacity to innovate and fill knowledge and data gaps. To support existing and future environmental policy objectives, the dialogue between science and policy, as well as monitoring of the environment and progress in policy implementation, needs to be strengthened. Innovation and technology, including Earth observation, big data backed by artificial intelligence analysis, and developments in digitalisation and citizen science, offer great opportunities for the pan-European region to step up the process of expanding the knowledge base to complement existing monitoring.

1. Increased use of technology and innovation to support systems thinking, Decision-making can benefit from a closer science-policy interface, supported by innovation and data-driven technologies. Digitalisation in all domains, while respecting individual rights, will be critical to improve understanding of the complex processes and interactions between human needs, environmental and

social impacts and planetary boundaries.
2 Utilising existing knowledge and potential new sources Utilising existing knowledge, tools and systems is beneficial not only from an economic point of view, but also for sustainability reasons. The ECE and OECD environmental performance review programmes, SEIS, various UNEP assessments and the EEA reports "European Environment: State and Prospects" are examples of existing knowledge products and tools in the pan-European region. Their further development and harmonisation with emerging policy needs should be supported. Use of the revised ECE
The Guidelines for the Application of Environmental Indicators and the ECE Set of Environmental Indicators in line with SEIS principles and the updated Recommendations on Enhancing the Effective Use of Electronic Media adopted by the Meeting of the Parties to the Aarhus Convention will contribute to sound policymaking. At the same time, improved environmental monitoring and reporting will facilitate reporting on Sustainable Development Goal indicators.
D. Developing and strengthening partnership initiatives and cooperation at the regional and subregional levels To achieve the Sustainable Development Goals and other global and regional policy goals, Governments, the private sector, academia and citizens must join forces. In the pan-European region, various forms of cooperation, partnerships, institutional information exchange and citizen engagement have contributed to improved environmental protection in certain areas. However, challenges remain in many areas, including in building partnerships on emerging policy themes.
1. Strengthening existing partnerships to address regional challenges
Governments should promote co-operation at all levels to address transboundary environmental problems, including integrated water resources management, prevention of industrial and chemical accidents, environmental impact assessment and establishment of environmental information systems in accordance with the principles and basic provisions of CEIS.
2. Developing new partnerships on emerging policy themes Governments and other actors should consider developing new partnerships on emerging and urgent policy themes, including the circular economy, sustainable infrastructure, resource efficiency and waste management.

## List of references used

1 Adderley, B., J. Reducing the cost of post-combustion carbon dioxide capture to 2030. 2016. Battiston, S. Accounting for finance - key to climate mitigation pathways. Science, pp.918-920

2 Adderley, B., J. Carey, J. Gibbins, M. Lukjaud, and R. Smith, 2016. Carbon dioxide capture following combustion

3 Battiston, S., Monasterolo, I., Riahi, C., and van Ruijven, B.J., 2021. Accounting for finance - key to developing climate mitigation pathways. Science, 372(6545), pp.918920.

4 Brutschin, E. 2021. Multivariate feasibility assessment of low-carbon scenarios. Environmental Research Letters, 16(6), .064069. Reducing costs to 2030 and beyond, Faraday Discussion on CCS.

5 Bauer, C., Trayer, K., Multivariate assessment of the feasibility of low-carbon scenarios. Environmental Research Letters, 16(6), p.064069.pp.66-75.

6 Bühler R., Pucher J., editors (2021a). Cycling for sustainable cities. Cambridge, MA: MIT Press (mitpress.mit.edu/books/cycling-sustainable-cities).

7 Buhler R., Pucher J. (2021b). COVID-19 Impacts on Cycling, 2019-2020. Transp Rev. 4:1-8. doi:10.1080/01441647.2021.1914900.

8 Buehler R, Pucher J, Bauman A (2020). Physical activity from walking and cycling for daily trips in the United States, 2001-2017: Demographic, Socioeconomic, and Geographic Variation. J Transp Health. 16:100811. doi:10.1016/j.jth.2019.100811.

9 Bundesministeriums für Verkehr und digitale Infrastruktur [German Federal Ministry of Transport and Digital Infrastructure] (2017). Mobilität in Tabellen [Mobility in Tables] [website]. Berlin: Bundesministeriums für Verkehr und digitale Infrastruktur (https://mobilitaet-in-tabellen.dlr.de/mit/login.html?brd ,) (in German).

10 Bundesamt für Statistik [Swiss Federal Bureau of Statistics] (2012). Mikrozensus Mobilität und Verkehr 2010 [Microcensus Mobility and Transport 2010]. Neuchâtel, Bundesamt für Statistik (https:// www.bfs.admin.ch).

11 Bundesamt für Statistik [Swiss Federal Bureau of Statistics] (2015). Strassenverkehrsunfälle: beteiligte Objekte nach Objektart [Road traffic accidents: involved objects and types crashes] [website]. Neuchâtel: Bundesamt für

Statistik (https://www.pxweb.bfs.admin.ch/pxweb/en/px-x-1106010100_105/- /px- x-1106010100_105.px/) (in German).

12 Bundesamt für Statistik [Swiss Federal Bureau of Statistics] (2017).

Tagesdistanz, Tagesunterwegszeit und Anzahl Etappen mit Velo und E-Bike nach Verkehrszweck [Daily distance travelled, daily travel time and number of segments where bicycles and electric bicycles were used depending on the purpose of the trip].
[website]. Neuchâtel: Bundesamt für Statistik. (https://www.bfs.admin.ch/
13 Buning RJ, Lulla V (2021). Bicycle use by visitors: tracking spatio-temporal visitor behaviour using big data. J Sustain Tour. 29(4):711-731. doi:10.1080/09669582.2020.1825456.
14 Bunn F, Colleir T, Frost C, Ker K, Roberts I, Wentz R (2003). Traffic calming for road traffic injury prevention: a systematic review and meta-analysis. Inj Prev. 9(3):200-204. doi:10.1136/ip.9.3.200.
15 Cabral L, Kim AM, Shirgaokar M (2019). Low-load cycling connectivity: Assessment of the Network Build-Out in Edmonton, Canada. Case Stud Transp Policy. 7(2):230-238. doi:org/10.7939/r3-ef3w-9397.
16 Cairns J, Warren J, Garthwaite K, Greig G, Bambra S (2015). Drive slowly: An umbrella review of the impact of 20mph zones and speed limits on health and health inequalities. J Public Health (Oxf). 37(3):515-520. doi:10.1093/pubmed/ fdu067.
17 Cairns S et al. (2008). The sensible choice: Assessing the potential to achieve traffic reduction through soft measures. Transp Rev 28(5):593-618.
doi:10.1080/01441640801892504.
18 Calvo M, Marquez R (2020). How Seville became a city of cyclists [website]. Vision Zero Cities Journal (https:// medium.com/vision-zero-cities-journal/how-seville-became-a-city-of-cyclists-fba864b4be66).
19 Cameron TA (2010). Euthanasia of the value of statistical life. Rev Environ Econ Policy, 4(2):161-178. doi:10.1093/ reep/req010.
20 Carlson JA, Steel C, Bejarano CM, Beauchamp MT, Davis AM, Sallis JF, et al (2020). Walking school bus programmes: Implementation Factors, Implementation Outcomes, and Student Outcomes, 2017-2018. Prev Chronic Dis.17.
doi:10.5888/pcd17.200061.
21 Carlson K., Ermagun A., Murphy B., Owen A., Levinson D. (2019). Safety in Numbers for Bicyclists at Urban Intersections. Transp Res Rec. 2673(6):677-684. doi:10.1177%2F0361198119846480.
22 Castro A, Haupp-Berghausen M, Dons E, Standaert A, Laeremans M, Clark A et al (2019). Physical activity of electric bicycle users compared to conventional bicycle users and non-cyclists: Insights from health and transport data from an online survey in seven European cities. Transp Res Interdiscip Perspect, 1:100017. doi:10.1016/j.trip.2019.100017.

23 Castro A, Kalmeier C, Getschi T (2018). Exposure-adjusted cycling and walking mortality rates in European countries. London: International Transport Federation, Paris: Organisation for Economic Co-operation and Development (https://www.itf-oecd.org/ exposure-adjusted-road-fatality-rates-cycling-and-walking-european-countries ).
24 Castro A, Künzli N, Götschi T (2017). Health benefits of reduced exposure to PM10 and NO2 after implementation of an air cleaning plan in the Lausanne-Morge agglomeration. Int J Hyg Environ Health. 220(5):829-839. doi:10.1016/j. ijheh.2017.03.012.
24 Celis-Morales CA, Lyall DM, Welsh P, Anderson J, Steell L, Guo Y, et al (2017). Association between active commuting and incidents of cardiovascular disease, cancer and mortality: a prospective cohort study. BMJ. 357.
doi:10.1136/bmj.j1456.
25 Cherp, A. 2021. National dynamics of wind and solar energy growth versus growth required to meet global climate goals. Nature Energy, 6(7), pp.742-754.
26 Chen C-F, Huang C-Y (2021). An investigation of the impact of bike sharing for tourism on tourist experience and its implications. Curr Issues Tour. 24(1):134-148 doi:10.1080/13683500
27 Chimba D, Mbuya C (2019). Modelling the impact of traffic calming strategies.
Centre for Transportation Research Reports. 42 (https:// scholarworks.wmich.edu/transportation-reports/42).
28 CHIPS Project (2022). Degree of separation from road transport [website]. Lille: Interreg Northwest Europe ( https://cyclehighways.eu/index.php?id=225).
29 Choi K, Park HJ, Dewald J (2021). The impact of a mix of transport options on residential property values: The synergistic effect of walkability. Cities. 111:103080. doi:10.1016/j.cities.2020.103080.Department of Traffic and Public Space City of Amsterdam (2017). Long-term bicycle plan. Amsterdam: City of Amsterdam
(https://bikecity.amsterdam.nl/documents/14/Long-term_Bicycle_Plan_2017-2022_web.pdf).
30 Colmer J (2020). What is the meaning of (statistical) life? Benefit-cost analyses in the time of COVID-19. Oxf Rev Econ Policy. 36:S56-S63.
doi:10.1093/oxrep/graa022.
31 Combs TS, Pardo CF (2021). COVID-19 Changing Streets mobility data: Insights from a global dataset and research agenda for transport planning and

policy. Transp Res Interdiscip Perspect, 9:100322. doi:10.1016/j.trip.2021.100322.
32 Conrow L, Mooney S, Wentz EA (2021). The relationship between house prices, cycling infrastructure and travel volume. Urban Stud, 58(4):787-808. doi:10.1177%2F0042098098020926034.
33 Cooper A., Page A., Bourne J. (2020). How coronavirus made 2020 the year of the electric bicycle. London: The Conversation (https://theconversation.com/how- coronavirus-made-2020-the-year-of-the-electric-bike-143158).
34 Cooper AR, Tibbits B, England C, Procter D, Searle A, Sebire SJ, et al (2018). The potential of electric bicycles to improve the health of people with type 2 diabetes: a feasibility study. Diabet Med. 35(9):1279-1282. doi:10.1111%2Fdme.13664.
35 Creutzig F, Roy J, Lamb WF, Azevedo IML, deBruine WB, et al (2018). Towards demand-based solutions for climate change mitigation. Nat Clim Change. 8:4, 8(4):260-263. doi:10.1038/s41558-018-0121-1.
36 TOWNSHIP (2021). Guidelines for the design of cycling. Netherlands: CROW Platform. ( https://crowplatform.com/product/design-manual-for-bicycle-traffic/) 37 Cuenot F, Fulton L, Staub J (2012). Perspectives on modal shifts in passenger transport worldwide and their impact on energy consumption and CO2 emissions. Energy Policy. 41:98106. doi:10.1016/j.enpol.2010.07.017.
38 Davies A (2005). Transport and health - what is the link? A study of conceptions of health held by chairmen of highways committees in England. Transp Policy. 12(4):324-333. doi:10.1016/j.tranpol.2005.05.005.
39 Davies A. L., Aubrey D. (2020). Equality of restraint: Reframing road safety through the ethics of private motorised transport. J Transp Health. 19:100970.
doi:10.1016/j.jth.2020.100970.
40 DEKRA (2019) Ermittlung der Helmtragequote bei Nutzer/innen von Fahrrädern, Pedelecs und (E)-Scootern in europäischen Hauptstädten [Determining the prevalence of helmet use among users of bicycles, electric bicycles and electric scooters in European capitals] Stuttgart: DEKRA (https://www.dekra- roadsafety.com/media/47-studie-helmtragequote-hauptstaedte.pdf ) (in German).
41 Delso J, Martín B, Ortega E (2018). Potentially substitutable car trips: Assessing a potential modal shift towards active transport modes in Vitoria-Gasteiz. Sustainability. 10(10):3510. doi:10.3390/su10103510.
42 Department for Transport (2018). Guidance on transport analysis.

London: UK Government ( https://www.gov.uk/guidance/transport-analysis-guidance-tag).
43 Department for Transport (2019). Recorded road accidents in the UK: annual report 2019. London: UK Government
(https://www.gov.uk/government/statistics/reported-road-casualties-great-britain- annual-report-2019).
44 Departement für Umwelt, Verkehr, Energie und Kommunikation [Federal Department for the Environment, Transport, Energy and Communications] (2018). Bundesbeschluss Velowege [Federal law on cycle paths] [website]. Bern.
(https://www.uvek.admin.ch/uvek/de/home/uvek/abstimmungen/velo-vorlage.html).
45 Dill J, McNeil N (2013). Four types of cyclists? Transp Res Rec. 2387:129138. doi:10.3141%2F2387-15.
46 Dill J, Smith O, Howe D (2017). Promoting active transportation among state departments of transportation in the United States. 5:163-171. doi:10.1016/j.jth.2016.10.003.
47 Dinu M, Pagliai G, Macchi C, Sofi F (2019). Active commuting and various health indicators: A Systematic Review and Meta-Analysis. Sports Med. 49:437452. doi:10.1007/s40279-018-1023-0.
48 Directorate-General for Mobility and Transport (2021a). 1.8 Cycle Streets [website]. Brussels: European Commission
(https://transport.ec.europa.eu/transport-themes/clean-transport-urban-transport/cycling/guidance-cycling-projects-eu/cycling-measures/18-cycle-streets_en).
49 Directorate-General for Mobility and Transport (2021b). 1.7 Mixed-use zones [website]. Brussels: European Commission
(https://transport.ec.europa.eu/transport-themes/clean-transport-urban-transport/cycling/guidance-cycling-projects-eu/cycling-measures/17-mixed-use-zones_en)
50 Directorate-General for Mobility and Transport (2021c). 1.5 Crossroads [website]. Brussels: European Commission
(https://transport.ec.europa.eu/transport-themes/clean-transport-urban-transport/cycling/guidance-cycling-projects-eu/cycling-measures/15-intersections_en).
51 Dons E, Rojas-Rueda D, Anaya-Boig E, Avila-Palencia I, Brand C, ColeHunter T, et al (2018). Transport mode choice and body mass index: CrossSectional and Longitudinal Evidence from a European-Wide Study. Environ Int. 119:109-116. doi:10.1016/j.

envint.2018.06.023.
52 Doorley R, Pakrashi V, Szeto WY, Ghosh B (2020). Designing bicycle networks to maximise health, environmental and travel time impacts: An optimisation approach. Int J Sustain Transp. 14(5):361-374. doi:10.1080/15568318.2018.1559899.
53 Doorley R, Pakrashi V, Ghosh B (2015). Quantifying the health impacts of active travel: Assessment of Methodologies. Transp Rev.35(5):559-582. doi:10.1080/01441647.2015.1037378
54 Dora S (1999). Another route to health: the implications of transport policy. BMJ. 318(7199):1686. doi:10.1136%2Fbmj.318.7199.1686
55 Dora C., Phillips M., WHO Regional Office for Europe (2000). Transport, Environment and Health, edited by Carlos Dora and Margaret Phillips. Copenhagen: WHO Regional Office for Europe. (https://apps.who.int/iris/handle/10665/107336).
56 Elvik R (2001). Urban traffic calming schemes at the neighbourhood scale: a meta-analysis of safety effects. Accid Anal Preven. 33(3):327-336. doi:10.1016/s0001- 4575(00)00046-4
57 Elwick R (2009). Risk nonlinearity and the advancement of sustainable transport. Accid Anal Preven. 41(4):849-855. doi:10.1016/j.aap.2009.04.009.
58 Eren E, Uz VE (2020). Bicycle sharing survey: Factors influencing demand for bicycle sharing. Sustainable Cities and Society. 54:101882. doi:10.1016/j.scs.2019.101882.
59 Euro (2020) cities. COVID-19 - Urban dialogue on mobility measures - Highlights. Brussels: Eurocities (https://eurocities.eu/latest/covid-19-city-dialogue-on-mobility-measures-highlights/).
60 European Environment Agency (2020). Train or aeroplane? Copenhagen: European Environment Agency (https://www.eea.europa.eu/publications/transport-and-environment-report-2020).
61 European Commission (2016). Emissions in transport [website]. Brussels: European Commission. ( https://ec.europa.eu/clima/policies/transport_en).
62 European Commission (2019). The European Green Deal [website]. Brussels: European Commission (https://ec.europa.eu/info/strategy/priorities-2019- 2024/european-green-deal_en ).
63 European Cycling Federation (2014). SWITCHING: WHO PAYS THE BILL? Brussels: European Cycling Federation (https://ecf.com/groups/commuting-who-pays-bill).
64 European Cycling Federation (2016a). ELECTROMOBILITY FOR ALL

Financial incentives for e-cycling. Brussels: European Cyclists' Federation ( https://ecf.com/groups/report-electromobility-all-financial-incentives-e-cycling). 65 European Cycling Federation (2016b). Cycling delivers on global goals. Brussels: European Cycling Federation ( https://ecf.com/groups/cycling-delivers- global-goals ).
66 Federal Ministry of the Republic of Austria (2018). Declaration "Starting a new era: clean, safe and affordable mobility for Europe". Informal Meeting of Environment and Transport Ministers, Graz, Austria - 29-30 October 2018.
(https://civitas.eu/news/european-ministers-adopt-graz-declaration-for-clean-)
67 Feleke R, Scholes S, Wardlaw M, Mindell JS (2018). Comparative mortality risk for different modes of mobility by age, gender, and deprivation.Transp Health.8:307-320. doi:10.1016/j.jth.2017.08.
68 Ferenchak NN, Marshall W (2018). Bicyclist safety trends by age, 1985-2015. 97th Annual Meeting of the Transportation Research Board, Washington, DC, 1-11 January 2018. In: TRID, TRIS and ITID database ( https://trid.trb.org/view/1494803).
69 Fiorello D, Martino A, Zani L, Christidis P, Navajas-Cawood E (2016). Mobility data in 28 EU member states: results of a large CAWI survey. Transp Res Proc. 14:1104-1113. doi:10.1016/j.trpro.2016.05.181. Licence: Creative Commons CC-BY-NC-ND.
Fishman E (2016). Bikeshare: A Review of Recent Literature. Transp Rev, 36(1):92-113. doi:10.1080/01441647.2015.1033036.
70 Fishman E., Washington S., Haworth N. (2013). Bike sharing: a synthesis of the literature. Transp Rev, 33(2):148-165. doi:10.1080/01441647.2013.775612.
71 Flanagan E., Lachapelle W., El-Geneidy A. (2016). Riding in tandem: Do investments in bicycle infrastructure reflect gentrification and privilege in Portland, Illinois and Chicago, Illinois? Res Transp Econ. 60:14-24. doi:10.1016/j.retrec.2016.07.027
72 Flemming C (2019). The Netherlands pays people to cycle to work [website]. Geneva: World Economic Forum
https://www.weforum.org/agenda/2019/02/the-netherlands-is-giving-tax-breaks-to- cycling-commuters-and-they-re-not-the-only-ones).
73 FLOW Project (2016). The role of walking and cycling in reducing congestion: A portfolio of measures. Brussels (http://h2020-flow.eu/uploads/tx_news/FLOW_REPORT_-.
_Portfolio_of_Measures_v_06_web.pdf).

74 Forster P (2020). For the UK to achieve carbon neutrality, the next five years are crucial - here's what needs to happen. London: The Conversation (https://theconversation.com/for-a-carbon-neutral-uk-the-next-five-years-are-critical-heres-what-must-happen-151708).
75 Furth PG, Mekuria MC, Nixon H (2016). Network Connectivity for Low-Stress Bicycling. Transp Res Rec. 2587:41-49. doi:10.3141%2F2587-06.
76 Fyhri A, Sundf0r HB, Bj0rnskau T, Laureshyn A (2017). Safety in numbers for cyclists - Insights from an interdisciplinary study of seasonal changes in interaction and conflict. 105:124-133. doi:10.1016/j.aap.2016.04.039.
77 Garcia L, Johnson R, Johnson A, Abbas A, Goel R, Tatah L (2021). Health impacts of changes in travel patterns in Greater Accra Metropolitan area, Ghana. Environ Int. 155:106680. doi:10.1016/j.envint.2021.106680.
78 Garrard J, Handy S, Dill J (2012). Women and cycling. In Pucher, J and Buehler, R (eds), City Cycling, MIT PRESS. 211-234.
79 Garrard J, Rose G, Lo SK (2008). Promoting cycling for women: the role of cycling infrastructure. Prev Med. 46(1):55-59. doi:10.1016/j.ypmed.2007.07.010.
80 Gascon M, Götschi T, de Nazelle A, Gracia E, Ambros A, Márquez S et al (2019). Correlates of walkability for travelling in seven European cities: The PASTA project. Environ Health Perspect. 127(9). doi:10.1289/EHP4603.
81 Gehrke SR, Akhavan A, Furth PG, Wang Q, Reardon TG (2020). A cyclist-centred accessibility tool to support connectivity of regional bicycle networks. Transp Res D Transp Environ. 85:102388. doi:10.1016/j.trd.2020.102388.
82 de Geus B, De Bourdeaudhuji I, Jannes C, Meeusen R (2008). Psychosocial and environmental factors associated with bicycle use as transport among the working population . Health Educ Res. 23(4):697-708. doi:10.1093/her/cym055.
83 Giallouros G, Kouis P, Papatheodorou SI, Woodcock J, Tainio M (2020). Long-term effects of restricting cycling and walking on days of high air pollution on all-cause mortality: a health impact assessment study. Environ Int. 140:105679. doi:10.1016/j.envint.2020.105679.
84 Goel R, Goodman A, Aldred R, Nakamura R, Tatah L, Totaro-Garcia LM, et al (2021). Cycling behaviour in 17 countries on 6 continents: level of cycling, who cycles, who cycles, for what purpose and how far? Transp Rev, 42(1):1-24.
doi:10.1080/01441647.2021.1915898.

85 Goodman A, Fridman Rojas I, Woodcock J, Aldred R, Berkoff N, Morgan M, et al (2019). Cycling to school travel scenarios in England and associated health and carbon impacts: Application of the Cycling Propensity Tool. J Transp Health. 12:263-278. doi:10.1016/j.
jth.2019.01.008.
86 Goodman A, Cheshire J (2014). Inequalities in London's bike sharing system: implications of extending the scheme to poorer neighbourhoods but subsequent price doubling. J Transp Geogr. 41:272-279. doi:10.1016/j.jtrangeo.2014.04.004.
87 Goodman A, Sahlqvist S, Ogilvie D (2014). New walking and cycling routes and increased physical activity: one and two year results from the iConnect UK study. A J Pub Health. 104(9):e38-e46. doi:10.2105%2FAJPH.2014.302059.
88 Gössling S, Schröder M, Späth P, Freytag T (2016). Urban space allocation and sustainable transport. Transp Rev, 36(5):659-679. doi:10.1080/01441647.2016.1147101.
89 Gössling S, Choi AS, Dekker K, Metzler D (2019). Social costs of car, cycle and pedestrian traffic in the European Union. Ecol Econ. 158:65-74.doi:10.1016/j.ecolecon.2018.12.016.
89 Gössling S, Choi AS (2015). Transport crossings in Copenhagen: A comparison of car and bicycle costs. Ecol Econ. 113:106-113. doi:10.1016/j.ecolecon.2015.03.006.
90 Götschi T (2011). Costs and benefits of investing in cycling in Portland, Oregon. J Phys Act Health, 8(Suppl 1):S49-S58. doi:10.1123/jpah.8.s1.s49.
91 Götschi T, de Nazelle A, Brand C, Gerike R, PASTA Consortium (2017). Towards a Comprehensive Conceptual Framework of Active Travel Behaviour: a Review and Synthesis of Published Frameworks. Curr Environ Health Rep. 4(3):286-295. doi:10.1007/s40572- 017-0149-9.
92 Götschi T, Kahlmeier S, Castro A, Brand C, Cavill N, Kelly P, et al (2020). Comprehensive assessment of the impacts of active travel: Extending the scope of the Health Economic Assessment Tool (HEAT) to walking and cycling. Int J Environ Res Public Health. 17(20). doi:10.3390/ijerph17207361.
93 Götschi T, Garrard J, Giles-Corti B (2016). Cycling as part of everyday life: A Review of Health Perspectives. Transp Rev. 36(1):45-71. doi:10.1080/01441647.2015.1057877.
94 Götschi T, Hadden Loh T (2017). Advancing project-scale health impact modelling for active transport: A user survey and health impact calculation of 14 routes in the USA. J Transp Health. 4:334-347.

doi:10.1016/j.jth.2017.01.005.
95 Grabow ML, Spak SN, Holloway T, Stone B, Mednick AC, Patz JA (2011). Air quality and exercise-related health benefits of reducing car travel in the Midwestern United States. Environ Health Perspect. 120(1):68-76. doi:10.1289/ehp.1103440.
96 Griffiths S (2020). Why your internet habits aren't as clean as you think - BBC Future. London: British Broadcasting Corporation (https://www.bbc.com/future/article/20200305-why-your-internet-habits-are-not- as-clean-as-you-think ).
97 Gudz EM, Fang K, Handy S (2016). When a Diet Prompts a Gain: Impact of a Road Diet on Bicycling in Davis, California. Transp Res Rec. 2587(1):61-67.
doi:10.3141%2F2587-08.
98 Guerra E, Zhang H, Hassall L, Wang J, Cheyette A (2020). Who and where commutes to work by bicycle? A comparative multilevel analysis of urban commuter travel in the US and Mexico. Transp Res D Transp Environ. 87:102554. doi:10.1016/j.trd.2020.102554.
99 Guthold R, Stevens GA, Riley LM, Bull FC (2018). Global trends in physical inactivity from 2001 to 2016: pooled analysis of 358 population-based studies with 1-9 million participants. Lancet Glob. Health. 6(10):e1077-e1086. doi:10.1016/S2214-109X(18)30357-7.
100 Guthold R, Stevens GA, Riley LM, Bull FC (2020). Global trends in physical inactivity among adolescents: pooled analyses of population-based studies with 1-6 million participants. Lancet Child Adolesc. Health. 4(1):23-35. doi:10.1016/S2352-4642(19)30323-2.
101Haas T, Sander H (2020). Decarbonisation of transport in the European Union: Emission efficiency standards and prospects for a European Green Deal. Sustainability. 12(20):8381. doi:10.3390/su12208381.
102 Hamer M, Chida Y (2008). Active commuting and cardiac vascular risk: A meta-analytic review. Prev Med. 46(1):9-13. doi:10.1016/j.ypmed.2007.03.006.
103 Hendriksen IJ, Simons M, Galindo Garre F, Hildebrandt VH (2010). The association between cycling and sickness absence. Prev Med. 51(2):132-135. doi:10.1016/j.ypmed.2010.05.007.
104 Hillman CH, Erickson KI, Kramer AF (2008). Be smart, train your heart: the effects of exercise on the brain and cognition. Nat Rev Neurosci 2008 9:1, 9(1):58-65. doi:10.1038/nrn2298.
105 Hosford K, Firth C (2021). The impact of road pricing on transport and health equity: a review. Transp Rev. 6:766-787.

doi:10.1080/01441647.2021.1898488.
106 Howland S, McNeil N, Broach J, Macarthur J, Dill J (2018). Bike Share and Equity in Low-Income Communities of Colour: What Opportunities Are There There to Include Older Adults? Transportation Research Board 97th Annual Meeting, Washington DC, 1-11 January 2018. In: TRID, TRIS and ITID database (https://trid.trb.org/view/1496588).
107 Huertas JA, Palacio A, Botero M, Carvajal GA, van Laake T, Higuera-Mendieta D, et al (2020). Classification based on transport stress levels: A cluster approach for Bogotá, Colombia. Transp Res Part D Transp Environ. 85:102420. doi:10.1016/j.trd.2020.102420.
108 Hunter RF, Garcia L, de Sa TH, Zapata-Diomedi B, Millett C, Woodcock J, et al (2021). Impact of COVID-19 response policies on pedestrian behaviour in US cities. Nat Commun. 2021, 12:3652. doi.org/10.1038/s41467-021-23937-9.
109 International Energy Agency (2020). Global EV Outlook 2020 Are we entering the decade of electric drive? Paris: International Energy Agency ( https://www.iea.org/reports/global-ev-outlook-2020, accessed 6 October 2021).
110 International Energy Agency (2021). Changes in transport behaviour during the Covid-19 crisis - Analysis [website]. Paris: International Energy Agency.
(https://www.iea.org/
112 International Transport Forum, Organisation for Economic Co-operation and Development (2021). Reversing car dependence. Paris: International Transport Forum, Copenhagen: Organisation for Economic Co-operation and Development ( https://www. itf-oecd.org).
113 Jacobsen PL (2003). Safety in numbers: more pedestrians and cyclists - safer walking and cycling. Inj Prev. 9(3):205-209. doi:10.1136/ip.9.3.205
114 Jaffe E (2015). The complete business case for converting street parking into bike lanes [website]. New York: Bloomberg
(https://www.bloomberg.com/news/articles/2015/every-study-ever-conducted-on- the-impact-converting-street-parking-into-bike-lanes-has-on-businesses)
115 Jarrett J, Woodcock J, Griffiths UK, Chapabi Z, Edwards P, Roberts I, et al (2012). The impact of increased active travel in urban areas in England and Wales on National Health Service costs. Lancet. 379(9832):2198-2205. doi10.1016/s0140- 6736(12)60766-1.
116 Johansson C, Lövenheim B, Schantz P, Wahlgren L, Almström P, Markstedt A et al (2017). Air pollution and health impacts of switching from

car to bicycle. Sci Total Environ. 584-585:55-63. doi:10.1016/j.scitotenv.2017.01.145.

117 Johansson R (2009). Vision Zero - realising road safety policy. Saf Sci. 47(6):826-831. doi:10.1016/j.ssci.2008.10.023.

118 Johnson T. (2002). Guidance on Selected Algorithms, Distributions, and Databases Used in Exposure Models Developed by the Office of Air Quality Planning and Standards. Washington D.C.: United States Environmental Protection Agency (https://www.epa.gov/fera/guide-selected-algorithms-distributions-and-databases- used-exposure-models-developed-office-air).

119 Kahlmeier S, Racioppi F, Cavill N, Rutter H, Oja P (2010). Health in All Policies in Practice: Guidelines and tools for quantifying the health effects of cycling and walking. J Phys Act Health. 7(s1):S120-S125. doi:10.1123/jpah.7.s1.s120.

120 Kahlmeier S, Castro A, Brand C (2017). Health Economic Assessment Tool (HEAT) for Walking and Cycling Methods and User Guide for Physical Activity, Air Pollution Injuries and Carbon Exposure Assessment. Copenhagen: WHO Regional Office for Europe ( https://apps.who.int/iris/handle/10665/344136).

121Khashir B.O.,/ Khashir B.O. Financial management in the world economy Textbook with the griffin of UMO - Krasnodar:, LLC "Publishing House-Yug". KubGTU, 2010. 326c.

122Khashir B.O.,/ Khashir B.O. Investment attractiveness of regional economic development projects of the forest sector. Proceedings of VI Mezinternationalni vedeko-prakticheskii konferentsii "Vedetskii porok na rozmezi tisitsileti 2010" Dill 8. Ekonomicke vedy/ Izdatelstvo "Obrazovanie i nauka" s.r.o. Praha. 2010. C.18-21.

123Khashir B.O., Krivonosov P.B. Characteristics of breed composition and reconstruction of recreational areas of the Southern Federal District Materials of the VII mezinarodnaya vedetsko-prakticheskaya konferencija "Predni vedetschke novinki -2011". Dil 2 Economic Sciences. Publishing house "Education and Science" s.r.o. Prague 2011. C.17-21.

124Khashir B.O., Khadzhuova S.K. Methodology of complex assessment of forest recreational resources. Materials of VII Mesinaroydni vedeko-prakticheskaya konferentsii "Predni vedeke novinki -2011" Dil 2 Economic Sciences. Publishing house "Education and Science" s.r.o. Prague 2011. C.61-64.

125Khashir B.O., / Khashir B.O. Methodology of technological assessment of territory sustainability of forest recreational landscapes. Materials for VII International Scientific Conference "Novini na nauchnia progress-2011"

Ikonomiki "Byal GRAD-BG "OOD Sofia 2011". C.32-35
126Khashir B.O.,/ Khashir B.O. Trends of regional forest management and use in the world economy. Study guide with the grfom UMI. - Krasnodar:, LLC "Publishing House-Yug" KubGTU, 2012. 200c.
127Khashir B.O.,/ Khashir B.O., Shakhanova D.A. Market and resource-potential approaches to strategic management of the forest complex. Scientific journal "Scientific Review" M:, № 6, 2013. C. 160-163.
128Hashir B. O.,/ Hashir B. O., Apsalyamova S. O. Medical aspects of nutritional and therapeutic value of forest plant products. Scientific journal "Scientific Review" M:, vol. 6, 2013. C. 15-18
129Khashir B.O., / Khashir B.O. Effective utilisation of forest resources. Collection of scientific works "Economics and efficiency of production organisation" v.18. Bryansk. BGITA. 2013. C.23-27
130Khashir B.O.,/ Khashir B.O., Shakhanova D.A. Analyses and prospects for the development of regional forest policy strategy. XIV International Scientific and Technical Internet Conference "Les-2013" Bryansk. 2013. C.
142-146
131Khashir B.O.,/ Khashir B.O., Apsalyamova S.O. Formation of economic, medical and social systems in the sphere of effective forest management. LLC "Publishing House - Svetoch". Krasnodar 2014 296 p.
132Khashir B.O.,/ Khashir B.O. Conceptual approaches to improving the system of regulation of sustainable development of the forest sector of the regional economy. Scientific journal "Scientific Review" M:, vol.
1, 2014. C. 173-178.
133Khashir B.O.,/ Khashir B.O., Apsalyamova S.O. Aspects of effective application of investment projects in the forest industry. Scientific edition "Lesotechnicheskiy zhurnal". Voronezh. VGLTA. Vol. 4 No. 1 (13). 2014 C. 236243
134Khashir B.O.,/ Khuazhev O.Z. Tendencies of the process of functioning and development of economic systems of forest resources management. Scientific edition "Lesotechnicheskiy zhurnal". Voronezh. VGLTA. Vol. 4 No. 1 (13). 2014. C. 243-253.
135Khashir B.O., Khut R.A. Conceptual approaches to improving the system of regulation of sustainable development of the forest sector of the regional economy. Materials of the international scientific and practical conference "I European Forestry Forum of Youth". Voronezh. VGLTA. Vol. 4 No. 1 2014. C. 243- 253
136Khashir B.O.,/ Khashir B.O., Kufanova S.K. Formation of the mechanism of regulation of sustainable economic development of the forest sector. Materials of the international scientific-practical conference "I European forestry forum of youth". Voronezh. VGLTA. Vol. 8 No. 1 (15).
2014. C. 283- 293

137Khashir B.O.,/ Khashir B.O. Socio-economic aspects of forecasting, reproduction of natural resources and ensuring medico-ecological safety in the development of the forest sector. LLC "Publishing House "Ecoinvest", Krasnodar. 2015.14 p.l.
253
138Khashir B.O.,/ Khashir B.O. Organisational and economic mechanisms of investment attractiveness of forest sector enterprises LLC "Publishing House "Ecoinvest", Krasnodar. 2015. 10 p.l.
139Hashir B.O.,/ Hashir B.O. Economic Mechanisms of Competitiveness in Nature Management, Environmental Protection and Medical-Ecological Safety. BBRA - Biosciences, Biotechnology Research Asia (India, ISSN 09731245, Scopus) Vol. 12(2), 2015. P. 1345-1349.
140Hashir B.O.,/ Hashir B.O. Green economy of ecosystems in forestry services / Green economy of ecosystems in forestry services, BBRA - Biosciences, Biotechnology Research Asia (India, ISSN 0973-1245, Scopus) September 2015. Vol. 12(Spl. Edn. 2), p. 643-649
141Khashir B.O.,/ Khashir B.O. Organisational and economic mechanisms for monitoring indicators of the processes ensuring sustainable development of the forest sector. /
Organisational and economic mechanisms for monitoring processes ensuring sustainable development of the forestry sector. BBRA - Biosciences, Biotechnology Research Asia (India, ISSN 0973-1245, Scopus) Vol. 12(2), 2015. P. 1345-1349
142Hashir B.O.,/ Hashir B.O. Legal aspects of ecosystem services of effective forest management / Legal aspects of ecosystem services associated with effective forest management. Journal of environmental management and tourism. University of Craiova, Romania Volume VI Issue 1(11) ASERS Publishing, 2015. P.53-61
143Hashir B.O.,/ Hashir B.O. Economic aspects of payments for forest ecosystem services/ Economic value of forest ecosystem services Journal of Environmental Management and Tourism. University of Craiova, Romania Volume VI Issue 1(11) ASERS Publishing, Winter 2015. P. 291-297
144Khashir B.O.,/ Khashir B.O. Evaluation of investment attractiveness of forest sector enterprise. Scientific journal "Scientific Review" M:, № 17, 2015. C. 425-433
145Khashir B.O.,/ Khashir B.O. Dynamic models of profit forecasting in the production of forest products. Scientific edition "Lesotechnicheskiy zhurnal". Voronezh. VGLTA. Vol. 5 No. 2 (18) 2015. C.254263
146Khashir B.O.,/ Khashir B.O. Formation of the concept of strategic

development of forestry. LLC "Publishing House "Ecoinvest", Krasnodar. 2016. 12p.l
147Khashir B.O.,/ Khashir B.O. "Green" economy in the formation of socio-economic services of medico-ecological systems of effective forest management. LLC "Publishing House "Ecoinvest", Krasnodar. 2016. 12p.l.
148Khashir B.O.,/ Khashir B.O. Tendencies of development of socio-economic forms of medico-ecological safety in the sphere of services of effective nature management. RIO "KUGTU" Krasnodar.2016. 12.5 p.l.
149 Khashir B.O., / Khashir B.O. Aspects of medico-ecological safety at effective nature management. RIO "KubGTUt" Krasnodar. 2016. 12.5 p.l.
150Khashir B.O.,/ Khashir B.O. Institutional aspects of forecasting and organisation of forest management. Journal of environmental management and tourism. University of Craiova, Romania Volume VI Issue 1(11) ASERS Publishing House, 2016. T. 7. № 2 (14). C. 195-205.
151Khashir B.O.,/ Khashir B.O. Tendencies of modern development of the forest sector of the economy. / Trends of modern development of forest sector of economy. Quality - access to success. Bucharest. Romania. T.17, №154. October 2016. C. 55-60
152Hashir B.O.,/ Hashir B.O. Legal and policy framework for the development of effective forest management / Legal and policy framework for effective forest management. Man In India, 96 (10) New Delhi. India. 2016. C. 3605-3625
153Hashir B.O.,/ Hashir B.O. Methodology for forecasting scenarios of effective forest management / Methodology for forecasting scenarios of effective forest management. International Journal of Entrepreneurial Knowledge (IJEK) Ostrava. Czech Republic. 13(6). 2016. C. 2541-2558 ISSN 0972-9380
154Khashir B.O.,/ , Apsalyamova S.O., Khuazhev O.Z., Zyza V.P. Institutional aspects of forecasting and organisation of forest management. Journal of Environmental Management and Tourism. Scopus. 2016 C. 53-61. www.asers.eu/journals/jemt/
155Khashir B.O. S.O. Apsalyamova, O.Z. Khuazhev, A.N. Drozdov, Y.V. Leshova. Trends of modern development of the forest sector of the economy. Quality - the way to success. Bucharest. Romania. T.17, №154. October. Scopus. 2016. C. 55-60
156Khashir B.O.,/ Apsalyamova S.O., Khuazhev O.Z. Methodology of forecasting scenarios of effective forest management. International Journal of Economic Research (IJER). Scopus. 2016. C. 83-85 http://serialsjournals.com

157Khashir B.O.,/ S.O. Apsalyamova, O.Z. Khuazhev Legal and Political Foundations of Effective Forest Management. Man in India. Scopus. 2016. C. 3605-3625 http://serialsjournals.comBAK
158Khashir B.O.,/ Khashir B.O. Formation of the concept of socio-economic development of the forest sector. Scientific journal "Economics and Entrepreneurship" M: Volume 1, (part 2) (66-2) 2016. C. 966-1005.
159Khashir B.O.,/ Khashir B.O. Assessment of the impact of investment processes on natural systems. Scientific Journal "Economics and Entrepreneurship" M: No. 3 4.2 (68-2) 2016 (Vol. 10 Vol. 3-2) P 494-499
160Hashir B.O.,/ Hashir B.O. Technological parameters economically efficient forest management Scientific Journal of Economics and Entrepreneurship M: No. 6 (71) 2016 (Volume 10 Number 6) P 575-579.
161Hashir B.O.,/ Hashir B.O. Aspects of economically efficient, plantation cultivation of non-timber forest products. Scientific journal "Economics and Entrepreneurship" M: No. 6 (71) 2016 (Volume 10 Number 6) P 336-341
162Khashir B.O.,/ Khashir B.O. Assessment of the impact of investment processes on natural systems. M. Scientific journal "Economics and Entrepreneurship". 2016. C. 1216-1224. www.intereconom.com
163Hashir B.O.,/ Hashir B.O., Technological parameters for economically efficient forest management. M. Scientific journal "Economics and Entrepreneurship", 2016. C. 1224-1230. www.intereconom.com
164Khashir B.O.,/ Khashir B.O. Formation of the concept of socio-economic development of the forest sector. M. Scientific journal "Economics and Entrepreneurship". 2016. C. 1230-1238. www.intereconom.comabCTBO".
165Khashir B.O., Khashir B.O. Aspects of effective formation of information base of forest management. Materials of the international scientific and practical conference "Actual directions of scientific researches of XX1 century: Theory and practice" Voronezh. VGLTU. No. 1 (21) (Volume 4, Issue 1) 2016 P.217-222
166Khashir B.O.,/ Khashir B.O. Trends of effective planning of forestry organisation. Materials of the international scientific-practical conference "Actual directions of scientific researches of XX1 century: Theory and practice" Voronezh. VGLTU. No. 1 (21) (Volume 4, Issue 1) 2016 P.222-227
167Khashir B.O.,/ Khashir B.O. Trends and directions of development of the regional forest complex. Collection of scientific papers "Actual problems of forest complex" Bryansk. BGITA. 2016. C.26-29
168Khashir B.O./Khashir B.O. Aspects of rational use of forests. Collection of scientific papers "Actual problems of forestry complex" Bryansk BGITA 2016 P.29-32
169Khashir B.O., /22 Khashir B.O. Trends and directions of development of the regional forest complex. Bryansk. BGITA. 2016. C. 72-75. www.science-bsea.bgita.ru

170Khashir B.O.,/ Khashir B.O., Kolomeets Y.V. Tendencies of effective planning of forestry organisation. Voronezh. VGLTU. 2016. C. 12 -16. www conf_vglta.vrn.ru
171Khashir B.O.,/ Khashir B.O., Apsalyamova S.O., Drozdov A.N., Khuazhev O.Z. Legal bases of sustainable forest management and use based on world experience. RIO "KubGTU. 2017. 230 c.
172Khashir B.O.,/ Khashir B.O., Apsalyamova S.O., Khuazhev O.Z. Formation of the regional concept of strategic development of medico-ecological safety in the sphere of sustainable forest management services. Krasnodar. RIO "KubGTU". 2017. 187c.
173Khashir B.O.,/ Khashir B.O., Khuazhev B.A., Apsalyamova S.O., Khuazhev O.Z. Conceptual forms of domestic and world forecasts of medico-ecological systems of healthy lifestyle on the basis of effective forest management. Krasnodar. RIO "KubGTU". 2017. 179c.
174Khashir B.O.,/ Khashir B.O., Khuazhev B.A., Apsalyamova S.O., Khuazhev 0.3. Formation of scientific and research programmes of medical and socio-economic services in the creation of healthy lifestyle systems, on the basis of effective forest management. Krasnodar. RIO "KubGTU". 2017. 218c.
175Khashir B.O.,/ B.O. Kashir, S.O. Apsalyamova, O.Z. Khuazhev, A.N. Drozdov, Y.V. Leshova. Trends of modern development of the forest sector of the economy. Quality - the way to success. Bucharest. Romania. Vol. 17, October. Web of Science 2017. C. 155-160
176Khashir B.O.,/ B.O. Kashir, S.O. Apsalyamova, O.Z. Khuazhev, Institutional aspects of forecasting socio-economic systems in the organisation of forest management in the Russian Federation. Academy of Strategic Management Journal. Volume 16, special issue 1, published by Jordan Whitney Enterprises, Inc, P.O Box 1032, Weaverville, NC 28787, USA. Scopus. 2017 C. 218-227 www alliedacademies.org
177Khashir B.O.,/ B.O. Kashir, S.O. Apsalyamova, O.Z. Huazhev Strategic development of recreational technologies in forestry. E-SdPTCONICIT - Espacios (ISSN07981015-Caracas Venezuela -Scopus), 2 (10) economics 2017. 606748 C.11-17 www.revistaespacios.com
178Khashir B.O.,/ B.O. Kashir, S.O. Apsalyamova, O.Z. Khuazhev Development of efficient production and processing of forest products. EEC-EM - Ecology, Environment and Conservation (0971765X-India-Scopus), 2017. 23 (3), 657461 C. 1774-1780 www envirobiotechjournals.com/
179Khashir B.O.,/ B.O. Kashir, S.O. Apsalyamova, O.Z. Khuazhev. Aspects of forecasting Russian and world markets of forest products. JARLE-ASERS Publishing House - Journal of Advanced Research in Law and

Economics(ISSN2068696X-Romania-Scopus) 2017. C.53-61. www.asers.eu
180Khashir B.O.,/Khamnp B.O., Bondarenko T.I., Zyza V.P., Styagun A.B. Russian and world experience of economically efficient organisation of forest management. M. Scientific journal "Economics and Entrepreneurship". №6. 2017. C. 339-345. www.intereconom.com
181Khashir B.O.,/ Khashir B.O., Bondarenko T.N., Kravtsova J.V., Zyza V.P. Certification of sustainable forest management system. M. Scientific journal "Economics and Entrepreneurship". №6. 2017. C. 990-995. www.intereconom.com
182Hashir B.O.,/Khamnp B.O., Bolik A.V., Shilovich O.B., Bgane Y.K. Structure of world trade in forestry products. M. Scientific journal "Economics and Entrepreneurship". №6. 2017. C. 1044-1051. www.intereconom.com
183Khashir B.O.,/ Khashir B.O., Styagun D.I., Styagun A.V. Production trends in the market of forest board materials. M. Scientific journal "Economics and Entrepreneurship". №6. 2017. C. 436-444. www.intereconom.com
184Khashir B.O.,/ Khashir B.O., Bondarenko T.N., Zyza V.P., Styagun A.V. Trends of economically efficient organisation of the Russian and global
257
on forest management. M. Scientific journal "Economics and Entrepreneurship". №6. 2017. C. 158-1164. www.intereconom.com 185 Hashir B.O.,/ Hashir B.O., Bolik A.V., Shilovich O.B., Bgane Y.K. Forest tenure system and timber distribution on public lands. M. Scientific journal "Economics and Entrepreneurship". №6. 2017. C. 1025-1029. www.intereconom.com
186Hashir B.O.,/ Hashir B.O., Bolik A.V., Shilovich O.B., Kravtsova J.V. Ecologically sustainable forest management. M. Scientific journal "Economics and Entrepreneurship". № 6. 2017. C. 1005-1013. www.intereconom.com
187Khashir B.O.,/ Khashir B.O., Martynova T.A., Cherminskaya L.G. "Green", economics world experience of payment for ecosystem services. M. Scientific journal "Economics and Entrepreneurship". №7. 2017. C. 1211-1217. www.intereconom.com
188Khashir B.O.,/ Khashir B.O., Thagapso M.B., Khalyapina O.G. Formation of the system of payment for ecosystem services in the process of transition to a "green" economy. M. Scientific journal "Economics and Entrepreneurship". №7. 2017. C. 1224-1230. www.intereconom.com
189Khashir B.O.,/ Khashir B.O., Khuazhev B.A., Apsalyamova S.O., Khuazhev 0.3. Legal regime of forest tenure, payments for ecosystem and medico-ecological services. M. Scientific journal "Economics and Entrepreneurship". № 9. 2017. C. 915-921. www.intereconom.com

190 Khashir B.O.,/ Khashir B.O., Khuazhev B.A., Apsalyamova S.O., Khuazhev 0.3. Variants of banking and compensation services of medico-ecological nature management. Scientific journal "Economics and Entrepreneurship". M. № 9. 2017. C. 939-945. www.intereconom.com 191 Khashir B.O.,/ Khashir B.O., Khuazhev B.A., Apsalyamova S.O., Khuazhev 0.3. Tendencies of development of paid medical and ecological services by effective forest use. Scientific journal "Economics and

Entrepreneurship." M. № 9. 2017. C. 976-981. www.intereconom.com 192 Khashir B.O.,/ Khashir B.O., Chitanava N.B., Ostapenko O.A.. External and internal threats to the economic security of the state and directions of their reduction. Scientific journal "Economics and Entrepreneurship". M. №10. 2017. C. 1031-1033. www.intereconom.com

193 Khashir B.O.,/ Khashir B.O., Saprunova E.V., Khalyapina O.G., Galitskaya Y.N. Aspects of economically efficient, plantation cultivation of non-timber forest products. M. Scientific journal "Economics and Entrepreneurship". M. № 10. 2017. C. 224-230. www.intereconom.com 194 Khashir B.O.,/ Khashir B.O. Social aspects of the role of the population whose livelihood depends on forests. Materials of the international scientific and practical internet conference "Economics and efficiency of production organisation" Bryansk. BGITA. NO. 25 2017. C. 65-71. www.science-bsea.bgita.ru

195 Khashir B.O.,/ Khashir B.O. Research of the market of non-wood forest products. Materials of the international scientific and practical internet conference "Actual problems of forest complex" Bryansk. BGITA. NO. 48 2017. C. 109-113. www.science-bsea.bgita.ru

196 Khashir B.O.,/ Khashir B.O. Legal aspects of forest management organisation. Materials of the international scientific-practical internet-conference "Actual directions of scientific researches of XX1 century: theory and practice". Voronezh. VGLTU. 2017. C. 132 -138. www conf_vglta.vrn.ru

197 Khashir B.O.,/ Khashir B.O., Apsalyamova S.O., Khuazhev 0.3. Innovative forms of effective medico-ecological forest management. Modern problems of public health and medical statistics. LLC "BelMedInvest" Volume 4 M 2017 P.17-32

198 Khashir B.O.,/ Khashir B.O. Aspects of rational use of forests. Bryansk BGITA 2017. P.12-15. www.science-bsea.bgita.ru

199 Khashir B.O., / Khashir B.O. Aspects of effective formation of information base of forest management. Voronezh. VGLTU. 2016. C. 13 -18. www conf_vglta.vrn.ru

200 Khashir B.O.,/ Khashir B.O. Market research of non-wood forest products. Bryansk. BGITA. 2017. C. 109-113. www.science-bsea.bgita.ru

201 Khashir B.O.,/ Khashir B.O. Ways to increase labour productivity in the forestry complex of the region. Materials of the scientific conference Krasnodar. KubGTU 2017 P.423-427

202 Khashir B.O., Apsalyamova S.O., Khuazhev O.Z. Aspects of development of the sphere of services of medico-ecological systems of agro-forestry economically effective nature management. Krasnodar. OOO "Publishing house-"Print-Terra". 2018. 209 c.
203 Khashir B.O.,/ Khashir B.O., Apsalyamova S.O., Khuazhev O.Z. Socio-economic monitoring of medico-ecological service management systems in the implementation of the concept of sustainable management of natural resources of the agro-.forestry sector of the economy of the Russian Federation. Krasnodar. LLC "Publishing house-"Print-Terra". 2018. 189 c.
204 Hashir B.O.,/ Hashir B.O., Huaj O.Z., Aps S.O. Medico-ecological safety in the development of nature management. Palmarium Academic Publishing - OmniScriptum Group. Riga. Latvia. 2018. 302 pp. www.omniscriptum.com 205 Khashir B.O.,/ Khashir B.O., Huazh O.3., Styagun A.B., Bondarenko T.P., Styagun D.I., Zyza V.P., Lesnikova N.E. Tendencies of economic development of social systems of effective forest management. Scientific journal "Economics and Entrepreneurship". M. № 12. 2018. C. 508-514. www.intereconom.com
206 Khashir B.O.,/ Khashir B.O., Huazh O.Z., Styagun A.V., Bondarenko T.I., Styagun D.I., Zyza V.P., Lesnikova N.E. Social aspects of "green economy" on forest ecosystem management. Scientific journal "Economics and Entrepreneurship". M. № 12. 2018. C. 205-211. www.intereconom.com
207 Khashir B.O.,/ Khashir B.O., Khuazhev 0.3. Methodological bases of monitoring of systems of realisation of the concept of sustainable management on agro-forest territories. Materials of the international scientific-practical internet-conference "Actual directions of scientific researches of XX1 century: theory and practice". Voronezh. VGLTU. №37 (1). 2018. C. 106 -115. www conf_vglta.vrn.ru
208 Khashir B.O.,/ Khashir B.O., Khuazhev O.Z. Tendencies of development of organisational and economic mechanism of agro-forestry productions. Materials of the international scientific-practical internet-conference "Actual problems of forest complex" Bryansk. BGITA. NO. 27. 2018. C. 21-25. www.science-bsea.bgita.ru
209 Khashir B.O.,/ Khashir B.O., Khuazhev O.Z. Strategic analysis of forest use in preserving the natural environment. Materials of the international scientific-practical internet-conference "Actual problems of forest complex" Bryansk. BGITA. NO. 27. 2018. C. 25-29. www.science-bsea.bgita.ru
210 Khashir B.O., Khuazhev O.Z. Strategy of forest management based on the development plans of agrarian and forestry. Materials of the international scientific-practical internet-conference "Actual problems of forest complex" Bryansk. BGITA. NO. 27. 2018. C. 32-36. www.science- bsea.bgita.ru .
211 Khashir B.O.,/ Khashir B.O., Khuazhev O.Z. Socio-economic and natural-resource potential of development of agrarian, forest-steppe areas of Krasnodar Krai. Eighth International Symposium "Steppes of Northern Eurasia (Steppe Forum of RGO)". Orenburg. IS Ural Branch of the Russian Academy of Sciences. 2018. C.1048-1051. www.orensteppe.org.

212 Hashir B. O.,/ Hashir B. O., Aps S. O., Huaj O. Z. Development of physical activity in the system of nature management. Palmarium Academic Publishing - OmniScriptum Group. Riga. Latvia. 2019. 197c. www.omniscriptum.com
213 Khashir, B.O.; Apsalyamova, S.O.; Kade, A.K.; Huaj, O.Z.; Zyza, V.P. Mapping as a part of medical-ecological services. /Medico-environmental mapping as a component of the complex of medico-environmental services. International Journal of Engineering and Advanced Technology (IJEAT) ISSN:2249-8958, SCOPUS Impact Factor -5.97 Volume 9 Issue-1, Bhopal (M.P.), India. October 2019.
214 Khashir, B.O.; Apsalyamova, S.O.; Huazh, O.Z.; Shtygun, A.V. Medico-ecological assessment of carcinogenic risk formation from air pollution in megacities/ Medico-ecological assessment of carcinogenic risk formation from air pollution in megacities. International Journal of Engineering and Advanced Technology (IJEAT) ISSN:2249-8958, SCOPUS impact factor -5.97 Volume 9 Issue-1, Bhopal (M.P.), India. October 2019.
215 Khashir B.O.,/Khamnp B.O., Zyza V.P., Apsalyamova S.O., Huazh O.Z. Formation of socio-economic systems of employment development in forestry. Scientific journal "Economics and Entrepreneurship". M. № 1 (102). 2019. C. 573-579. www.intereconom.com
216 Khashir B.O.,/ Khashir B.O., Apsalyamova S.O., Huazh O.Z., Bolelova M.M. Trends in the development of socio-economic forms of employment in forestry. Scientific journal "Economics and Entrepreneurship". M. № 1 2019 C. 1212-1218. www.intereconom.com
217 Khashir B.O.,/ Apsalyamova S.O., Khashir B.O. Development of the mechanism of strategic management of the complex. Collection of scientific papers. Issue 54. - Bryansk: BGITU, 2019. C. 282- 286. ISSN 2310-9335 www.science-bsea.bgita.ru
218 Khashir B.O.,/ Khashir B.O. Social mechanisms of labour remuneration of green jobs in forestry. Collection of scientific papers. Issue 54. - Bryansk: BGITU, 2019. C. 286-290. ISSN 2310-9335 www.science-bsea.bgita.ru 219 Khashir B.O.,/ Khashir B.O., Khuazhev 0.3. Aspects of modernisation of working conditions and profitable part of forest business. Collection of scientific works. Issue 54. - Bryansk: BGITU, 2019. C. 290- 293. ISSN 2310-9335 www.science- bsea.bgita.ru
220 Khashir B.O.,/ Khashir B.O., Khuazhev 0.3. Tendencies of development of effective forest use. Collection of scientific papers. Issue 54. - Bryansk: BGITU, 2019. C. 293- 297. ISSN 2310-9335 www.science-bsea.bgita.ru 221 Khashir B.O.,/ Khashir B.O., Khuazhev 0.3. Investment and institutional mechanisms of land use regulation in the forest-steppe zone. Materials of the international scientific conference "Zapovednoe delo: achievements, problems and prospects", №15. Orenburg, IS Ural Branch of the Russian Academy of Sciences, 2019 P. 332-337. www.orensteppe.org.
222Khashir B.O.,/ Khashir B.O., Apsalyamova S.O., Huazh 0.3. Sustainable

management of development of innovative medico-ecological systems of agro-industrial forestry services cluster. Palmarium Academic Publishing - OmniScriptum Group. Riga (Latvia)-Saarbrucken (Germany). 2020. 209 pp. www.omniscriptum.com
223Khashir B.O.,/ Khashir B.O., Apsalyamova S.O., Huazh 0.3 Monitoring of management systems for the implementation of the concept of sustainable management of natural resources. Palmarium Academic Publishing - OmniScriptum Group. Riga (Latvia)-Saarbrucken (Germany). 2020. 194c. www.omniscriptum.com
224Khashir B.O.,/ Khashir B.O., Apsalyamova S.O., Huazh 0.3 Legal aspects of production and consumption waste management with the system of nature management. Khashir B.O., Huazh O.Z., Apsalyamova S.O. Legal aspects of production and consumption waste management with the system of nature management. Jour of Adv Research in Dynamical & Control Systems, Vol. 12, Issue-06, Kansas City, USA. 2020. p.1275-1282 ISSN 1943023x. www jardcs.org
225Khashir B.O.,/ Khashir B.O., Apsalyamova S.O., Huazh 0.3 Aspects of medico-ecological services in the system of effective nature management B.O.. Hashir, O.Z. Huazh, S.O. Apsalyamova Aspects of medico-environmental services in the system of natural water bodies. International journal of pharmaceutical research Volume 12. Issue 4. Bengaluru - Salem. India. 2020. p. 702-712. ISSN 0975 - 2366. www.ijpronline.com
226Hashir B.O.,/ B.O. Hashir, O.Z. Huaj, S.O. Apsalyamova MEDICAL AND ECOLOGICAL SERVICES IN THE SYSTEM OF EFFECTIVE MANAGEMENT OF NATURAL RESOURCES Journal of Critical Reviews ISSN- 2394-5125 Vol 7, Issue 13, Kuala Lumpur, Malaysia. 2020. p.2894-2899. www jcreview.com
227Hashir B.O.,/ B.O. Hashir, O.Z. Huaj, S.O. Apsalyamova CRITERIA AND INDICATORS OF MEDICAL AND ECOLOGICAL SERVICES IN REGIONAL NATURAL RESOURCE MANAGEMENT Journal of Critical Reviews ISSN- 2394-5125 Vol 7, Issue 13, Kuala Lumpur, Malaysia. 2020. p. 2887-2893 www jcreview.com
228Khashir B.O.,/ Khashir B.O., Basamygina I.N., Zyza V.P., Huazh O.Z., Apsalyamova S.O. Trends in the global development of the market of forest products and services. Scientific journal "Economics and Entrepreneurship". M. № 4 (117). 2020. C. 573-579. www.intereconom.com
229Khashir B.O.,/ Khashir B.O., Basamygina I.N., Zyza V.P., Huazh O.Z., Apsalyamova S.O. Trends in the development of medico-environmental services in the creation of green jobs in the forestry sector. Scientific journal "Economics and Entrepreneurship". M. № 4 (117). 2020. C. 579-585. www.intereconom.com

230Khashir B.O.,/ Khashir B.O., Apsalyamova S.O., Huazh 0.3 Forest condition monitoring in the system of environmental protection cpenu.The Scientific Heritage - Global science LP (Prague-Budapest) #43-3(43). 2020. C.63-69. www.tsh- journal.com
Apsalyamova S., Hashir B., Huazh O. MONITORING of forest condition in the
ENVIRONMENTAL PROTECTION SYSTEM
231Hashir B.O.,/ Hashir B.O., Apsalyamova S.O., Huaj 0.3 Measuring socio-economic returns of effective forest management. Scientific heritage - global science LP (Prague-Budapest) No. 43-3(43). 2020. C.55- 62. www.tsh-journal.com
232Khashir B.O.,/ Khashir B.O., Apsalyamova S.O., Huazh 0.3 Trends in the development of biological diversity. Materials of the international scientific forum "Science and Innovations-modern concepts". M. Infiniti. 2020. P.7-15 www nauchoboz.ru
233Khashir B.O.,/ Khashir B.O., Apsalyamova S.O., Huazh 0.3 Aspects of development of ecosystem (biome) and natural landscape diversity. Proceedings of the international scientific forum "Science and Innovations-modern concepts". M. Infiniti. 2020. P.15-24 www nauchoboz.ru
234Khashir B.O.,/ Khashir B.O., Apsalyamova S.O., Huazh 0.3 Importance of biodiversity and ecosystem services in forest management system. Proceedings of the international scientific forum "Science and Innovations-modern concepts". M. Infiniti. 2020. C. 24-32 www nauchoboz.ru
235Khashir B.O.,/ Khashir B.O., Apsalyamova S.O., Huazh 0.3 Medico-ecological services of ecosystem functions of human life support. Materials of the international scientific forum "Science and Innovations - modern concepts". M. Infiniti. 2020. P.32-40 www nauchoboz.ru 236 Huazh O.Z., Apsalyamova S.O., Khashir B.O. Innovative medico-ecological systems of nature management. - Aspects of models and technologies of prevention in the development of the concept of medical-ecological services of nature management. Palmarium Academic Publishing - OmniScriptum Group. Riga (Latvia) - Saarbrucken (Germany). 2021.186s. www.omniscriptum.com.
237Huazh O.Z., Apsalyamova S.O., Khashir B.O. Physical activity in the system of medical ecological services. - Trends in the development of screening in the system of medical ecology of nature management. Palmarium Academic Publishing - OmniScriptum Group. Riga (Latvia) - Saarbrucken (Germany). 2021.179 c. www.omniscriptum.com
238Huazh O.Z., Apsalyamova S.O., Khashir B.O. Fundamentals of medical ecology in the formation of a healthy lifestyle. - Trends in the development of

medical ecological services cluster based on the rational use of natural resources. Palmarium Academic Publishing - OmniScriptum Group. Riga (Latvia) - Saarbrucken (Germany). 2021.199 c. www.omniscriptum.com
239Khashir B.O., Stygun D.I., Stygun A.V. Aspects of technological modernisation of forestry enterprise. Journal of Contemporary Issues in Business and Government, Melbourne (Australia) 2021, Volume 27, Issue 2, Pages 36383644 WoS. Doi: 10.47750 / cibg. 2021.27.02.374. https://cibg.org.au/
240Hashir B.O., Apsalyanova S.O., Kade A.H.. Optimisation of medical and environmental services using TPP therapy. Journal of complementary medicine research. Nashville, USA. E-ISSN 2577-5669. WoS. doi: 10.5455 / jcmr.2021; 12 (2): P 21-28 www.jocmr.com
241Hashir B.O., Huazh O.Z., Apsalyamova S.O., KaScreening of regional health and environmental recreational services. Journal of complementary medicine research. Nashville, USA. E-ISSN 2577-5669. WoS. doi: 10.5455 / jcmr.2021; 12 (2): P 21-28 www.jocmr.com
242Hashir B.O., Huaj O.Z., Apsalyamova S.O., Kadeh A.H., Trends in screening health and environmental services in TPP therapy system. Journal of complementary medicine research. Nashville, USA. E-ISSN 2577-5669. WoS. doi: 10.5455 / jcmr.2021; 12 (2): P 21-28 www.jocmr.com
243Khashir B.O., Huazh O.Z., Stiagun D.I., Stiagun A.V., Khuazhev A.A. Trends in the development of human capital in the conditions of digitalisation of the economy. Journal "Modern Problems of Business and Management". Melbourne (Australia) 2021, Volume 27, Issue 2, P. 3645-3654. WoS. DOI: 10.47750 / cibg.2021.27.02.375 https://cibg.org.au/
244Hashir B.O., Huaj O.Z., Apsalyamova S.O., Kade A.H. Aspects of wellness and environmental services using TPP therapy. Journal of complementary medicine research. Nashville, USA. E-ISSN 2577-5669. WoS. doi: 10.5455 / jcmr. 2021; 12 (2): P 21-28 www jocmr.com.
245 Khashir B.O., Huaj O.3., Khashir B.O., Apsalyamova S.O. Khashir E.A. Formation of scenarios for the development of carbon neutrality in the system of nature management. Scientific journal "Economics and Entrepreneurship". M. № 10. 2022. C. 970- 976. www.intereconom.com 246 Khashir B.O.,/ Huazh O.Z., Khashir B.O., Apsalyamova S.O., Khashir E.A. Trends in the development of carbon neutrality in the system of nature management. Scientific journal "Economics and Entrepreneurship". M. № 10. 2022. C. 426-433. www.intereconom.com 247 Khashir B.O.,1 Khashir E.A., Apsalyamova S.O., Huazh O.Z. Integration of health-saving technologies in the system of nature management/ Screening medical and

ecological technologies of health protection in the system of environmental development. Lambert Academic Publishing - OmniScriptum S.R.L. Chisinau (Moldova) - London (UK). 2023. 220c. www.lap-publishing.com LAP ISBN 978-620-6-78863-8
248 Khashir B.O., Khashir E.A., Apsalyamova S.O.,Huazh O.Z. Formation of medical-ecological systems of screening of non-communicable diseases for cost-effective npnpoflono4b3OBaHM.Formation of medical-ecological systems of screening of non-communicable diseases for cost-effective nature management. UDC 001.1 BBK 1 III International Scientific and Practical Conference "Theoretical and Practical Perspectives of Modern Science", 01-02 August 2023, Stockholm. Sweden. 64 c. ISBN 978-91-65423-27-5 DOI https://doi.org/10.5281/zenodo. 8221145 Publisher: "SK. Scientific Conferences ". https://sconferences.com
249 Katsis P, Papageorgiou T, Ntziachristos L (2014). Modelling the effect of trip length distribution on CO2 emissions of electrified vehicles. 4(1A):57-64. doi:10.5923/s.ep.201401.05.
Kazemzadeh K, Loreshin A, Winslot Hyselius L, Ronchi E (2020). Expanding the scope of the cyclist level of service concept: A Review of the Literature. Sustainability. 12(7):2944. doi:10.3390/su12072944.
250 Keith DR, Houston S, Naumov S (2019). Fleet turnover and the future of fuel economy. Environ Res Lett. 14(2):021001. doi:10.1088/1748-9326/aaf4d2. 251 Kelly P, Kahlmeier S, Götschi T, Orsini N, Richards J, Roberts N et al (2014). A systematic review and meta-analysis of the reduction in all-cause mortality from walking and cycling and the shape of the dose-response relationship. Int J Behav Nutr Phys Act. 11(1):132. doi:10.1186/s12966-014-0132-x.100
252 Kelly P, Williamson C, Baker G, Davis A, Broadfield S, Coles A et al (2020). Beyond cycle paths and large-scale infrastructure: A review of initiatives that groups and organisations can implement to promote cycling for the Cycle Nation project. Bri J Sports Med. 54(23):1405-1415. doi:10.1136/bjsports-2019- 101447.
253 Kraus S, Koch N (2021). COVID-19 pre-infrastructure induces a large and rapid increase in cyclicity. Proceedings of the National Academy of Sciences of the United States of America, Prot Natl Acad Sci USA. 118(15):e2024399118. doi:10.1073/pnas.2024399118.
254 Krauß S, Ruhl S, Richter T (2016). Geschwindigkeitsverhalten bei Tempo-30- Beschilderungen aus Laermschutzgruenden in den Nachtstunden [Traffic speed at 30 km/h limit to reduce night-time noise].
Straßenverkehrstechnik [traffic flow control technology]. 60(3):159-66

(https://www.baufachinformation. de/geschwindigkeitsverhalten-bei- tempo-30-beschilderungen-aus-laermschutzgruenden-in-den-nachtstunden/z/2016039024028) (in German).
255 Kriit HK, Williams JS, Lindholm L, Forsberg B, Sommar JN (2019). Health economic evaluation of a scenario for promoting cycling as active transport in Stockholm, Sweden. BMJ Open. 9:e030466. doi:10.1136/ bmjopen-2019-030466. 256 Krizek KJ (2018). Measuring the wind in your hair? Unravelling the positive utility of cycling. Res Transp Bus Manag. 29:71-76.
doi:10.1016/j.rtbm.2019.01.001.
257 Kroesen M, De Vos J (2020). Does active travel make people healthier or are healthy people more likely to be active travellers? Transp Health 16:100844 doi:10.1016/j.jth.2020.100844
258 Kuhnimhof T, Armoogum J, Buehler R, Dargay J, Denstadli JM, Yamamoto T (2012). Men shape the trend in lower car use among young adults - evidence from six industrialised countries. Transp Rev. 32(6):761-779. do i:10.1080/01441647.2012.736426.
259 L'Agència de Salut Pública de Barcelona [Barcelona Public Health Agency] (2022) Salut als Carrers. Avaluació dels àmbits Superilles [Health in the streets. Development of super neighbourhoods] [website].
Barcelona: L'Agència de Salut Pública de Barcelona ( https://www.aspb.cat/documents/salutalscarrers/) (in Catalan).
260 Lamu AN, Jbaily A, Verguet S, Robberstad B, Norheim OF (2020). Is expanding the cycling network cost-effective? An economic evaluation of cyclists' health in Oslo. BMC Pub Health, 20:1869. doi:10.1186/s12889-020-09764-5.
261 Lancet Global Burden of Disease (2020). Global health indicators: Low physical activity - risk level 2. Volume 396, 17 October 2020. Lancet (https://www.thelancet.com/pb-assets/Lancet/gbd/summaries/risks/low-physical- activity.pdf).
262 Lee I-M, Shiroma EJ, Lobelo F, Puska P, Blair SN, Katzmarzyk PT, et al (2012). The impact of hypodynamia on major noncommunicable diseases worldwide: analyses of disease burden and life expectancy. Lancet. 380(9838):219-229. doi:10.1016/S0140-6736(12)61031-9.
263 Lee RJ, Sener IN, Jones SN (2017). Understanding the role of equity in active transportation planning in the United States. Transp Rev. 37(2):211-226.
doi:10.1080/01441647.2016.1239660.
264 Lewis A, Moller SJ, Carslaw D (2019). Non-exhaust emissions from

road traffic. United Kingdom: Defra (https://uk-air.defra.gov.uk/assets/documents/reports/cat09/1907101151
265
265 Leyland L-A, Spencer B, Beale N, Jones T, van Reekum CM (2019). Effects of cycling on cognitive function and well-being in older adults. PLoS One. 14(2):e0211779. doi:10.1371%2Fjournal.pone.0211779.
266 Li, W., & Joh, K. (2016). Investigating the synergistic economic benefits of improving neighbourhood cycling accessibility and public transport accessibility based on property transactions: Urban Stud. 54(15), 3480-3499. doi: 10.1177/0042098016680147.
267 Lieske SN, van den Nouwelant R, Han JH, Pettit C (2021). A new hedonic price modelling approach for estimating the impact of transport infrastructure on property prices. Urban Stud. 58(1):182-202. doi:10.1177%2F0042098019879382.
268 Lilly C (2022) Electric car market statistics. Bristol: The next 'green' car www.nextgreencar.com
269 Lim SS, Vos T, Flaxman AD, Danaei G, Shibuya K, Adair-Rohani H, et al (2012). Comparative risk assessment of the burden of disease and injury associated with 67 risk factors and clusters of risk factors in 21 regions during 1990-2010: a systematic review for the Global Burden of Disease. 2010. Lancet. 380(9859):2224-2260. doi10.1016/S0140- 6736(12)61766-8.
270 Litman, T. (2013). Transport and public health. Annu Rev Pub Health. 34(1):217-233. doi:10.1146/annurev-publhealth-031912-114502.
271 Lowry M, Loh TH (2017). Quantifying bicycle network connectivity. Prev Med. 95 Suppl:S134-S140. doi:10.1016/j.ypmed.2016.12.007.
272 Lowry MB, Furth P, Hadden-Loh T (2016). Prioritising new cycle facilities to improve low-load network connectivity. Transp Res Part A Policy Pract.
86:124-140. doi:10.1016.
273 Lozzi G, Rodrigues M, Marcucci E, Teoh T, Gatta V, Pacelli V (2020). Research for the TRAN Committee - COVID-19 and urban mobility: impact and perspectives. Brussels: European Parliament, Policy Department for Structural and Cohesion Policies ( https://www. europarl.europa.eu/thinktank/en/document/IPOL_IDA(2020)652213).
274 Lusk AC, (2011). Risk of injury when cycling on cycleways and on streets. Inj Prev. 17: 131-135. doi:10.1136/ip.2010.028696.
275 Ma L, Ye R (2019). Does daily commute to work matter for labour productivity? J Transp Geog. 76:130-141. doi:10.1016/j.jtrangeo.2019.03.008.

276 Ma L, Ye R (2021). Walking and cycling to work makes commuters happier and more productive. London: The Conversation (https://theconversation.com/walking-and-cycling-to-work-makes-commuters- happier-and-more-productive-117819).
277 Maizlish N, Linesch NJ, Woodcock J (2017). Health and GHG benefits of ambitious expansion of biking, walking, and transit in California. J Transp Health. 6:490-500. doi:10.1016/j.jth.2017.04.011.102
278 Mäki-Opas TE, Borodulin K, Valkeinen H, Stenholm S, Kunst AE, Abel T, et al (2016). The Contribution of Travel- Related Urban Zones, Cycling and Pedestrian Networks and Green Space to Commuting Physical Activity Among Adults - A Cross-Sectional Population-Based Study Using Geographical Information Systems. BMC Public Health. 16(1):760. doi:10.1186/s12889-016- 3264-x.
279 Marqués R, Hernández-Herrador V (2017). On the impact of cycleway networks on cycling risk. The example of Seville. Accid Anal Prev. 102:181-190. doi:10.1016.
280 Marsden G., Frick K. T., May A. D., Deakin E. (2011). How do cities approach policy innovation and policy learning? A study of 30 policies in Northern Europe and North America. Transp Policy. 18(3):501-512. doi:10.1016/j.
tranpol.2010.10.006.
281 Marshall WE, Ferenchak NN (2019). Why cities with high levels of cycling are safer for all road users. J Transp Health. 13:100539. doi:10.1016/j.jth.2019.03.004.
282 Matz CJ, Egyed M, Hocking R, Seenundun S, Charman N, Edmonds N (2019). Human health impacts of traffic-related air pollution (TRAP): A scoping review protocol. Syst Rev. 8(1):1-5. doi.10.1186/s13643-019-1106-5.
283 McNeil N, Dill J, MacArhtur J, Broach J (2018). Bikeshare for Everyone? Views of residents of colour in low-income communities. 97th Annual Meeting of the Transportation Research Board, Washington, DC, 1-11 January 2018. In: TRID, TRIS and ITID database ( https://trid.trb.org/view/1495936).
284 Melendez S (2021). Companies subsidise e-bikes as workers return to offices. New York: Fast Company. (https://www.fastcompany.com/90659189/subsidized-e-bikes-back-to-the-office-commute).
285 Mizdrak A, Blakely T, Cleghorn CL, Cobiac LJ (2019). The potential of active transport to improve health, reduce health care costs, and reduce

greenhouse gas emissions: A modelling study. PLoS ONE. 14(7):e0219316. doi:10.1371%2Fjournal.pone.0219316.
286 Mobilitätsagentur Wien [Vienna Mobility Agency] (2022). Schulstraße [School Streets] [website]. Vienna:
287 Mobilitätsagentur Wien Mobility (www.wienzufuss.at/schulstrasse ) (in German).
Molloy J, Schatzmann T, Schomann B, Chervenkov S, Hintermann B, Axhausen KV (2021a). Observed effects of the first wave of Covid-19 on travel behaviour in Switzerland based on a large GPS panel. Transp Pol. 104:43-51.
doi:10.1016/j.tranpol.2021.01.009.
288 Molloy JB, Castro Fernandez A, Götschi T, Tchervenkov C, Tomic U, Hintermann B, et al (2021b). A national mobility pricing experiment using GPS tracking and online surveys in Switzerland: Response rates and survey method results. Arbeitsberichte Verkehrs- und Raumplanung. 1555.
doi:10.3929/ethz-b-000441958.
289 Muller N., Rojas-Rueda D., Cole-Hunter T., de Nazel A., Dons E., Gericke R. et al. (2015). Health impact assessment of active transport: A systematic review. Prev Med. 76:103-114. doi:10.1016/j.ypmed.2015.04.010.
290 Muller N, Rojas-Rueda D, Salmon M, Martinez D, Ambros A, Brand C et al (2018). Health impact assessment of the expansion of the cycling network in European cities. Prev Med. 109:62-70. doi:10.1016/j.ypmed.2017.12.011. RightsLink licence number: 5157590818857
291 Muller N, Rojas-Rueda D, Heris H, Chirach M, Andres D, Ballester J, et al (2020). Changing urban design of cities in favour of health: the superblock model. Env Int. 134:105132. doi:10.1016/j.envint.2019.105132
292 Mulley C, Tyson R, McCue P, Rissel C, Munro C (2013). Assessing the value of active travel: Incorporating the health benefits of sustainable transport into transport appraisal systems. Res Transp Bus Manag. 7:27-34.
doi:10.1016/j.rtbm.2013.01.001.
293 Mytton OT, Panter J, Ogilvie D (2015). Longitudinal associations of active travel to work with well-being and sickness absence. Prev Med. 84:19-26.
doi:10.1016/j.ypmed.2015.12.010.
294 Nanda A (2020). Super neighbourhoods: Barcelona's car-free zones could prolong life and boost mental health. London: The Conversation (https://theconversation.com/superblocks-barcelonas-car-free-zones-could-extend- lives-and-boost-mental-health-123295).

295 National Association of City Transportation Officials (2019). Don't give up at the crossroads. [website]. New York: National Association of City Transportation Officials ( https://nacto.org/publication/dont-give-up-at-the-intersection ). de Nazelle A, Bode O, Orjuela
296 New York City Department of Transportation (2013). The economic benefits of sustainable streets. New York: New York City Department of Transportation (https://www.nyc.gov/).
297 Nabavi Niaki M, Saunier N, Miranda-Moreno LF (2016). Methodology for quantifying gaps in the bicycle network: A case study in Montréal boroughs. Paper presented at the 95th Annual Meeting of the Transportation Research Board, Washington, DC.
(https://www.researchgate.net/publication/324201128_Methodology_to_quantify_
discontinuities_in_a_cycling_network_Case_study_in_montreal_boroughs).
298 Nicola S, Behrmann E (2018). Car Ownership Declining: 'Peak Car' And The End Of An Industry [website]. Mumbai: BloombergQuint
(https://www.bloombergquint.com/business/-peak-car-and-the-end-of-an-industry). 299 Nilsson JH (2019). Urban cycling tourism: path dependencies and innovation in Greater Copenhagen. J Sustain Tour. 27(11):1648-1662. doi:10.1080/09669582.2019.1650749.
300 Organisation for Economic Co-operation and Development (2016). Zero Road Deaths and Serious Injuries: Leading a Paradigm Shift to a Safe System [website]. Paris: Organisation for Economic Co-operation and Development
(https://www.oecd.org/publications/
zero-road-deaths-and-serious-injuries-9789282108055-en.htm).
301 Orozco LGN, Battiston F, Iñiguez G, Szell M (2019). Data-driven strategies for optimal growth of bicycle networks. R Soc Open Sci. 7(12):201130-201130.
doi:10.1098/rsos.201130
302 Otero I, Nieuwenhuijsen MJ, Rojas-Rueda D (2018). Health impacts of bike-sharing systems in Europe. Env Int. 115:387-394.
doi10.1016/j.envint.2018.04.014.
303 Panik RT, Morris EA, Voulgaris CT. (2019). Does more walking and cycling mean less physical activity? Evidence from the United States and the Netherlands. J Transp Health. 14:100590. doi:10.1016/j.jth.2019.100590.Gro Petrunoff N, Rissel C, Wen LM (2016). Impact of workplace-based active mobility interventions on driving to work: A systematic review. J Transp Health. 3(1):61-76. doi:10.1016/j 304 Pisoni E, Thunis P, Clappier A (2019). Application of SHERPA source-receptor relationships based on the EMEP

MSC-W model to evaluate air quality policy scenarios. Atmos Environ X. 4:100047.
doi:10.1016/j.aeaoa.2019.100047.
305 Pojani E, Van Acker V, Pojani D (2018). The car as a status symbol: Young people's attitudes towards sustainable transport in a post-socialist city. Transpo Res Part F Traffic Psychol Behav. 58:210-227. doi:10.1016/j.trf.2018.06.003.
306 Porter AK, Kontou E, McDonald N, Evenson K (2020). Perceived barriers to cycling to work and exercise among US adults: the National Household Travel Survey 2017. J Transp Health, 16:100820. doi:10.1016/j.jth.2020.100820.
307 Pritchard R, Fr0yen Y (2019). Location, location, location: how office relocation from the suburbs to the inner city affects walking and cycling. Eur Transp Res Rev. 11(1):14. doi:10.1186/s12544-019-0348-6.
308 Pritchard R, Fr0yen Y, Snizek B (2019). Cyclists' level of service for route choice - a GIS evaluation of four existing indicators using empirical data.
ISPRS Int J Geo-Inf. 8(5):214. doi:10.3390/ijgi8050214.
309 PTV Group Traffic (2016). PTV Vissim and Viswalk: 5 modes of transport with 200 people each - focusing on space utilisation [website]. In: YouTube, PTV Group Traffic (https://www.youtube.com/watch?v=g_ILtWzH3Ko).
310 Pucher J, Buehler R (2012). Urban cycling (Pucher J, Buehler R, eds.). Cambridge, MA; London: MIT Press (https://mitpress.mit.edu/books/city-cycling).
311 Putta T, Furth PG (2019). A method for identifying and visualising barriers in a low-load cycling network. Transp Res Rec. 2673(9):452-460.
doi:10.1177%2F0361198119847617.
312 Raser E, Gaupp-Berghausen M, Dons E, Anaya-Boig E, Avila-Palencia I, Brand C, et al (2018). European cyclists' travel behaviour: Differences and similarities between seven European cities (PASTA). J Transp Health. 9:244-252. doi:10.1016/j.jth.2018.02.006.
313 Reid C (2018). People who walk and cycle spend more in London shops than motorists. Jersey City: Forbes.
(https://www.forbes.com/sites/carltonreid/2018/11/16/cyclists-spend-40-more-in- londons-shops-than-motorists/?sh=50ec8d36641e).
314 Rérat P (2021). The emergence of the e-bike: Towards an expansion of cycling practices? Mobilities, 16(3):423-439. doi:10.1080/17450101.2021.1897236.

315 Rodrigues PF, Alvim-Ferraz MCM, Martins FG, Saldiva P, Sá TH, Sousa SIV (2020). Economic valuation of health in the transition to active transport. Environ Pollut. 258:113745. doi:10.1016/j.envpol.2019.113745.
316 Ruffino P, Jarre M (2021). Evaluation of bicycle and pedestrian projects. In: Adv in Transp Pol Plann. 7:165-203. doi:10.1016/bs.atpp.2020.08.005.
317 Ruiz-Hermosa A, Álvarez-Bueno C, Cavero-Redondo I, Martinez-Vizcaino V, Redondo-Tébar A, Sánchez-López M (2019). Active travelling to and from school, cognitive performance and academic achievement in children and adolescents: a systematic review
And a meta-analysis of observational studies. Int J Environ Res. 16(10)1839. doi:10.3390/ijerph16101839.
318 Rupprecht S, Brand L, Böhler-Baedeker S, Brunner LM, Rupprecht Consult.
(2019). Guidelines for the development and implementation of a sustainable urban mobility plan (2nd edition). European Platform for Sustainable Urban Mobility Plans.
Cologne: Rupprecht Consult
- Forschung and Beratung GmbH (https://www.eltis.org
319 Saelens BE, Handy SL (2008). Correlates of walking in the built environment: a review. Med Sci Sports Exerc. 40(7 Suppl):S550-66.
doi:10.1249%2FMSS.0b013e31817c67a4.
320 Sahlqvist S, Goodman A, Cooper AR, Ogilvie D (2013). Changes in active mobility and changes in recreational and total physical activity in adults: longitudinal results from the iConnect study. Int J Behav Nutr Phys Act. 10(1):28.
doi:10.1186/1479-5868-10-28.
321 Saunders L (2021). What are "healthy streets"? [website]. In: Healthy Streets (https://www.healthystreets.com/what-is-healthy-streets).van Schalkwyk MCI, Mindell JS (2018). Current issues in the health impacts of transport. Br Med Bull. 125(1):67-77. doi:10.1093/bmb/ldx048.
322 Scharnhorst E (2018). Quantified Parking - Comprehensive Parking Inventories for Five Major U.S. Cities, Mortgage Bankers Association [website]. (https://www.mba.org/2018-press-releases/july/riha-releases-new-report- quantified-parking-comprehensive-parking-inventories-for-five-major-us-cities).
323 Schepers P, Hagenzieker M, Methorst R, van Wee B, Wegman F (2014). A conceptual framework for road safety and mobility as applied to cyclist safety. Accid Anal Preven. 62:331-340. doi:10.1016/j.aap.2013.03.032.
324 Schepers P, Klein Wolt K, Helbich M, Fishman E (2020). Safety of e-

bikes compared to conventional bicycles: What role does cyclists' health status play? J Transp Health. 19:100961. doi:10.1016/j.jth.2020.100961.
325 Schroten A, van Wikngaarden L, Brambilla M, Maffii S, Trosky F, Kramer H, et al (2019a). A review of (costs and expenditure on transport infrastructure.
Luxembourg: Publications Office of the European Union (https://op.europa.eu/en/publication-detail/-/publication/7ab899d1-a45e-11e9- 9d01-01aa75ed71a1).
326 Schroten A, Scholten P, van Wikngaarden L, van Essen H, Brambilla M, Gatto M, et al (2019b). Transport taxes and charges in Europe. Luxembourg: European Union Publications Office (https://op.europa.eu/en/publication-detail/-/publication/4de76a04-a385- 11e9-9d01-01aa75ed71a1 ).
327 Shoup D (2018). Parking and the City.NY: Taylor and Francis.doi:10.4324/9781351019668.
328 Singleton PA (2019). Walking (and cycling) to well-being: Modal and other determinants of subjective well-being during the commute. Travel Behav and Soc. 16:249-261. doi:10.1016/J.TBS.2018.02.005.
329 Smith M, Hosking J, Woodward A, Witten K, MacMillan A, Fiels A, Baas P et al (2017). A systematic review of the literature on environmental influences on physical activity and active transport - an update and new evidence on health equity. Int J Behav Nutr Phys Act. 14(1):158. doi:10.1186/s12966-017-0613-9.
330 Standen C, Greaves S, Collins AT, Crane M, Rissel C (2019). The value of slow journeys: Economic evaluation of cycling projects using a logarithmic measure of consumer surplus. Transp Res Part A Pol Pract. 123: 255-268.
doi:10.1016/j.tra.2018.10.015.
331 Strain T, Brage S, Sharp SJ, Richards J, Tainio M, Ding D (2020). Using the proportion of deaths averted for a population to determine deaths averted by the existing prevalence of physical activity: a descriptive study. Lancet Glob Health.
8(7):e920-e930. doi:10.1016/S2214-109X(20)30211-4.
332 Street Plans Collaborative, John S. and James L. Knight Foundation, NACTO, Vision Zero Network (2016). Tactical Urbanism Materials and Design Guide. New York: The Street Plans Collaborative (http://tacticalurbanismguide.
com/guides/tactical-urbanists-guide-to-materials-and-design/).
333 Stylianou N, Guibourg C, Briggs H (2019). Climate change food calculator: What is the carbon footprint of your diet? - BBC News [website].

London: British Broadcasting Corporation (https://www.bbc.com/news/science-environment- 46459714).
334 Sugiyama T, Carver A, Koohsari MJ, Veitch J (2018). Benefits of public green spaces in promoting community health. Landsc Urban Plan 178: doi:10.1016/j.landurbplan.2018.05.019
335 Sustrans (2014). Sustrans design guide. Bristol: Sustrans(https://www.eltis.org/sites trainingmaterials/sustrans_handbook_for_cycle-friendly_design_11_04_14.pdf).
336 Sustrans (2020) What are the economic impacts of increasing space for walking and cycling? [website]. Bristol: Sustrans (https://www.sustrans.org.uk/our blog/opinion/2020/may/) what-are-the-economic-impacts-of-making-more-space-for-walking-and-cycling).
337 Swiss Federal Council (2018a). Direct counterproposal to the "Bike Initiative" [website]. Bern: Swiss Federal Council ( https://www.admin. ch/gov/en/start/documentation/votes/20180923/ bundesbeschluss-ueber-die-velowege-sowie-die-fuss--und-wanderweg.html).
338 Swiss Federal Council (2018b). Bundesbeschluss über die Velowege [Federal law on cycle paths] [website]. Youtube. Bern ( https://www.youtube.com.
339 Synek S, Koenigstorfer J (2018). Exploring the determinants of adoption of tax-subsidised company-rented bicycles from the perspectives of German employers and employees. Transp Res A: Policy and Pract. 117:238-260. doi:10.1016/j. tra.2018.08.011.
340 Szarata A, Nosal K, Duda-Wiertal U, Franek L (2017). Impact of car restrictions in city centre on the quality of public space. Transp Res Proc. 27:752-759. doi:10.1016/j.trpro.2017.12.018.
341Tainio M, de Nazelle A, Götschi T, Kahlmeier S, Rojas-Rueda D, Nieuwenhuijsen MJ et al (2016). Can air pollution negate the health benefits of cycling and walking? Preventive Medicine. 87:233-236. doi: 10.1016/j. ypmed.2016.02.002. Licence: Creative Commons CC-BY.107
342 Tainio M, Andersen ZJ, Nieuwenhuijsen MJ, Hu L, de Nazelle A, An R et al (2021). Air pollution, physical activity and health: A mapping review of the evidence. Environ Int. 147:105954. doi:10.1016/j.envint.2020.105954.
343 Teschke K, Harris MA, Reynolds CCO, Winters M, Babul S, Chipman M et al (2012). Road infrastructure and bicyclist injury risk: a cross-sectional study. Am J Public Health. 102(12):2336-2343. doi:10.2105/AJPH.2012.300762.

344 Government of the Grand Duchy of Luxembourg (2015). Declaration on cycling as a climate-friendly mode of transport. Informal meeting of EU Transport Ministers, Luxembourg, Luxembourg, 7 October 2015. (http://www.eu2015lu.eu/en/actualites/communiques/2015/10/07-info-transports- declaration-velo/07-Info-Transport-Declaration-of-Luxembourg-on-Cycling-as-a-climate-friendly-Transport-Mode---2015-10-06.pdf)
345 Thaler R, Eder M (2007). Klimaaktiv mobil [website] (in German) Vienna: Klimaaktiv ( https://www.klimaaktiv.at/mobilitaet/).
346 Thaler R., Eder M. (2015a). Masterplan for the development of cycling in Austria. Vienna: Klimaaktiv (https://www.klimaaktiv.at/service/publikationen/mobilitaet/mprad2015englisch.ht ml).
347 Thaler R, Eder M (2015b). Masterplan "Walking on foot" [Walkable Masterplan]. (in German) Vienna: Klimaaktiv (https://www.klimaaktiv.at/dam/jcr:de62856d-6fc9-434c-b67c-9a21d0de4253/MP- Gehen_final_forWeb.pdf).
348 PEP (2020). Mobility Management - A Guide to International Best Practices. Geneva: United Nations Economic Commission for Europe ( https://thepep.unece.org/node/805).
349 PEP (2021). Pan-European masterplan for the development of cycling. Geneva: United Nations Economic Commission for Europe. (https://thepep.unece.org/node/825).
350 PEP (2021a). Action toolkit for the promotion of cycling based on best practices in the Pan-European region. Geneva: UN Economic Commission for Europe ( https://thepep.unece.org/node/826).
351THE PEP (2021b). Recommendations for Green and Healthy Sustainable Transport - Building Forward Better Geneva: United Nations Economic Commission for Europe ( https://thepep.unece.org/index.php/node/823).
272
352 PEP (2022). Pan-European Transport-Health-Environment Programme. Geneva: United Nations Economic Commission for Europe ( https://thepep.unece.org/).
353 Torres-Barragan CA, Cottrill CD, Beecroft M (2020). Spatial inequalities and media representations of cyclist safety in Bogotá, Colombia. Transp Res Interdiscip Perspect 7:100208. doi:10.1016/j.trip.2020.100208.
354 Transport for London (2018) Street Appeal London:transport of London. content.tfl.gov.uk
355 (2018). The spatial footprint of urban transport: how much space is used by transport in the city? [website]. Brussels: Wavestone .

(https://www.transportshaker-wavestone.com/urban-transports-spatial-footprint- much-space-used-transports-city/).
356Tucker B, Mano K (2018). Bicycle equity in Brazil: Access to safe cycling routes in different neighbourhoods of Rio de Janeiro and Curitiba. Int J Sustain Transp. 12(1):29-38. doi:10.1080/15568318.2017.1324585.
357 TOnnesen A, Knapskog M, Uteng TP, 0ksenholt KV (2020). Integrating active travel and public transport into Norwegian policy packages: A study of 'access, egress and transfer' and their positioning in two tiered contractual arrangements. Res Transp Bus Manag. 40:100546. doi:10.1016/j.rtbm.2020.100546. 358 Uhr A, Hertach P (2017). Verkehrssicherheit von E-Bikes mit Schwerpunkt Alleinunfälle. Beratungsstelle für Unfallverhütung [Road safety of E-Bikes with a Focus on Single-Vehicle Crashes] Bern: Beratungsstelle für Unfallverhütung. DOI 10.13100/bfu.2.340.01 [Swiss Accident Prevention Advisory Centre] (https://www.bfu.ch/ (https://www.bfu.ch/ media/cvud2vwz/bfu_2-340-01_bfu-report-nr-75- verkehrssicherheit- von-e-bikes-mit-schwerpunkt-alleinunfaelle. pdf).
359 United Nations (2016) Habitat III Conference, Quito, Ecuador, 17-20 October 2016 [website] ( https://habitat3.org/).
360 UN (2018). World Urbanisation Prospects The 2018 Revision. New York: United Nations Department of Economic and Social Affairs (https://www.un.org/development publications/ 2018-revision-of-world-urbanisation-prospects.
361 United Nations (2022) Streets for Life [website]. As part of Road Safety Week. New York: United Nations (www. unroadsafetyweek.org/en/streets-for-life).
362 United Nations Economic Commission for Europe (2021). Vienna Declaration: Transforming towards clean, safe, healthy and inclusive mobility and transport for happiness and prosperity for all. Preparatory Meeting for the Fifth High-level Meeting on Transport, Health and Environment 25 January 2021 (https://thepep.unece.org).
363 United Nations in Western Europe (2022). Cycling for the Global Goals [website]. Brussels: United Nations (https:// unric.org/en/cycling-for-the-global-goals/).
364 United Nations / Framework Convention on Climate Change, 2015. Adoption of the Paris Agreement, 21st Conference of the Parties, Paris: United Nations.
365 United Nations / Framework Convention on Climate Change, 2021. Glasgow Climate Pact, 26th Conference of the Parties, Glasgow: United

Nations.

366 United Nations Economic Commission for Europe, 2019. United Nations resource classification framework - 2019 update. Geneva: United Nations.
367 United Nations Economic Commission for Europe, 2020. A framework for achieving carbon neutrality in the region of the United Nations Economic Commission for Europe Economic Commission for Europe (ECE) by 2050 - note by the Task Force on Carbon Neutrality. Geneva: United Nations.
368 United Nations Economic Commission for Europe, 2020. Pathways to sustainable energy. Geneva: United Nations.
369 United Nations Economic Commission for Europe, 2020. Solar and wind energy for cross-border energy co-operation in beneficiary countries. Geneva: United Nations.
370 United Nations Economic Commission for Europe, 2020. United Nations Resource Classification Framework for Commercial Valuations - Update. In UNECE (Ed.). (p. 25). Geneva: United Nations.
371 United Nations Economic Commission for Europe, 2020. United Nations Resource Management System: Overview of concepts, objectives and requirements. Geneva: United Nations.
372 United Nations Economic Commission for Europe, 2020. United Nations Resource Classification Framework. Case study of Finland/Estland, Sweden and Norway - Norcalk limestone and Forsand sand and gravel mines. Geneva: United Nations.
373 United Nations Economic Commission for Europe, 2021. The Triple Commitment. Geneva: United Nations.United Nations Economic Commission for Europe, 2021. A Push to Pivot - Delivering the 2030 Agenda and the Paris Agreement. Geneva: United Nations.
374 United Nations Economic Commission for Europe, 2021. Summary of carbon capture, utilisation and storage technologies. Geneva: United Nations.
375 United Nations Economic Commission for Europe, 2021. Geological CO2 Storage in Eastern Europe, the Caucasus and Central Asia: Initial Potential and Policy Analysis. Geneva: United Nations.United Nations Economic Commission for Europe, 2021. Hydrogen Technology Brief. Geneva: United Nations.
376 United Nations Economic Commission for Europe, 2021. Life cycle assessment of generation options electricity. Geneva: United Nations.
377 United Nations Economic Commission for Europe, 2021. Nuclear Energy Technology Brief. Geneva: United Nations.United Nations Economic Commission for Europe, 2021. United Nations resource classification

framework for commercial assessments. An introductory guide. Geneva: United Nations.
378 United Nations Economic Commission for Europe, 2022. Building a sustainable energy system in the ECE region. Geneva: United Nations.
379 United Nations Economic Commission for Europe, 2022. Draft United Nations resource management system: Principles and requirements. Geneva: United Nations.
380 United Nations Environment Programme, 2021. Emissions gap report. New York: United Nations.
381 United Nations Statistical Commission, 2011. International Recommendations for Energy Statistics (IRES). New York: United Nations.
382 United Nations, 2021. Transforming extractive industries for sustainable development. In U. S. General (Ed.), (p. 18). New York: United Nations.
383 U.S. Department of Transportation (2021). Complete Streets [website]. Washington: U.S. Department of Transportation (https://www.transportation.gov/mission/health/complete-streets).
384 Venter ZS, Barton DN, Gundersen V, Figari H, Nowell MS (2021). Back to nature: Norwegians support increased recreational use of urban green spaces months after the COVID-19 outbreak. Landsc Urban Plan, 214:104175.
doi:10.1016/j.lurbplan.2021.104175
385 Voulgaris CT, Taylor BD, Blumenberg E, Brown A, Ralph K (2017). Synergies between neighbourhoods and travel behaviour: A travel analysis of 30,000 US neighbourhoods. JTLU. 10(1):437-461. doi: 10.5198/jtlu.2016.840.109 References
386 Wanner M, Götschi T, Martin-Diener E, Kahlmeier S, Martin BW (2012). Active transport, physical activity, and body weight in adults: a systematic review. Am J Prev Med. 42(5):493-502. doi:10.1016/j.amepre.2012.01.030.van Wee B, Börjesson M (2015). How to make CBA more appropriate for cycling policy evaluation. Transp Policy. 44:117-124.
doi:10.1016/j.tranpol.2015.07.005
387 Wegman F, Aarts L, Bax S (2008). Promoting sustainable safety. National road safety forecast for the Netherlands 2005-2020 Saf Sci 46(2)323-343 doi:10.1016/j.ssci.2007.06.013
388 Weiss M, Dekker P, Moreau A, Scholz H, Patel MK (2015). On the electrification of road transport - a review of the environmental, economic and social performance of electric two-wheelers. Transp Res D Transp Environ. 41:348-366. doi:10.1016/j.trd.2015.09.007.

389 Welle B, Li W, Adriazola-Steil CA (2016). What Makes Cities Safer by Design? A review of evidence and research on practices to improve traffic safety through urban and street design. 95th Annual Meeting of the Transportation Research Board, Washington, DC,
10-14 January 2016. In: TRID, TRIS database and ITID ( https://trid.trb.org/view/1393567).
390 WHO Regional Office for Europe (2014). WHO Expert Meeting: Methods and tools for assessing air pollution risks to health at local, national and international levels. Copenhagen: 391 WHO Regional Office for Europe ( https://apps.who.int/iris/handle/10665/143712).
392 WHO Regional Office for Europe (2015). European facts and global status report on road safety 2015. Copenhagen: WHO Regional Office for Europe ( https://apps.who.int.
393 Winters M, Fischer J, Nelson T, Fuller D, Whitehurst DGT (2018). Equity in Spatial Access to Bicycling Infrastructure in Mid-Sized Canadian Cities. Transp Res Rec. 2672(36):24-32. doi.org/10.1177/0361198118791630.
394 Winters M, Buehler R, Götschi T (2017). Policies to promote active travel: Evidence from Reviews of the Literature. Curr Environ Health Rep. 4(3):278-285. doi: 10.1007/s40572-017-0148-x.110
395 Wittwer R, Hubrich S, Wittig S, Gerike R (2018). Development of a new method for harmonising household travel survey data. Transp Res Proc. 32:597- 606.doi:10.1016/j.trpro.2018.10.017.
396 Woodcock J, Tainio M, Cheshire J, O'Brien O, Goodman A. (2014). Health impacts of London's bike-sharing system: a health impact modelling study. BMJ. 348. doi:10.1136/bmj.g425.
397 World Health Organisation (2013). 8th Global Conference on Health Promotion, Helsinki, Finland, 10-14 June 2013 [website].
(https://www.who.int/teams/health-promotion/enhanced-wellbeing/eighth-global- conference ).
398 World Health Organisation (2013a). Global action plan for the prevention and control of NCDs 2013-2020. Geneva:
(https://www.who.int/publications/i/item/9789241506236).
399 World Health Organisation (2018). Global State of Road Safety Report 2018.
Geneva: World Health Organisation
(https://www.who.int/publications/i/item/9789241565684).
400 World Health Organisation (2018a). Global network of age-friendly cities and communities. Geneva,

(https://www.who.int/publications/i/item/WHO- FWC-ALC-18.4 ).
401 World Health Organisation (2018b). Global action plan for physical activity 2018-2030: more active people for a healthier world. Geneva: (https://apps.who.int).
402 World Health Organisation (2020a). WHO recommendations on physical activity and sedentary behaviour: a brief review. Geneva: WHO ( https://apps.who. int/iris/bitstream/handle/10665/337001/9789240014909-rus.pdf)
403 World Health Organisation (2020b). Cyclist safety: an information resource for decision-makers and practitioners. Geneva: (https://www.who.int/publications/i/item/cyclist-safety-an-information-resource- for-decision-makers-and-practitioners).
404 World Health Organisation (2020c). Personal interventions and risk communication for air pollution. Geneva: (https://www.who.int/publications/i/item/9789240000278).
405 World Health Organisation (2020e). WHO manifesto for a healthy recovery from COVID-19. Geneva: (https://www.who.int/publications/m/item/who- manifesto-for-a-healthy-recovery-from-covid-19).
406 Wu Y, Rowangould D, London J (2018). Modelling health equity in active transport planning. Transp Res D Transp Environ. 67: 528-540. doi.org/10.1016/j.trd.2019.01.011.
407 Yao S, Loo BPY (2016). Safety in numbers for cyclists beyond national and city level data: a study of risk non-linearity in Hong Kong city. Inj Prev, 22(6):379-385. doi: 10.1136/injuryprev-2016-041964.
408 Zahabi SAH, Strauss J, Manaugh K, Miranda-Moreno LF (2011). Assessing the potential effects of speed limits, built environment, and other factors on the severity of pedestrian and cyclist injuries in road traffic crashes. Transp Res Rec. 2247(1):81-90. doi:10.3141/2247-10.
409 Zhao Y, Hu F, Feng Y, Yang X, Li Y, Guo C et al (2021). Association of cycling with risk of all-cause mortality and cardiovascular disease: A Systematic Review and Dose-Response Meta-analysis of Prospective Cohort Studies. Sports Med, 51(7):1439-1448. doi: 10.1007/s40279-021-01452-7.
410 Zuo T, Wei H (2019). Prioritising cycleways to increase bicycle network connectivity and connect bicycles to transport: A multi-criteria decision analysis approach. Transp Res Part A Policy Pract. 129:52-71. doi: 10.1016/j.tra.2019.08.003.

411 2018 Physical Activity Guidelines Advisory Committee (2018). 2018 Physical Activity Guidelines Advisory Committee Scientific Report. Washington D.C.: U.S. Department of Health and Human Services (https://health. gov/our-work/nutrition- physical-activity/ physical-activity-guidelines/current-guidelines/scientific-report).

GLOSSARY

**A blue economy** is an economy that includes a number of economic sectors and associated policies that together determine whether the use of ocean resources is sustainable.

**Climate neutrality** refers to the idea of achieving an overall zero level of GHG emissions by balancing these emissions in such a way that they are equal to the emissions that are removed by natural uptake on Earth.

**Coastal resilience - the** ability of a community to recover from hazardous events such as hurricanes, coastal storms, and flooding, rather than simply reacting to impacts.

**Conservation** agriculture is a system of farming that promotes minimal soil disturbance (i.e. no-tillage), maintenance of permanent soil cover and diversification of plant species. It improves biodiversity and natural biological processes above and below the land surface, which contributes to increased water and nutrient use efficiency and improved and sustainable crop production.

**Vital** raw materials (VNRM) are raw materials that are important for the current and future economy and whose availability is associated with high risk due to absolute scarcity, market characteristics or strong regional concentration. Based on two main parameters - importance for the economy and supply risk - a list of FICRs has been compiled for the European Union. The specific list of raw materials that are essential and therefore should be categorised as LLDCs depends on the region and sector.

**Decarbonisation** is the reduction of carbon dioxide emissions through the use of low-carbon energy sources, resulting in less GHG emissions to the atmosphere.

**Energy balance** is the allocation of primary energy sources to final energy consumption in a given geographical region. **Eutrophication** is the process by which a water body is enriched with dissolved nutrients (e.g. phosphates) that stimulate the growth of aquatic plants, usually resulting in the depletion of dissolved oxygen.

**E-waste**, or waste in the form of waste electrical and electronic equipment (WEEE), is electrical and electronic equipment that the owner disposes of, intends to dispose of, or is required to dispose of. This may be because the equipment is no longer satisfactory to the owner or is no longer functional. The e-waste category includes any appliance with 278

electrical power supply when it reaches the end of its useful life. This includes large technical appliances such as washing machines, small appliances such as toasters, IT and telecommunication equipment such as computers and telephones, and household equipment such as radios, lighting and other technical devices. **Flame retardants** are chemicals added to materials or applied as coatings to products or components to increase the fire resistance of flammable products.

**Food safety** is the assurance that food will not cause harm to the consumer and will provide the expected nutritional value when prepared and/or eaten as intended.

Food security exists when all people at all times have physical, social and economic access to sufficient, safe and nutritious food to meet their caloric needs and food preferences for an active and healthy life.

**Fossil** fuels are carbon-based fuels from fossil hydrocarbon deposits, including coal, peat, oil and natural gas.

**Greenhouse gases** (GHGs) covered by the UN Framework Convention on Climate Change are carbon dioxide (CO2), methane (CH4), nitrous oxide (N2O), hydrofluorocarbons (HFCs), perfluorocarbons (PFCs), sulphur hexafluoride (SF6) and nitrogen trifluoride (NF3). **Illegal, unreported and unregulated** (IUU) fishing includes all fishing activities, is committed in violation of fisheries laws or occurs outside the scope of fisheries laws and regulations.

**Industrial symbiosis** describes synergistic networks between traditionally separate industrial enterprises. Participants jointly manage material or energy resources and share infrastructure, capacity or know-how. One common element is the high-value valorisation of by-products and waste by another company in the network. Industrial symbiosis goes beyond traditional waste management, being a coordinated effort of several entities to harmonise their activities and needs in order to find mutually beneficial solutions. Industrial symbiosis increases the efficiency of resource utilisation in a cost-effective way, thereby both increasing the profitability of economic activity and reducing the negative impact on the environment.

**Land withdrawal from turnover** means land previously used for growing agricultural crops or 279

pasture/grazing areas, but no longer fulfil agricultural functions and at the same time have not been purposefully converted to forest areas or artificial areas.

**Malnutrition** essentially means "poor nutrition". It includes both overnutrition and undernutrition. It refers not only to the quantity and quality of food (inadequate, excessive or unbalanced intake), but also to the body's response to a wide range of infections that result in impaired nutrient absorption or an inability to utilise nutrients properly to maintain health.

**Municipal Solid Waste** (MSW) is waste from households and waste generated from other sources that is similar in nature and composition to household waste. This also includes trade and small business waste. This category also includes waste from a number of municipal services such as parks and gardens, street cleaning and public waste bins. **Nationally Determined Contributions** (NDCs) are set by the parties to the Paris Agreement, describing each country's national efforts to reduce emissions at the national level and adapt to the impacts of climate change.

Natural infrastructure refers to strategically planned and managed networks of natural lands, waters and soils, such as forests and wetlands, working landscapes and other open spaces, that maintain or enhance ecosystem values and functions and provide co-benefits for people.

**Nature-based solutions** (NBS) are measures to protect, sustainably manage and restore natural or modified ecosystems that contribute to effective and adaptive solutions to social problems, while ensuring human well-being and benefits for biodiversity. (Source: International Union for Conservation of Nature).

No-tillage (or no-tillage) is a simple technique of applying seed to the soil without prior land preparation. No-tillage is one of the technical components of conservation agriculture, but is not only used by proponents of conservation agriculture.

**Overeating** is the daily intake of calories in an amount consistently higher than energy needs, leading to overweight or obesity. Obesity is associated with the risk of developing chronic diseases such as high blood pressure, diabetes, etc. Thus, children and adults whose body weight is significantly higher than their normal weight over a long period of time are overeating.

**Persistent organic pollutants** (POPs) are a group of organic compounds that are resistant to degradation in the environment, i.e. demonstrate high stability under the influence of chemical, biological and photolytic processes occurring in the environment. Examples are polycyclic aromatic hydrocarbons (PAHs), polychlorinated biphenyls (PCBs) and brominated flame retardants. Most POPs are halogenated organic compounds with high fat solubility and bioaccumulative properties and consequently high risk of harmful effects on the environment and human health (e.g. cancer, endocrine disruption, effects on the immune system). Most POPs are of artificial origin. They are or have been used, for example, as pesticides, flame retardants

in plastics and electrical goods, heat-exchange fluids or condensers. Others, such as dioxins, are furans, unintended by-products of high-temperature processes, including combustion.

**The Pollutant Release and Transfer Register** (PRTR) is a publicly available database that creates a pollution inventory by documenting chemicals or pollutants released from industrial and other facilities to air, water and soil and transported off-site for treatment. A set of defined activities and pollutants is under consideration.

**Polycyclic aromatic hydrocarbons** (PAHs) are aromatic hydrocarbons whose chemical structure contains several aromatic rings from the PAH group. Human exposure to PAHs causes cancer, cardiovascular diseases and foetal developmental disorders. Bioaccumulation (gradual accumulation of substances in a living organism) is a particular problem.

**Recycling is a** material processing operation that extracts secondary raw materials from waste, including the processing of organic materials through composting or anaerobic digestion. The recycling rate is calculated by dividing the weight of (recyclable) material delivered to recycling facilities by the total weight of (separately) collected (recyclable) material. The amount of waste collected (or recyclables collected) is not equivalent to the amount of waste generated (or recyclables received) because some of the waste generated does not enter the collection systems. The recycling rate refers only to the quantity collected.

**Major refurbishment is the** process of bringing a product up to standards and into a more satisfactory working condition or making it look more attractive. Commonly used measures include replacing obsolete components, such as in computer equipment, and cosmetic changes to improve the appearance of the item (e.g. painting, changing the surface finish).

Products sold on the market after major repairs often have a warranty that covers the entire product (unlike products after minor repairs). Unlike a refurbished product, a product after a major repair usually has a level of performance that is not equivalent to the original unit.

**Remanufacturing** is a product life extension programme carried out on an industrial scale, either by the original manufacturer or by a remanufacturing company. This involves returning an already used product to the parameters specified by the original manufacturer, usually using some combination of reused, refurbished and new parts. A prerequisite for remanufacturing is that a programme is in place to return the specific product to the remanufacturer/rebuilder. Products are disassembled and components are returned to their original condition; the reassembled product is extensively tested. Remanufactured products are delivered in "like new" condition; they meet the same consumer expectations as new products. The warranty is usually at least equal to that of the original product. Examples from different industries are collected by the European Remanufacturing Network.

**A minor repair** is an operation to correct a product malfunction. It can be carried out privately or by using the services of an appropriate company. Repairs are usually carried out without warranty for the product as a whole.

Reuse means any situation in which it is achieved that a non-waste product or its components are used again for their original purpose, that is, for the same purpose for which they have already been used at least once. Where products or components are reused but for a purpose other than their original purpose, reuse occurs. Reuse is part of waste prevention measures. In contrast, "preparation for reuse" is part of waste management and depends on the availability of appropriate infrastructure and procedures for waste collection and treatment. Preparation for reuse refers to inspection, cleaning or repair operations by which products or components of products that have become waste are prepared so that they can be reused without any other pretreatment403. Preparation for reuse is a scheme waste valorisation. Both reuse and preparation for reuse are programmes to extend the life of products. Reproduction, recovery and repair are important elements of reuse programmes.

**Soil carbon sequestration** is a biogeochemical process by which soil absorbs and retains carbon. Soil carbon sequestration is a climate change mitigation option with a wide range of synergistic effects. By increasing soil carbon concentration through more efficient tillage practices, this option provides benefits for soil biodiversity, soil fertility and productivity, and the soil's ability to store water. In addition, soil carbon sequestration stabilises and increases food production, reversing land degradation and restoring the 'health' of ecological processes.

**Soil erosion** - in geology, erosion is defined as a process that slowly shapes hillsides, allowing soil cover to form as a result of weathering of rocks and from alluvial and colluvial deposits. Anthropogenic erosion as a consequence of thoughtless exploitation of the environment leads to an increase in surface runoff and a decrease in arable layers and crop yields.

**Soil organic** carbon (SOC) is the carbon contained in soil, expressed as a percentage by weight (gC/kg soil). Climatic shifts in temperature and precipitation strongly influence the decomposition process and the amount of SOC stored in the ecosystem and released to the atmosphere. The amount of SOC stored in the ecosystem depends on the quantity and quality of organic matter returned to the soil matrix, the capacity of the soil to hold organic carbon (depending on its texture and cation exchange capacity), and the biotic effects of temperature and precipitation.

**Sustainable infrastructure systems** (sometimes referred to as green infrastructure) are systems that are planned, designed, constructed, managed and decommissioned in a way that ensures economic and financial, social, environmental (including climate change resilience) and institutional sustainability throughout the life cycle of the infrastructure. Sustainable infrastructure can include built infrastructure, natural infrastructure or hybrid infrastructure containing elements of both.

**Total final energy consumption** - primary and secondary energy consumption in manufacturing, construction and non-fuel mineral extraction, transport and other sectors (agriculture, forestry and fisheries, trade and public services, households and other consumers).

**The triple planetary crisis** comprises the interrelated and sequential manifestations of climate change, biodiversity loss and pollution.

The **waste management hierarchy** or waste hierarchy prioritises waste management options in order of environmental optimality. The waste management hierarchy used in the European Union has five levels: waste prevention; preparation for reuse; recycling; other forms of recovery; and disposal.

In other regions or contexts, alternative versions of the waste management hierarchy exist, including prioritisation at more than five levels. In all cases, waste prevention is identified as the top priority, while recycling is the least favoured waste management option.

**Waste** means any substance or object that the owner disposes of, intends to dispose of, or is required to dispose of. They are not equal to residues. In manufacturing, the latter refers to materials that have not been purposefully consumed in the production process; such residues may or may not be waste.

**A by-product** is material left over from the production process that is not categorised as waste.Waste prevention includes activities and measures to prevent products, substances or materials from becoming waste. Waste prevention can be achieved by reducing the amount of materials used in products, for example through eco-design, or the amount of materials used to provide services; by improving the efficiency of product use, for example by sharing products instead of buying them; and by introducing schemes to extend the life of products, such as reuse and minor and major repairs.406 Changes in the lifestyles of citizens towards more intangible consumption patterns and the dematerialisation of the economy, for example by increasing the share of services, tourism and culture, also contribute to waste prevention.

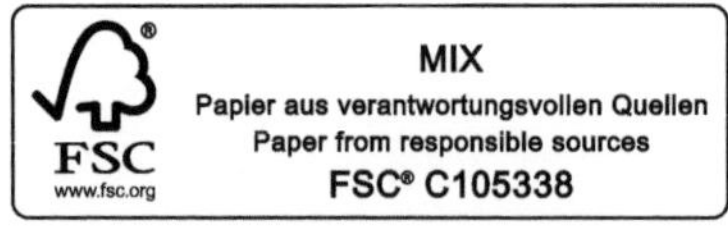


Printed by Books on Demand GmbH, Norderstedt / Germany